Who's Watching?

Who's Watching?

Daily Practices of Surveillance
among Contemporary Families

Edited by
Margaret K. Nelson and
Anita Ilta Garey

Vanderbilt University Press

Nashville

© 2009 by Vanderbilt University Press
Nashville, Tennessee 37235
All rights reserved

13 12 11 10 09   1 2 3 4 5

This book is printed on acid-free paper.
Manufactured in the United States of America

Library of Congress Cataloging-in-Publication Data

Who's watching? : daily practices of surveillance among
contemporary families / edited by Margaret K. Nelson,
Anita Ilta Garey.
p. cm.
Includes bibliographical references.
ISBN 978-0-8265-1671-8 (cloth : alk. paper)
ISBN 978-0-8265-1672-5 (pbk. : alk. paper)
1. Home detention—United States. 2. Electronic
surveillance—United States. 3. Families—United States. I.
Nelson, Margaret K., 1944– II. Garey, Anita Ilta, 1947–
HV9469.W53 2009
649'.1—dc22
2008052793

To the new families,
Sam and Lani
and
Jeff, Becca, Maya, and Sadie
—MKN

To TyAnn Alys Garey,
who prompts me to think about these issues anew
—AIG

Contents

Guide to Topics

Family Formation

Gender

Kinship Networks

Law Enforcement

The Market

New Technology

Parenthood

Race/Ethnicity

Schools

Sexuality

Acknowledgments

Although she has probably forgotten, after hearing three of the chapters in this book presented as papers at an Eastern Sociological Society conference in 2006, Julia Wrigley suggested editing a book around the issues those papers raised. And so we have.

We are grateful to the authors of the chapters in this book for bearing with us as we asked for draft after draft after draft. We hope the final product lives up to their expectations.

Both volume editors had previously worked with Michael Ames, Director of Vanderbilt University Press, and thus already knew that he is an editor who cares about the books he publishes and who responds quickly and thoughtfully to questions and requests. It's been a privilege to work with him.

Toward the end of the process of editing this book, Valerie Benka agreed to give the chapters one more careful read. She made many invaluable suggestions for improvement. Jessie Hunnicutt at Vanderbilt University Press improved the manuscript still further with her insightful copyediting. Thanks also to Shel Sax for technical assistance and to Middlebury College for its financial support.

Margaret K. Nelson is grateful to Anita Ilta Garey for coming on board and for the talents and efforts she directed at this project. Anita Ilta Garey is grateful to Margaret K. Nelson for inviting her to participate and for the talents and efforts *she* directed at this project. Both authors cherish the friendship forged through this collaboration.

Who's Watching?

Who's Watching?

An Introductory Essay

Margaret K. Nelson and Anita Ilta Garey

This volume of writings linking the field of surveillance studies and the field of family sociology is situated in the specific historical moment when issues of individual—and family—privacy are being reevaluated, and when the issue of individual rights (in conjunction with the countervailing issues of governmental and social good) is more in contention than usual.[1] Even if surveillance itself has not increased, this specific historical moment is also one in which the *technological* possibilities for monitoring (and for the invasion of privacy) have expanded in ways never before considered.[2] We are all subject to the technological expansion of monitoring in our daily lives, such as when we drive under cameras at traffic lights and use our discount cards in supermarkets. We also make use of the new technology within the family as we check computer histories for the Internet activity of our children and partners and observe what is happening in a child's day care through a video camera. Each of the two fields we link—that of surveillance and that of the family—is central to sociological concerns.[3]

Surveillance can serve a multiplicity of purposes, but the activity itself provides a connection between two people—sometimes between two people who might otherwise have no ties or affiliation, and sometimes between two people who are closely bound through kinship or friendship. The essays in this collection explore these linkages through an analysis of the many different ways in which family members monitor their own family and its borders as well as other families.

Although in this collection we do not examine the state as a direct agent of surveillance, we include essays that focus on occasions of monitoring by family members at the behest of outside agencies, including both the state and the market. Other contributions focus on monitoring that is connected to the strong notions people have about what a family should be and what family members should do; individuals "police" themselves and their neighbors with those notions in mind. Hence, we argue, monitoring goes on all the time—even (or maybe especially) when there seems to be no monitoring going on at all, such as when families and their members appear to meet normative judgments.

The essays are attentive to the wide range of ways in which individuals and groups "observe" and obtain information about other individuals and groups. Intentionally, we include traditional practices of information gathering as well as newer methods that rely on technology, and we also intentionally include both covert/invisible and overt/visible practices. We are similarly broad in our consideration of individuals relevant to family life. The definition of a "family" itself is in contention in the United States. We extend our interest here beyond even a broad definition to include members of kinship networks (whether "real" or "fictive" kin) and those "outsiders" who are central to the family work of caring for dependents, such as nannies and networks of caregivers.

Combining surveillance studies and family sociology enables us to see issues and problems that are otherwise invisible or obscured. Examining family practices through the lens of surveillance complicates and informs our understanding of family life. Similarly, expanding surveillance studies to include the realm of the family complicates and informs our understanding of surveillance.

Understanding Families through Studies of Surveillance

The issues raised in this volume are rarely covered explicitly, although we would maintain that concerns about monitoring and accounting for families are implicit subterranean themes in much of the existing literature on families. This set of issues is applicable whether the focus is on the relationship of individuals in the family to other social institutions, the interaction of people in their roles as family members with people outside their families, or the internal dynamics of families.

External Institutions and Families

Although the family is often portrayed as a private sanctuary, separate and autonomous from the "outside world," families and family members are constrained by outside authorities. Institutions outside the family determine the shape of the family itself: who can marry whom, what are acceptable reasons for divorce, who can adopt whom, and whether a woman can abort a fetus. Outside institutions also regulate the internal dynamics of the family, for example by requiring inoculations, prosecuting for child abuse or neglect, and mandating children's school attendance.

Some families, usually those with more economic resources, can deflect parts of this outside control by concealing more of their daily activities from observation. Families who live in crowded neighborhoods, who rely on state subsidies, or who enter the legal system have fewer options for privacy and thereby unwittingly reveal more of their internal dynamics to outside forces. To take a simple example, families paying privately for child care can hire whomever they want to care for their children; however, families relying on state support for child-care arrangements must choose among providers who meet specific criteria. Or, to take another example, a well-off woman who chooses to raise a child on her own can decide whether she wants to reveal the name of the father of that child; a woman relying on welfare is required to do so. Indeed, governmental monitoring of family life, including spending patterns, is a central component of reliance on state resources (Gilliom 2006). Of course, all families are subject to some constraints: teachers have to report suspicions of abuse no matter what the social class of the potential victim. However, suspicion may well rest on perceptions of social class, race, and ethnicity, and the standards used are biased in favor of some social groups over others (Lareau 2003; Nelson, Chapter 6).

Many of the issues concerning the impact of outside agencies on the family have been explored in other studies (Hays 2004; Reich 2005). The specific issue of how outside agencies affect the internal dynamics of the family has been less thoroughly examined. In this collection, contributors explore how agencies external to the family engage family members in a form of "nested responsibility" (Garey, Chapter 1), turn family members into agents of the state or "ancillary watchers" (Staples, Chapter 2), or substitute the family for the more coercive arm of the law (Moore and Haggerty, Chapter 3). The essays in Part I explore the dynamic issue of what happens when outsiders require or urge parents to monitor their dependents within the family.

Families and the Public

As individuals go about their daily lives and present themselves as members of a family, they and their family units are accountable, *as family members and as families,* to outside evaluation. "Accountability" refers to engaging in behavior that is at risk of assessment by others (*American Heritage Diction-*

ary 1985). West and Zimmerman's (1987) classic presentation of behavior at risk of assessment was about "doing gender," and it made clear that gender is social in two important senses. It emerges through interaction in particular institutional settings, and individuals are evaluated according to the norms that prevail in those settings: "Though it is individuals who do gender, the enterprise is fundamentally interactional and institutional in character, for accountability is a feature of social relationships, and its idiom is drawn from the institutional arena in which those relationships are enacted" (West and Zimmerman 2002, 13). Very much the same is true of "doing family" (Nelson 2006).

In the social world, families and individual family members are observed and assessed. Behavior that falls within the acceptable norms of the observer receives positive reinforcement through the observer's apparent lack of notice and the smooth interaction of people in public. Behavior that falls outside the acceptable norms becomes a catalyst for negative comment, stares, hostile avoidance, or unpleasant or awkward interactions. On some occasions this monitoring becomes intrusive, as when outsiders accost individuals and ask about their relationship to an adopted child of a different race or ethnicity (Jacobson, Chapter 4) or report on the behavior of a hired caregiver (Nelson, Chapter 6). On other occasions, the monitoring may be less intrusive but still convey a negative assessment, such as a disapproving look from another woman on a park bench (Blackford, Chapter 5). Families whose membership violates some groups' deeply held norms (for instance, gay or lesbian couples, interracial couples, and polygamous marriages) can be treated harshly—and even with violence. The essays in Part II explore how "private" family life is situated in the public sphere and subject to public assessments.

Family Boundaries and Family Dynamics

In order to understand the role of surveillance in family life, it is critical to look at the way in which family members themselves monitor the form and content of their families. Individuals engaged in such "border patrol" use a variety of methods to obtain information on which to base decisions, including traditional practices of common sense and instinct, gossip, and conversation as well as new technologies that provide information that might previously have been unattainable. The essays in Part III explore how individuals monitor others in order to make decisions about inclusion and exclusion with respect to family membership itself.

In large part, families are created by the decisions of individuals about appropriate membership. These decisions, in turn, rest on the close observation of others: individuals check out potential dates on the Internet (Andrejevic 2005), rely on ultrasounds to make decisions about moving forward with a pregnancy (Rapp 1988; Rapp, Chapter 7; Sandelowski 1994), and study the behavior of potential caregivers to determine who may care for their children (Hansen 2004; Hansen, Chapter 9; Uttal 1996). The family is also dissolved on the basis of monitoring. While private detectives are probably less common in daily life than fiction would have us believe, individuals do rely on surveillance to make decisions about the trustworthiness of partners (Stone 2007), children (Katz 2001; Moore and Haggerty, Chapter 3), and employees within the home (Romero 1992; Wrigley 1995). Indeed, a central part of "doing family" (Naples 2001; Nelson 2006; Roy and Burton, Chapter 10) involves patrolling the borders and making decisions about who is eligible for inclusion and whom to exclude.

Family borders expand to include new members (through birth, marriage, or genealogical searches) and contract to exclude former members (sometimes, though not necessarily, through divorce, betrayal, or failure to perform or reciprocate). Family borders are also permeable in less obvious ways. As Shapiro (1998, 282) notes, "Technologies such as the telephone, the Internet, and interactive television are bidirectional. They bring portions of the outside world into the home, but they also bring parts of the home into the outside world . . . [and thus] have the potential to confound historical conceptions of the boundary constituted by the home. . . . Thus individuals can interact with the large community while potentially free of any direct surveillance." This permeability is clearly of concern to parents who seek to impose rules about television and Internet use (Wang, Bianchi, and Raley 2005). Some parents rely on governmental controls, such as television filters and movie ratings, thereby accepting a form of state intrusion into the family.

Inside the family's borders, members monitor each other, simultaneously taking care of others and seeking to control them.[4] Indeed, care and control are so tightly interwoven that it is difficult to give primacy to one impulse over another or to describe actions using one term rather than the other. Tensions emerge when what one party views as care is viewed as control by another; this is clearly the case in relationships between adolescents and their parents. Looking at surveillance within the family makes evident the fact that all members do not have the same needs and interests—and some of these differing needs may be mutually exclusive. Parents' need for information about the activities of their teenage children, for example, conflicts with teenagers' need to maintain their privacy and be independent. These struggles now incorporate technologies such as cell phones and e-mail, which simultaneously enable more communication and create the potential for greater duplicity (Fotel and Thomsen 2004).

The chapters in Part IV focus on the dynamics of monitoring within the family when the impulse for that monitoring does *not* originate with an outside authority (as is the case in the chapters of Part I). Some of these chapters especially highlight how new technologies provide mechanisms for increased surveillance of dependents. Surveillance *within* the family entails varying amounts of labor and levels of finesse—the "work of monitoring." Kurz (Chapter 13) notes that parents "develop multiple strategies to monitor teens," and that the work involved in monitoring varies by social class, race/ethnicity, and employment status of the adults in a family. In describing the supportive behavior of family members in households where one member is subject to house arrest, Staples (Chapter 2) comments that "even if they gladly offer this assistance, 'back up' work is still work—emotional, mental, and physical labor." Some of the family work of care and control is the responsibility of individuals who stand outside the family circle: nannies and other child-care providers, for example, but also workers in nursing homes (Bowers 1990) and schools (Lareau 2000). Those individuals, in turn, may also become the subjects of monitoring.

In sum, monitoring is a lens through which to understand family dynamics. It enables us to explore how this process shapes family life, and how it does so differently depending on where families are located in the social structure.

The Issue of Family in Surveillance Studies: Shifting the Balance

The field of surveillance studies is considerably smaller and more recent than the field of family sociology. A number of edited collections now exist on the general topic of surveillance, but by and large these readers give short shrift to the particular issues of concern in this collection.[5] The field of surveillance studies concerns itself more with the intrusiveness of those operating on behalf of organizational structures outside the family—the government and corporations—than it does with the actions of private individuals. But Staples (2000, 153) argues that "as a general rule in sociology we should 'forget Big Brother'" because "surveillance power is bi-directional, and is more-often-than-not triggered by us." As individuals we watch other family members for purposes of care and control; we also watch those outside our families both because we believe their actions might have consequences for us directly (as when we ask others to care for our children) and because we believe their actions are violating (or shifting) social norms.

Marx (2007, 126) notes that the uses of surveillance "by *individuals* (e.g., in familial contexts or by voyeurs)" have been neglected in the field, along with "the interaction between agents and subjects." Gilliom (2006, 126) argues that the field of surveillance studies has been good at examining the "watchers . . . but not so good at the necessarily messier, less institutionalized, and exploratory but absolutely crucial job of studying the watched—the real people and real bodies who are the subjects of these systems." By looking within families, the chapters in this volume get closer to these "real people and real bodies": young children and teens who are the subject of parental surveillance, individuals enduring house arrest, nannies who themselves comment on their attitudes toward surveillance, and parents whose children appear in truancy court.

Looking at monitoring within the context of the family highlights the issue of care, which is often missing from debates about surveillance that focus on the "negative" and problematic, the violations of privacy, and the loss of autonomy. But surveillance, both from outside and within the borders of the family, might be motivated by an interest in care and protection; thus, some surveillance is clearly "positive" (Haggerty 2006, 35). For example, Kane (Chapter 12) notes that when parents monitor the dress and behavior of young children for the performance of gender, they are hoping to forestall negative feedback from outsiders, and Garey (Chapter 1) notes that truancy court judges monitor the behavior of truant children and their parents in the belief that if these children stay in school and get an education, they will be able to avoid poverty and misfortune. At the same time, because the family is itself relational, these "advantages" might not apply to all family members. By focusing on people in their relationships as family members, rather than as discrete individuals in relation to the state, we can explore how surveillance has different consequences for different individuals within the same family.

Four Themes

The kind of activities we examine in this collection affect people's daily lives and interactions in profound ways and make visible particular cultural assumptions that feed into the decisions made by state actors. Four major themes emerge from the analysis of the family as an arena of surveillance and of surveillance as it is practiced in families: (1) the dynamic interplay between care and control; (2) the relevance of technology; (3) the nature of resistance; and (4) the abiding significance of social location.

Care and Control Combined

Whether we are looking at surveillance from the level of those who stand outside the family and have power over it (the state, corporations) or from the level of the everyday internal workings of the family itself, we can identify two compelling interests that drive practices of monitoring: a desire to care for and protect those who are the objects of surveillance, and a desire to control and impose social order.[6] One of these stances—"care"—is usually viewed in a positive light (for example, parents care for their children, doctors care for their patients, and teachers care for their students). The other—"control"—is often seen in a negative light (as in how the state is too intrusive into our private lives [Donzelot 1979; Ehrenreich and English 1989] or how parents want to mold their children in their own image).

But it is not easy, and often not even possible, to know whether the actions of others are motivated by the desire to care or to control. Nor is it necessarily true that motivation and intention are the criteria that determine whether something constitutes care or control. For example, is it care (of children) or control (of parents and children) when family court judges sanction parents for not ensuring that their children attend school regularly (Garey, Chapter 1), or when strangers comment, through the Internet or on the playground, on the care provided within the family (Blackford, Chapter 5; Nelson, Chapter 6)? This confusion also occurs when we consider the actions of family members with regard to each other. When parents test their children for drug use, seek information about their children's friends, guide their children toward a traditional performance of gender, or communicate on a daily (or even hourly) basis through cell phone calls, can we tell which concern the impulse comes from—to care or to control? Nor can the motivations of care and control always be separated. For example, although it makes sense to characterize a parent's use of a baby monitor as an attempt to provide good care for an infant, this kind of action can easily slip into or merge with control (Nelson, Chapter 11).

A dichotomy between care and control overlooks the ways in which care itself can operate through mechanisms of control, including practices of inclusion and exclusion. Parents monitor the behavior of other family members in order to allow or restrict access to their children (Hansen, Chapter 9; Roy and Burton, Chapter 10), thus exercising a form of control in order to protect. Similarly, a decision about who to include within the family (Rapp, Chapter 7; Hertz, Chapter 8) necessarily means the exclusion of those seen as being "unfit." In short, care and control are in a dialectical relationship with each other, and not a simple dichotomous one.

Views of Technology

Two straw men guard the gates of debate about the role of technology: a technological determinist position that argues for the autonomous role of technology in producing and creating new sets of social relations, and a social determinist position that essentially reduces technological developments themselves (and often also their effects) to preexisting sets of social relationships. Most of those who walk through the gates to explore surveillance technology argue for a more nuanced and dynamic view that acknowledges both sides simultaneously.

A dynamic approach helps move discussions of surveillance beyond simple examinations of efficiency and trade-offs to probe the more subtle ways in which relationships are affected by the introduction of new technologies (Monahan 2006). The new technology of house arrests, for example, alters social relations *within* the family in ways that are not easily characterized as "side effects" (Monahan 2006, 12). Asking only whether house arrest is an effective strategy for purposes of social control would miss these alterations entirely.

The relevance of preexisting sets of social relations is a central theme in many discussions of surveillance (addressed more fully in our discussion of social location). For example, Hertz (Chapter 8) notes that thinking about how to categorize and make sense of donor siblings (children whose mothers both used the same donor for artificial insemination) involves working through "traditional" sets of family relationships and making assessments on the basis of deeply rooted social classifications (shared values, shared social class). Indeed, Hertz herself cannot talk about these new sets of relationships without referencing how they differ from more commonly recognized ones. In a chapter that explores consequences of Internet connections, Nelson (Chapter 6) argues that although the gossip enabled by a website differs from face-to-face gossip (for example, by allowing more anonymity), the gossip itself builds on and draws from familiar attitudes accompanying everyday stereotypes about race/ethnicity. Yet, in the same chapter, Nelson suggests that new technologies such as the Internet can help shift and rearrange the balance of power in preexisting relationships by, for example, allowing those who are gossiped about to use this medium to express their own point of view and thus to have a public voice they might not otherwise have.

In this volume we include both studies focusing on traditional methods of monitoring (assessing reputations and others' behavior through close observation and conversation) and studies focusing on technological approaches to these same practices. Along with the new technologies of surveillance come new ethical dilemmas: should one use these new technologies, and, if so, what should one do with the information thus acquired? Are there ethical and moral distinctions between talking with teens about their daily actions and relying on home drug tests to assess their drug use? Are different ethical issues raised in gossip via the Internet than are raised when we consider face-to-face transactions of social control and social approval?

Issues of Resistance

At the public level, resistance to being monitored may be limited because surveillance is frequently desired; while the public gripes about the surveillance that now makes plane travel more difficult, few question its necessity. The attractiveness of some surveillance devices, and the fascination with the technology on which they rest, may also serve to undermine resistance. In choosing to have cell phones, for example, teens trade off the possibility of greater parental control for access to ongoing communication with their peers. Even so, much of the monitoring that occurs—at every level explored in this book—provokes, at the minimum, ad hoc and unorganized resistance.[7]

Moore and Haggerty (Chapter 3) suggest that we have to conceive of this resistance broadly: "The notion of resisting surveillance brings to mind someone standing outside of the gaze, finding cracks and fissures where surveillance does not penetrate. Resisting surveillance, however, can also involve strategies that work creatively within the field of visibility through imaginative engagements with the particularities of an observational regime." With respect to "standing outside of the gaze," Roy and Burton (Chapter 10) describe how single mothers find it difficult to monitor the fathers of their children when those men can move to another state or easily return to their country of origin. Similarly, choosing not to register on a website listing sperm donor numbers can be seen as effort to stand outside of the gaze (Hertz, Chapter 8). Resistance *within* the field of visibility includes the strategies teens use to beat drug tests (Moore and Haggerty, Chapter 3) and the strategies developed by white parents with Chinese daughters to deal with intrusive comments from interested strangers (Jacobson, Chapter 4). Resistance stands in a complex relationship to compliance.

Social Location

Social location refers to how families and individuals are positioned in broader social hierarchies of race/ethnicity, social class, and gender (and also ability, sexuality, and age). Social location is highly relevant to a full range of concerns about monitoring and surveillance. Haggerty (2006, 29) reminds us that even as the "multiplication of the sites of surveillance ruptures the unidirectional nature of the gaze," surveillance nonetheless "continues to play an important role in establishing and reinforcing social inequalities." In a country in which racial profiling is an issue of widespread discussion and even the public is on the lookout for "terrorists" based on skin color and dress, this reminder simply underscores what we already know but often do not want to admit.

In various ways, race/ethnicity, social class, and gender can each alter the frequency, intensity, and focus of the surveillance gaze. Some groups are more vulnerable than others to surveillance itself, and that heightened vulnerability extends to issues that affect the entire family. For example, those in poverty are more often the objects of surveillance both because they are less able to secure privacy and because so many norms privilege middle-class behavior. The heightened vulnerability of African American and Latino youth to surveillance by the police can motivate parents to engage in tighter monitoring of their own children; surveillance on the outside thus affects internal family dynamics. Unexpected differences in race/ethnicity (and perhaps social class) can evoke vulnerability to intrusive surveillance (Jacobson, Chapter 4). Racial/ethnic difference is also a basis for strangers to make the assumption that caregivers are not family members, thus subjecting those caregivers to a particularly intense form of surveillance.[8] In addition, parents monitor their children's gender performance, with particular concern for boys' gender conformity (Kane, Chapter 12), and a child's gender shapes perceptions of vulnerability (Nelson, Chapter 6).

Social location also shapes access to the technologies of surveillance. As Haggerty (2006, 29) reminds us, groups of people "are differentially positioned to be able to exploit these surveillance potentialities, and their abilities to do so are often structured according to traditional social cleavages." Social class also shapes the kinds of resources used and thus the necessity for engaging in specific kinds of surveillance: for example, wealthy people often hire nannies and thus face the issue of how to monitor nanny behavior; poor women often need to rely on men who are themselves poor and thus face special issues of assessing one's ability to care; more dangerous neighborhoods require more parental monitoring; parents with less flexibility in their employment face special difficulties in attempting to monitor their children. Social location thus remains central to our understanding of the dynamics of surveillance.

Book Organization: Four Sites of Analysis

The issues and themes discussed above are organized into four different sections in this volume: external institutions and families, families and the public, family boundaries, and internal family dynamics. We understand, however, that some—if not all—of the chapters could easily find a home in a different section from the one in which we have placed them. For this reason, we also include a Guide to Topics designed to encourage alternative groupings of the issues raised in the individual chapters. Finally, we acknowledge that although we have tried to be inclusive in this volume, there are some populations (such as the elderly) and some topics (such as sexuality) that are not covered or are covered only briefly. We encourage further discussion and investigation of the important issues that emerge from consideration of monitoring families. We hope that the discussion of these issues will encourage readers to think about their own cultural assumptions and their own judgments of—or even interventions in—other people's lives.

Notes

1. Since the terrorist attacks of September 11, 2001, some people are more willing to put aside individual rights to privacy than they were in the not-so-distant past, but individual privacy remains highly valued in the United States in the first part of the twenty-first century. By contrast, at other times, even in the United States, private citizens easily accepted the involvement of the state, the church, and other members of the public in their own lives. Indeed, the current "animosity" toward state involvement in the family is a relatively recent phenomenon—as is the sense that the family is, and should be, private (Nock 1998; Berardo 1998).
2. It is impossible to know whether the degree to which individuals are under surveillance has increased or decreased over time. We know, for example, that during the Colonial Era, individuals were watched closely by neighbors, the church, and the state. A general loosening of restrictions regarding appropriate behavior might mean that some forms of surveillance have actually diminished over time.
3. In the introduction to a symposium on "surveillance studies" in *Contemporary Sociology*, the journal's editors commented that the specific field fit squarely within the discipline, both because it had been "a mainstay in both classic and contemporary sociology" and because surveillance itself was "a particularly compelling empirical window through which to examine a slew of interesting topics, including . . . the workings of the state and systems of inequality." What these editors said of surveillance studies is no less true of family studies. Not only is the study of the family itself a mainstay of sociology, but a focus on the family gives rise to a similar range of theoretical and empirical topics. Both in

writing this introduction and in determining which essays to include in the book, we used very broad definitions of monitoring and surveillance and made no sharp distinction between the two. The noun "surveillance" refers to close observation or the act of observing. One definition of the verb "to monitor" is to keep close watch over, to supervise. Monitoring, then, is the activity on which surveillance relies.

4. On a related point, see Lyon's (2001, 119) discussion of workplace surveillance with its closely linked functions of supervision and monitoring.

5. For example, Monahan's collection *Surveillance and Security: Technological Politics and Power in Everyday Life* (2006) has only one chapter that looks exclusively at issues affecting family dynamics, and Haggerty and Ericson's *The New Politics of Surveillance and Visibility* (2006) has no chapters on this topic.

6. Included in this latter goal is the surveillance of those individuals and groups who might harm others—hence the current surveillance techniques directed at "terrorists" and the Megan's Law monitoring directed at convicted pedophiles.

7. Lyon (2001, 126–40) describes two forms of resistance to monitoring: "regulative responses" that "enunciate how personal data should be handled," and "mobilizing responses," or "the popular non-government groups and movements that arise to challenge what they see as abuses and excesses within personal data-processing." Within families, the civil-liberties concerns that generate resistance via both regulation and mobilization have little place. For example, children cannot legally claim a "right to privacy" vis-à-vis their parents, and employers appear to have a right to monitor their employees, particularly within the context of the private home (Wrigley 1995).

8. Although none of the studies included here do so specifically, we might also consider how social location shapes the perception of resistance by others. In a study of the public health campaign to reduce SIDS (sudden infant death syndrome) by strongly encouraging parents to put their babies to sleep on their backs, Hackett (2007, 3) argues that "resistance to the official policy is framed differently by the media and health professionals: upper and middle class mothers are presented as rational actors making informed decisions, and lower-income, primarily African-American mothers who put their babies to sleep on their stomachs are portrayed as noncompliant resisters in need of more targeted messages and outreach."

References

American Heritage Dictionary. 1985. New college ed. Boston: Houghton Mifflin.

Andrejevic, Mark. 2005. The Work of Watching One Another: Lateral Surveillance, Risk, and Governance. *Surveillance and Society* 24 (4): 479–97.

Berardo, Felix M. 1998. Family Privacy: Issues and Concepts. *Journal of Family Issues* 19 (1): 4–19.

Bowers, Barbara. 1990. Family Perceptions of Care in a Nursing Home. In *Circles of Care: Work and Identity in Women's Lives*, edited by Emily K. Abel and Margaret K. Nelson, 278–89. Albany: State University of New York Press.

Ehrenreich, Barbara, and Deirdre English. 1989. *For Her Own Good: 150 Years of the Experts' Advice to Women*. Reissue ed. New York: Anchor.

Fotel, Trine, and Thyra Uth Thomsen. 2004. The Surveillance of Children's Mobility. *Surveillance and Society* 1 (4): 535–54.

Donzelot, Jacques. 1979. *The Policing of Families*. New York: Pantheon Books.

Gilliom, John. 2006. Struggling with Surveillance: Resistance, Consciousness, and Identity. In *The New Politics of Surveillance and Visibility*, edited by Kevin D. Haggerty and Richard V. Ericson, 111–40. Toronto: University of Toronto Press.

Hackett, Martine. 2007. I Am so Sick of Being Presented with Official Orders about How I Should Raise My Child: Parental Resistance to a Public Health Campaign. Paper presented at the Annual Meeting of the Eastern Sociological Society, March 15–18, Philadelphia.

Haggerty, Kevin D. 2006. Tear Down the Walls: On Demolishing the Panopticon. In *Theorizing Surveillance: The Panopticon and Beyond*, edited by David Lyon, 23–46. Portland, OR: Willan.

Haggerty, Kevin D., and Richard V. Ericson. 2006. *The New Politics of Surveillance and Visibility*. Toronto: University of Toronto Press.

Hansen, Karen V. 1994. *A Very Social Time: Crafting Community in Antebellum New England*. Berkeley: University of California Press.

———. 2004. *Not-So-Nuclear Families: Class, Gender and Networks of Care*. New Brunswick, NJ: Rutgers University Press.

Hays, Sharon. 2004. *Flat Broke with Children: Women in the Age of Welfare Reform*. New York: Oxford University Press.

Katz, Cindi. 2001. The State Goes Home: Local Hyper-vigilance of Children and the Global Retreat from Social Reproduction. *Social Justice* 28 (3): 47–56.

Lareau, Annette. 2000. My Wife Can Tell Me Who I Know: Methodological and Conceptual Problems in Studying Fathers. *Qualitative Sociology* 23: 407–33.

———. 2003. *Unequal Childhoods: Class, Race, and Family Life*. Berkeley: University of California Press.

Long, Jane. 2005. "Be [Net] Alert, But Not Alarmed"? Regulating the Parents of Generation MSM. *Media International Australia Incorporating Culture and Policy* 114: 122–34.

Lyon, David. 2001. *Surveillance Society: Monitoring Everyday Life*. Philadelphia: Open University Press.

———. 2006. The Search for Surveillance Theories. In *Theorizing Surveillance: The Panopticon and Beyond*, edited by David Lyon, 3–20. Portland, OR: Willan.

———. 2007. Sociological Perspectives and Surveillance Studies: "Slow Journalism" and the Critique of Social Sorting. *Contemporary Sociology* 36 (2): 107–11.

Marx, Gary T. 2007. Desperately Seeking Surveillance Studies: Players in Search of a Field. *Contemporary Sociology* 36 (2): 125–30.

Mele, Christopher, and Teresa A. Miller. 2005. *Civil Penalties, Social Consequences*. New York: Routledge.

Monahan, Torin. 2006. Questioning Surveillance and Security. In *Surveillance and Security: Technological Politics and Power in Everyday Life*, edited by Torin Monahan, 1–26. New York: Routledge.

————, ed. 2006. *Surveillance and Security: Technological Politics and Power in Everyday Life.* New York: Routledge.

Naples, Nancy A. 2001. A Member of the Funeral: An Introspective Ethnography. In *Queer Families, Queer Politics: Challenging Culture and the State*, edited by Mary Bernstein and Renate Reimann, 21–43. New York: Columbia University Press.

Nelson, Margaret K. 2006. Single Mothers "Do" Family. *Journal of Marriage and Family* 68: 781–95.

Newburger, Eric C. 2001. *Home Computers and Internet Use in the United States: August 2000.* Current Population Reports No. P23–207. Washington, DC: Department of Commerce, U.S. Census Bureau, September.

Nock, Seven L. 1998. Too Much Privacy? *Journal of Family Issues* 19 (1): 101–20.

Rapp, Rayna. 1988. Chromosomes and Communication: The Discourse of Genetic Counseling. *Medical Anthropology Quarterly* 24 (2): 143–57.

Reich, Jennifer. 2005. *Fixing Families: Parents, Power, and the Child Welfare System.* New York: Routledge.

Roberts, Dorothy. 1998. *Killing the Black Body: Race, Reproduction, and the Meaning of Liberty.* New York: Vintage.

Romero, Mary. 1992. *Maid in the U.S.A.* New York: Routledge.

Sandelowski, Margarete. 1994. Separate, but Less Unequal: Fetal Ultrasonography and the Transformation of Expectant Mother/Fatherhood. *Gender and Society* 8 (2): 230–45.

————. 1998. Looking to Care or Caring to Look? Technology and the Rise of Spectacular Nursing. *Holistic Nursing Practice* 12 (4): 1–11.

Shapiro, Stuart. 1998. Places and Spaces: The Historical Interaction of Technology, Home, and Privacy. *The Information Society* 14: 275–84.

Staples, William G. 2000. *Everyday Surveillance: Vigilance and Visibility in Postmodern Life.* Lanham, MD: Rowman and Littlefield.

Stone, Brad. 2007. Tell-All PCs and Phones Transforming Divorce. *New York Times*, September 15.

Torpey, John. 2007. Through Thick and Thin: Surveillance after 9/11. *Contemporary Sociology* 36 (2): 116–19.

Uttal, Lynet. 1996. Custodial Care, Surrogate Care, and Coordinated Care: Employed Mothers and the Meaning of Child Care. *Gender and Society* 10 (3): 291–311.

Wang, Rong, Suzanne M. Bianchi, and Sara B. Raley. 2005. Teenagers' Internet Use and Family Rules: A Research Note. *Journal of Marriage and Family* 67: 1249–58.

West, Candace, and Don H. Zimmerman. 1987. "Doing Gender." *Gender and Society* 1 (2): 125–51.

————. 2002. "Doing Gender." In *Doing Gender, Doing Difference: Inequality, Power, and Institutional Change*, edited by Sarah Fenstermaker and Candace West, 3–25. New York: Routledge.

Wrigley, Julia. 1995. *Other People's Children.* New York: Basic Books.

Zureik, Elia. 2007. Surveillance Studies: From Metaphors to Regulation to Subjectivity. *Contemporary Sociology* 36 (2): 112–15.

Part I

They're Watching You
Watch Each Other

A long tradition of scholarship has demonstrated that the "private" family is not so private after all, that public policies shape family life in multiple ways, and that the capacity of families to delineate their own realms of action depends on the resources available to them (see, for example, Jacques Donzelot, *The Policing of Families* [1979]; Nancy Folbre, *The Invisible Heart: Economics and Family Values* [2002]; and Barrie Thorne with Marilyn Yalom, *Rethinking the Family: Some Feminist Questions* [1982]). As we noted in our introductory essay, resource-rich families can easily hide themselves from public view, while resource-poor families have more aspects of their daily lives available to the public eye and subject to public condemnation or approval. And families whose members come in contact with the criminal justice system at any level or rely on state resources (such as Temporary Assistance for Needy Families) are subject to behavioral requirements from external agents.

The essays in this section raise issues about the role of outside authority in shaping family life. What distinguishes these chapters from most scholarship on outside intervention is that each considers how the external agent challenges the family to become more intensely involved in the monitoring *of its own members*.

1

"Nested Responsibility" and the Monitoring of Children and Parents in Family Court

Anita Ilta Garey

Parents often talk as if the decisions they make about raising their children are theirs alone and are nobody else's business, especially not anyone outside the immediate family. They are therefore surprised to discover that the state has the legal right to step in and assert control over families and their members. The state regulates the behavior of parents toward their children, and in cases of abuse, neglect, or endangerment of children, the state may temporarily remove children from their families or go so far as to take away a mother's and father's "parental rights," thereby permanently severing their legal familial status as "parent and child." There is understandable concern over the hand of the state in family life; nevertheless, most people agree that some sort of oversight of children is necessary for their safety (Reich 2005). In this chapter, I use the concept of "nested responsibility" to refer to the tiered framework in which some institutions or people are responsible for monitoring the responsibility obligations of others. In the United States, for example, parents or guardians are responsible for caring for the children in their keep. The state, however, by way of its various child protective agencies and family courts, is charged with the responsibility of monitoring families for abuse or neglect of their responsibility to care for their children. Responsibility in one realm is thus nested within the responsibility obligations of another.

The state, however, intervenes not only to protect children from others but also to protect others from children—and to protect children from themselves. In the United States, the judicial system has chosen to treat crimes and offenses committed by children in a special type of court that deals with juveniles—family court. Family courts deal with crimes committed by juveniles and also adjudicate cases involving juvenile "status offenses." A status offense is not a criminal act in and of itself, but is a legal offense only because the act is performed by people in a particular status—in this case, people under a certain age (usually those under eighteen years of age, but also those under sixteen for school truancy offenses or those under twenty-one for alcohol use). Running away from home, school truancy, tobacco and alcohol use, and "ungovernability" are common juvenile status offenses. Adults cannot be charged with a crime for running away from home, missing classes, or disobeying their parents—but children behaving in these ways are breaking the law and are at risk of being charged with a status offense.

Central to the adjudication of juvenile offenses is the issue of responsibility. Family court provides a setting in which to examine notions of responsibility for children in our society—not just the basic responsibility to care for and protect one's own children, but also responsibility for the actions of children themselves. Much discussion has surrounded the issue of how much, if any, legal responsibility parents should have for criminal actions by their children (Thurman 2003; Tomaszewski 2005; U.S. Department of Justice 1997). The position that parents should be legally and financially liable for crimes committed by their children rests on the belief that it is the responsibility of parents to train their children to behave appropriately and to monitor their children's behavior and activities; criminal activities by children therefore attest to the fact that their parents have failed in those responsibilities. In other words, the child committed the crime, but the parent allowed it to happen.

In this chapter I focus on the allocation of responsibility for children's status offenses and the way in which those responsibilities are framed and monitored by social institutions outside the family. The rationale for holding parents responsible for their children's status offenses is the same as for holding parents responsible for children's criminal offenses. In both types of offense, the argument for holding parents legally responsible for their children's actions rests on the proposition that parenting practices are a determining factor in children's behavior (Tomaszewski 2005, 583). Focusing solely on juvenile status offenses allows me to separate the issue of responsibility for children's actions from victim-centered concerns, such as restitution, that arise in criminal cases (Tomaszewski 2005, 582). This chapter thus examines notions of responsibility and processes of monitoring that apply to the mundane, everyday behaviors of parents and families and their interactions with outside institutions. I examine how parental responsibility is framed and monitored in a special unit of the family court that deals with the status offense of school truancy.

Truancy is a status offense, and in cases of excessive school absence a truancy petition may be filed against a child by a school district's truant officer. These cases are seen in family court, but since the late 1990s, many states have established special programs within the courts to deal with the problem. In the state in which I conducted my research, special "truancy courts" had been established. Modeled on drug courts and diversion programs, and part of the growing category of "problem-solving courts," truancy courts aim to monitor and manage the offender until the problem behavior is corrected, at which point the case may be successfully dismissed with nothing posted to the child's permanent juvenile record. Families may choose truancy court over adjudication in family court because of the convenience of its location in the school or the opportunity to get some needed assistance in dealing with their children, but the desire for the child to emerge with a clean record is the major inducement for most families.

The truancy courts in this study were presided over by family court magistrates but were physically located in the schools. The truancy court (black-robed magistrate, court clerk, court aide, court juvenile files, and flag) traveled from one school to the next, appearing in "School A" on Mondays, "School B" on Tuesdays, and so forth. Students against whom truancy petitions were filed were required to come to truancy court with a parent for their arraignment on a specified date. At that time, they could choose to remain in truancy court and be subject to weekly court monitoring or to have their case heard in family court, at which point, if found guilty of the alleged truancy, they would receive a penalty, usually probation, and enter "the system." All but two families among the more than three hundred arraignments I witnessed chose truancy court over having their case tried in the main family court.

In truancy court, a child's case is reviewed weekly in front of the judge. Both child and parent are required to attend the court review, at which the truancy office reports on the child's attendance since the previous court session and the school guidance counselor reports on the child's academic progress and behavior at school. After three or four weeks, if the child's attendance improves, the parent may be excused from attending the weekly court reviews. If attendance, grades, and behavior all improve, the child may be reviewed every two or three weeks instead of weekly. But if the child reverts to his or her previous habits of unexcused absences or poor grades, weekly reviews may resume and parents may be summoned back to court. Family, school, or individual problems that emerge over the course of the case may be addressed by the judge, who can issue a court order for family or individual counseling, testing for learning disabilities, psychological evaluation, and so forth. The goal is to get the child back on track and dismiss the case at the end of the school year. However, if progress is not made toward that goal, the court exerts its power and authority. I have observed cases in which the judge has temporarily removed children from their homes or has ordered home investigations by the state's child protective agency, and judges frequently order less dramatic but nonetheless family-intrusive consequences for continued school absence. A truancy petition thus brings children and their parents under the scrutiny (or surveillance) of the family court system.

Method

For almost three years between 2001 and 2004, I observed the proceedings of state truancy courts in three different school districts, covering seven middle schools (grades six through eight), in a New England state. Twenty to fifty cases are seen during each court's weekly four- to five-hour-long truancy session, and I observed about three hundred cases multiple times. My primary data are my field notes recording my observations of the court proceedings and the interactions of judges, court aides, school guidance counselors, teachers, principals, and children and their family members during and between cases. My field notes contain descriptions of interactions and people, verbatim exchanges taken down in my own style of shorthand, and paraphrases when the exchanges went too quickly for me to capture every word.

The three school districts vary in the degree to which they are ethnically and racially diverse. In one school district, the middle school population is predominantly white (83 percent); in another, it is 62 percent Hispanic, 28 percent white, and 10 percent African American; and in the third, it is 55 percent white, 25 percent Hispanic, and 22 percent African American. The socioeconomic status of children's families also varies widely between the three school districts and even more greatly between individual schools. In the only school in the study that served an upper-middle-class community, only 5 percent of the students qualified for the free lunch program, while in the school that served the poorest school district in the state, 99 percent of children were in the free lunch program. Although boys land in truancy court more often than girls, girls are by no means strangers to the court: 58 percent of the cases I observed were boys and 42 percent girls.

I use three cases to illustrate interactions between the courts, the schools, and the parents within a framework of nested responsibility. The dynamics of each case are representative of patterns of interaction between the judge, school counselors and principals, and parents that emerged from my data. In all three cases, the children are boys from white, working-class, native-born families. Gender, race/ethnicity, socioeconomic position, and immigrant status all play a part in shaping interactions and outcomes, but I have chosen to hold those categories constant in this chapter and to use cases of male students in white working-class families in order to focus primarily on the interactive dynamics in the courts. In these cases the parents not only share a similar social location, but that social location is treated as "the norm" in this school system. In the school districts in which this research is based, most white families were working class or lower middle class, and it was with this group that court and school personnel seemed to be most comfortable.[1] Correctly or not, the court personnel assumed that all white working- and lower-middle-class families shared values and characteristics that they understood. They also judged other family forms in terms of their understanding of this norm.

The concept of nested responsibility applies to all the cases that come before the truancy court, but the way in which this ideology is expressed and implemented is likely to differ across race/ethnicity, social class, and gender. The particular kind of treatment the students and families in these three cases received was linked to being white, working class, and, in the case of the truant students, male, but it is not the purpose of this chapter—nor is there space—to examine racial or ethnic differences in the ways that nested responsibility is applied. It is precisely because race/ethnicity, social class, and sex categories are crucial categories of analysis that I am holding them constant. These three cases do not represent some unmarked or "typical" pattern; they are marked by race/ethnicity (white), class (working class), and gender (male). In looking at the concept of nested responsibility across cases, I want to first examine the differences that emerge in cases when the differences are linked *not* to differential treatment on the basis of race/ethnicity, social class, or gender but rather to the patterns of parental responses. I observed the range of parental responses examined here among all types of families (as defined by race/ethnicity and social class) and for both male and female students.[2]

Monitoring Responsibility

In truancy court, children's behavior is monitored by the court on an ongoing basis, and parents are judged in terms of how well they are monitoring their children. Both children and parents are held accountable when a child does not "measure up" on specified criteria. Although the magistrate clearly tells each family at the arraignment that the petition is against the child, not the parent, and that it is the child who is the subject of the court proceedings, parents and family systems are also being scrutinized, judged, and held responsible by the court. For example, the judge not only issues court orders to the child, as when ordering detentions, community service, or house confinement, but often issues court orders to the parents. Parents may be court-ordered to appear in truancy court on particular dates, remove the computer from their house, or arrange for their child to get eyeglasses or medical care.

The child's failure is seen as a lack of individual responsibility, while parents are held to a court-defined standard of parental responsibility. Parents are blamed for making it possible for dependent children to act irresponsibly and are expected to make them act responsibly. For example, if a child skips school out of frustration at not being able to see the blackboard because of poor eyesight, the court considers it the parents' responsibility to provide the needed glasses. If a child stays up late playing on the computer and refuses to get out of bed in time for school in the morning, parents are advised to put ice down the back of the child's pajamas to force them out of bed. If parents fail in their duties—and the presence of their children in truancy court indicates to the court a failure of some kind—then the state may use its authority to monitor the parents' monitoring of their children. Thus, in terms of status offenses such as truancy, the responsibility for the monitoring of children is layered. The child is responsible for self-monitoring; parents are responsible for monitoring their children's self-monitoring; and the state is responsible for monitoring parents' monitoring of their children. However, as I will discuss in this chapter, this framework of nested responsibility can be both a sensible approach and one that can limit adequate solutions to real problems.

Parental Responses to Nested Responsibility

Parents' responses to the truancy court's authority to intervene in family life varied. In general, those families living in poverty or otherwise marginalized by race/ethnicity, immigration status, language facility, and so forth understood the power of the state in this regard more fully than those who were less vulnerable to state intrusion. Some parents, particularly but not exclusively parents from upper-middle-class families, contested the idea that the court had the right to dictate what decisions they should make regarding their child. One such mother expressed her outrage by saying, "How can the school department tell me, *as a parent*, when I can and can't keep my daughter home?!" Parents summoned to truancy court soon learned, however, that the state did have the authority to monitor parents' decisions about their children's school attendance as well their behavior in many other realms.

Parents negotiate this situation in various ways. Interactions run most smoothly when parents share the court's definition of the problem and not only accept but are also grateful for its intervention (or, at the very least, appear to be grateful). Although not a frequent response, some parents express relief that they are getting assistance in dealing with a problem that they are at their wits' end to solve. In these cases parents accept the responsibility for monitoring their children but admit that their monitoring has not been effective in bringing about the desired behavior in their children. The story of Richard's mother provides an illustration of a parent who has accepted the frame of nested responsibility and is working in concert with the truancy court.[3]

Richard was fourteen years old and repeating the eighth grade; he had been in truancy court for several months, during which time the judge ordered psychological testing for him. When Richard and his mother appeared in court for a review of his case, the school guidance counselor reported that although Richard had not been truant for the past two months, he was not passing any of his classes and had been suspended for eight days for being disrespectful to several teachers. In response to this news about Richard's recent behavior, the judge asked Richard's mother if Richard was still being tested. Richard's mother replied,

> He was tested. They gave me their response on Tuesday, but they said
> it will take three to four weeks to get the full file of the report together.
> Testing suggested ADD, and I've made an appointment for him with a
> physician, tutoring over the summer, and therapy for anger management,
> problem solving, self-esteem, and depression. The tester also said that the
> judge should call her if she [the judge] wants more information. I'm also
> looking into three different school programs for next year.

Through this response, Richard's mother is indicating to the judge that she is taking responsibility for dealing with Richard's problem behavior by actively pursuing multiple sources of assistance.

Because it is the end of the school year and Richard's case is unresolved, it is decided that he will be reviewed over the summer at the main courthouse. The judge asks Richard's mother what day would be good for her to come to court during the summer, adding, "We'll hold the case until *I* can see you. We'll call you." This way of scheduling a court date is unusual in two respects. First, the judge proactively tries to take the parent's schedule into consideration. Parents and their schedules are rarely taken into account in assigning court review dates, and when they are, it is in response to a request from a parent. Second, the judge wants to see this case through and does not want it assigned to another judge's calendar, indicating that she and the parent are working on something together. As the review ends, the judge says that Richard can go back to class, but Richard's mother reminds her that Richard is suspended and adds, "About the suspension. I understand why he is suspended, but why an out-of-school suspension? He just sits home and I don't see what he learns from this." The judge nods in agreement, explains that the schools have the problem of needing to use increasing consequences for repeated infractions, and adds that she is trying to set up a community service center for next year, where suspended students will have to go to work for eight hours a day.

Regardless of one's analysis of what transpired in the review of Richard's case, the interactions of the participants proceeded smoothly. The mother is articulate, talks in terms of process, shows deference, accepts the responsibility for monitoring her son, and acts on that responsibility. Because of these actions, the court's responsibility to monitor the mother's monitoring of her child can be manifested as "helping" rather than as "admonishing" her. However, while the court may decide what parents should do to make sure that children act responsibly, the monitoring of responsibility goes only in one direction. The judge, and the teachers working through the judge, may define what parents need to do to make sure their children act responsibly, but attempts by parents to question the monitoring actions or efficacy of the school or the court carry no weight. When Richard's mother respectfully questions the monitoring actions of the school in its decision to suspend her son, the judge acknowledges her concern about the point of suspension but does not challenge the principal's authority or wisdom in doing so. Richard's mother does not pursue the issue.

Some parents, like Richard's mother, accept the framework of nested responsibility but also try more directly to suggest ways in which the court or the school could do things that would help the parent to monitor the child. These attempts to work with the school or the court in ways other than their usual institutional procedures were generally not effective. The message given was that it was the parent and the child, not the institution, who needed to change. Peter's father provides an example. When Peter and his father appeared for a review of Peter's case, his guidance counselor reported that Peter had had no absences or tardies in a month and his behavior had been excellent, but he wasn't doing his schoolwork and was behind in all his classes. Peter's father wanted to know if he could get a report earlier in the process so that he would know whether Peter was doing his work before they got to the weekly truancy court hearing. In other words, Peter's father is asking the school to help him by providing the information he needs in order to effectively monitor his son's responsibility for doing his homework. The exchange between Peter's father, the guidance counselor, and the judge illustrates the way in which the nesting of responsibility is unidirectional.

> *Guidance Counselor:* He has a planner. The teacher signs it and the parent is supposed to sign it daily—and the parent can ask questions, but we need to get Peter to buy into it.
> *Father:* The planner is not working.
> *Guidance Counselor:* Well, we need to get Peter to buy into it. The planner is the most efficient way—so everyone is involved.
> *Judge:* But Father is saying that the planner is not working.
> *Guidance Counselor:* The planner is not working because Peter is not using it.
> *Judge:* I know, but—What is the issue, Peter? Why aren't you using your planner?
> [Peter doesn't answer.]
> *Father:* I'd like to have some kind of tool that works.
> *Guidance Counselor:* The problem is—the big problem is—the teacher has two minutes between classes. Other kids get their planners signed. There are reminders in class, but we're going to have to have Peter do his part.

Peter's father continued, conveying an earnest and dogged effort to find a way for him to more effectively monitor Peter's schoolwork. The guidance counselor remained a broken record on the subject of the planner and of Peter doing his part. Finally, the judge interrupted this circular exchange and said to Peter's father, "Revise the planner any way that works for you, but Peter needs to get his homework done. I'm ordering Peter into detention to do his homework."

Peter's father's attempt to get the school to take more responsibility for communicating with him about Peter's schoolwork is unsuccessful for two major reasons. First, although each nested box of responsibility has its own attendant area of accountability, they are arranged hierarchically. The court has authority, in specific realms, over the parent, the school, and the child; the school has authority, in specific realms, over the child, and although it does not have direct power over parents, it is not directly accountable to them; the parent has authority over the child.[4] The authority does not go in the other direction. Second, although they are arranged hierarchically, each nested box of responsibility has its own assigned turf. For example, one of the legal arguments used to challenge the right of the court to hold parents responsible for specific kinds of parenting is that "attempts to prescribe parent behavior may violate the established privacy right in child rearing" (U.S. Department of Justice 1997, 20). In Peter's father's attempt to get the school to take more responsibility in communicating homework assignments to him, the turf battle was not only the manifest one between Peter's father and the guidance counselor but also the latent one between the judge and the guidance counselor (as representatives, respectively, of the court and the school). The judge refrained from supporting Peter's father's request because to do so would be to challenge a procedure that fell within the school's turf. The same dynamic was evident when Richard's mother questioned the wisdom of using suspension from school as a punishment for Richard's behavior. Although the judge showed support for Richard's mother's position (and, indeed, privately agreed that suspensions were a counterproductive way to handle these problems), she defended the school's need to use suspension, while indicating that she was trying to find an alternative for the future.[5]

In most cases, parents' attempts to suggest new or nonstandard approaches to dealing with their children's problem behavior were framed by the court and the school as ways to shirk parental responsibility or to further mollycoddle children who were not being taught by their parents to take responsibility. Parents had to negotiate a situation that was defined by those in power as one in which the problem was with the child and in which they, as parents, were responsible for making the child behave responsibly regarding school attendance, behavior, and performance. A few parents, however, refused to accept this framework. Unlike Richard's mother or Peter's father, both of whom basically accepted the nested-responsibility framework, Roger's father rejected this definition of the problem.

At the beginning of the truancy court review, Roger's father is in the school "courtroom" with the judge, one of Roger's teachers, and the principal, while the guidance counselor tries to find Roger. The judge tells Roger's father that the guidance counselor has reported that Roger is still not doing his schoolwork. Roger's father replies, "He says he's been doing his work. I see him doing something—I don't know what he's doing." Roger's father then says he wants to move Roger to another school:

Principal: You think it's the school?
Father: Yes.
Principal: Where are you going to take him?
Father: We're moving to [nearby state]—to live with my sister.

Principal: When?
Father: As soon as I can arrange it.

Not convinced that Roger's father is really moving and concerned that Roger's situation will continue to deteriorate if Roger's father persists in trying to avoid the problem, the principal continues:

Principal: Roger is probably failing. He'll have to repeat eighth grade. He'll be another year older and still in the same grade.
Father: Let me be honest with you. The kid is fourteen years old. Out of all the schools he's been to, he's never had a problem until he came to this school.
Principal: He's been here for four years!

At this point, the judge intercedes and, with the authority of the court, moves up the chain of nested responsibility: "Respectfully, I'm going to send this to the chief judge [of the family court]. I think Roger needs in-patient assessment. Unless everyone shows a team approach, there is no point in staying here. I respect your decision, but I feel that in-patient would benefit Roger because he will find out he cannot use the same excuses and get away from it." In other words, if, in the eyes of the court, Roger's father fails to take parental responsibility for adequately monitoring his son, in terms of both Roger's care needs (e.g., psychological well being) and Roger's level of individual responsibility (e.g., completing his schoolwork), then the state, in its monitoring role, must step in. The principal tries one more time to mollify Roger's father and to enlist his cooperation: "As a father, you have a vested interest in your son and want his best interests. As a school, so do we. But I don't want to be sitting down in June and saying he's failed eighth grade."

At this point, Roger enters the room. The judge tells him that because he has not done his homework, she is referring him to the chief judge in the family court. Roger tells the judge that he did do the homework, and his father states firmly, "I believe him." Then, turning to his son, he says, "Don't worry. I think they're torturing you. We're going. Don't worry. As a matter of fact, we're going now." And Roger and his father walk out.

In this case, Roger's father refused to accept the school's assessment that Roger was not doing his homework (or that Roger had any problems at all). Nor was he willing to accept that, as Roger's father, he should be doing anything other than asking Roger and taking his word for it that the homework was being done. Whether he was correct in his assessment or not, he refused to categorize his child as the problem, and thus refused to become a team player or to accept the role of failed parent.

Conclusion

Parents respond to the framework of nested responsibility in various ways. The three cases presented in this chapter represent ideal types along the spectrum of parental responses.[6] The judge, guidance counselor, and principal respond to parents accordingly. As in Richard's case, they work cooperatively with parents who not only accept the framework but also display a willingness and ability to fulfill their responsibility in monitoring their children. As in Peter's case, they ignore or stonewall attempts by parents who suggest, however respectfully, that perhaps there should be changes in the way responsibilities are carried out by those higher up the monitoring chain, such as the schools or the court. And as in Roger's case, they assert the full power of their position in the monitoring chain toward parents who refuse to accept the legitimacy of the nested responsibility framework.[7]

In all three cases, excessive absence from school triggered the involvement of the family court, but as these cases progressed, all three of the boys began attending school as required. Thus, their problem was no longer truancy. The "problems" being addressed in the court became problems of responsibility—for passing courses, progressing to the next grade, being respectful to teachers, suppressing anger, and doing homework. There are, of course, cases in which the truancy problem that triggered court involvement reveals more serious issues within the lives of children and their families, such as drug abuse, clinical depression, family violence, bullying, and gang involvement. In these situations, the framework of nested responsibility could be seen as providing a safety net for children, by, for example, requiring parents to obtain psychological therapy for their children, to monitor their children by administering drug tests to them, or to modify their own behavior.

Nested responsibility could, however, also be seen as passing the buck back to individual families. Richard's mother, for example, complied completely with the court-ordered psychological testing of her son, but it would take another month before test results and recommendations were available. In the meantime, she was left with a child whose behavior had resulted in an eight-day suspension from school. Neither the school nor the court was exercising any responsibility for helping Richard while he was suspended. Richard's mother was also trying to line up some of the services that were recommended: a physician to manage his ADD medications, therapy for anger management and depression, enrollment in an alternative school. The judge told her that she did not want to dismiss Richard's case from truancy court until she knew that all these services were in place. Richard's mother responded to this by saying, "I'm working on it now. It's hard to do this from work. There are only so many phone calls I can make in a day. I need to arrange to go to the conference room to make a private call, and I probably can't reach everyone before a holiday weekend." None of the services recommended for Richard were set up or provided as part of the testing service, the court's monitoring, or the school's psychological or guidance counseling; the responsibility for finding and obtaining the services Richard needed belonged to Richard's mother.

I began this chapter with the observation that most parents think that, except in serious cases of child abuse or neglect, families and family life do and should fall outside the purview of state regulation and monitoring. The cases presented here, however, illustrate a situation in which children and parents are monitored and held accountable in situations that do not involve risk to the health of their child or restitution to someone their child has harmed. Rather, the activity being monitored is parental responsibility for making children act responsibly. The court defines and monitors what constitutes responsible activity on the part of the child: going to school, completing homework, being respectful to teachers, and so forth. These may seem like reasonable things to expect from children, but who should be held responsible if children do not perform adequately in these areas? What happens when school and court definitions of responsibility run up against family-centered definitions of responsibility, as, for example, when a child stays home to care for younger siblings or to translate for parents who do not speak English? The effects on the parent-child relationship of the court's intrusion into family life is something that needs further study (but see Ferguson 2001; Reich 2005). As Staples (Chapter 2) points out, however, there are "collateral consequences" when external authorities insert themselves into the day-to-day lives of families. One example of this is the disruption in parents' lives as they seek to fulfill court mandates; as Richard's mother indicated, her efforts to find help for her child had to be meshed with her responsibilities as an employee. Moreover, the truancy court creates a situation in which parents are perceived to be appropriately responsible only if they join forces with the legal and educational systems in getting their children to behave according to certain normative standards regarding school performance and behavior. If they fail, or appear to fail, in their cooperation, the court can use its power to force parents and children to comply and to punish them if they refuse. Distinguishing themselves from the adjudication role of the family court, truancy courts aim to solve problems and help children and families, but failure to comply with their mandates can have serious consequences for family integrity.

Notes

1. Children of upper-middle-class families were much more likely to attend private schools or a few select public schools in other areas of the state.
2. In my larger project, I am examining family-school-court interactions across race/ethnicity, social class, gender, family form, and immigrant status.
3. The names used in this chapter are pseudonyms.
4. For example, the school is not accountable to the parent for its systems, rules, and processes unless it violates the law, in which case the parent can call on the legal system to exert its authority to make the school accountable. Families do not have any direct authority over the school.
5. The judge could, and sometimes did, order the school to take particular actions, such as testing a student for learning disabilities even if the student didn't meet the school's guidelines for testing. The family court, however, was not the venue for reviewing school processes or procedures. The judge could respectfully ask principals or guidance counselors whether they could make accommodations for a particular student, but to do more would risk the "team" relationship (Goffman 1959) between the judge and the school's personnel.
6. Other cases differ in their details, arrange themselves in different places on this continuum, and raise different issues, but for the purpose of illustrating the framework of nested responsibility that underlies much of the dynamic between these adult representatives of family, educational, and judicial systems, the cases of Richard, Peter, and Roger capture the ends and middle of that continuum.
7. In Roger's case, his father threatened to remove him from the state, which would remove Roger from the authority of the truancy court as well as from the broader family court. However, in most other cases of impasse between the court and the parent that I witnessed, the court removed children from their homes, mandated in-patient psychological testing, sent the case to family court for prosecution, or committed other acts of authority over the parent and child.

References

Ferguson, Ann Arnett. 2001. *Bad Boys: Public Schools in the Making of Black Masculinity*. Ann Arbor: University of Michigan Press.

Goffman, Erving. 1959. *Presentation of Self in Everyday Life*. New York: Doubleday.

Reich, Jennifer A. 2005. *Fixing Families: Parents, Power, and the Child Welfare System*. New York: Routledge.

Thurman, Tammy. 2003. Parental Responsibility Laws: Are They the Answer to Juvenile Delinquency? *Journal of Law and Family Studies* 99.

Tomaszewski, Amy L. 2005. From Columbine to Kazaa: Parental Liability in a New World. *University of Illinois Law Review*, pp. 573–99.

U.S. Department of Justice, Office of Justice Programs, Office of Juvenile Justice and Delinquency Prevention. 1997. *Juvenile Justice Reform Initiatives in the States: 1994–1996. ojjdp/ncjrs.org/pubs/reform.*

2

"Where Are You and What Are You Doing?"

Familial Back-Up Work as a Collateral Consequence of House Arrest

William G. Staples

It's not just me doing the house arrest, but [members of my family] feel *they're* on house arrest . . . and that's unfair to them for what, you know, me being punished, they're being punished also, by the phone ringing, by being woke up in the middle of the night to make sure that I am up and I am on the phone so I don't get in trouble and have the police coming out here to get me.

—Jeff, on living under house arrest

Between August and October 2001, I interviewed twenty-three people living under house arrest in a midwestern metropolitan area.[1] Jeff is one of these individuals. A twenty-four-year-old European American who works as a plastics fabricator, Jeff was convicted of driving under the influence of alcohol (DUI) and a number of misdemeanors, including violating the conditions of his parole. This is his second experience with house arrest. Altogether, he has spent more than a month being electronically monitored

Portions of this chapter first appeared as William G. Staples, "The Everyday World of House Arrest: Collateral Consequences for Families and Others," in *Civil Penalties, Social Consequences*, edited by Christopher Mele and Teresa Miller, 139–59 (© 2005 by Taylor & Francis Group LLC–Books). Reproduced by permission of Taylor & Francis Group LLC–Books; permission conveyed through Copyright Clearance Center, Inc.

at home, this time following a three-month stint in a residential treatment center. Once released from the residential program, Jeff moved in with his father and grandmother. Being on house arrest means that Jeff must respond within the first three rings to random phone calls from a Department of Corrections computer to verify that he is home when he is scheduled to be. There is a small computerized unit attached to the family's only home phone line. When the Department of Corrections calls Jeff's phone, he must answer the phone and blow into an alcohol tester built into the machine. While he is doing this, the device takes his picture and compares it to a reference photograph stored on a central computer.

For Jeff and many of the other house arrest "clients" with whom I spoke, a sentence to house arrest is characterized, for a variety of reasons, as "better" than the alternative of sitting in the county jail. Yet during our interview, Jeff expressed frustration and anger at several aspects of his treatment by corrections officials, and especially at how his house arrest means that his family is being, in his words, "punished" for something he did. In fact, nearly all individuals with whom I spoke reported that their spouses, lovers, immediate family, roommates, relatives, or others close to them are affected, in various ways, by *their* sentence to house arrest. These secondary effects, or "collateral consequences" (Mele and Miller 2005; Mauer and Chesney-Lind 2002), of a house arrest sentence are wide-ranging, including the inconvenience of not being able to have alcohol in the house, the disruption of frequent phone calls, and increased tension and stress in relationships. Through an examination of these offender narratives, we can see how the penalty of house arrest is made meaningful and has an impact on the daily experiences of the clients and those who share their domestic worlds.[2]

In this chapter, I explore two types of collateral consequences associated with a sentence to house arrest. The first is the various forms of emotional, mental, and physical labor, what I call "back-up work," in which family members and others often engage because of their relationships with the offenders. I show how, through their actions and behaviors in "support" of those on house arrest, these significant others may end up functioning as ancillary "watchers," keeping an eye on the offender's behavior and prodding him or her to stay in compliance with program demands. In this way, family members and intimates are turned into agents of the state within their domestic worlds (Donzelot 1979; see also Garey, Chapter 1). The second collateral consequence I identify is what I call the "co-experience" of house arrest for family and intimates of the arrestee. The focus here is on the stress, the tension, and the feeling among these significant others that they, too, are being disciplined and controlled by house arrest. Through these collateral consequences, significant others who have not been convicted of a crime experience monitoring by the state while they become monitors themselves.

Doing Time at Home

The original, commonly used method of electronically monitoring someone at home involves a small radio transmitter, typically attached to the ankle of the offender. A monitoring box is placed in the home or apartment, and the arrestee cannot stray beyond approximately 150 feet from the box without a violation being recorded by a central computer. Sometimes called "tagging," the idea is credited to a New Mexico district court judge who was supposedly inspired by the use of a similar device in a 1979 Spiderman comic strip (Klein-Saffran 1993). House arrest was first used on nonviolent felony offenders on parole from prison. In the mid-1990s, it began to proliferate and be used among various levels of offenders, as well as those at nearly every point in the justice process. Currently, house arrest programs tether more than seventy thousand individuals to central monitoring systems in the United States (Harrison and Karberg 2003), and there are similar programs in Australia, Canada, the Netherlands, New Zealand, Sweden, and the United Kingdom (Newman 1999).

House arrest with electronic monitoring emerged as one of the community-based "intermediate sanctions" associated with the "new penology" (Feeley and Simon 1992) of the 1980s. This ideological and policy shift emphasized a new rationality centered on the sorting and classifying of offenders into finer categories of risk and dangerous. Classification was set along a continuum between high-cost incarceration for those who pose the greatest risks, such as violent offenders, and lower-cost methods of surveillance for low-risk offenders. Intermediate sanctions, including boot camps, intensive supervision, community service, work-release, restitution, day-reporting centers, and day fines, were conceived as incremental punishments along the continuum between the extremes of probation at one end and prison at the other. They were therefore viewed as better suited to individuals classified as lower risk or marginally dangerous.

The bulk of academic literature dealing with house arrest has focused either on determining whether the treatment is effective at reducing recidivism or on assessing its relative cost when compared to other sanctions (see Maxfield and Baumer 1990; Glaser and Watts 1992; Jolin and Stipak 1992; Lilly et al. 1993; Sandhu, Dodder, and Mathur 1993; Jones and Ross 1997; Courtright, Berg, and Mutchnick 1997a, 1997b, 2000; Ulmer 2001). By contrast, I am interested in investigating the broader social-control implications of the use of this kind of technology, as well as how it actually operates and is experienced in routine, everyday ways. I see house arrest as one of a plethora of contemporary, disciplinary practices and technologies—technologies that I contend are constituted by and indicative of conditions of postmodernity (Staples 1994, 2000).

Only a few studies (Holman and Quinn 1992; Payne and Gainey 1998; Gainey and Payne 2000; Maidment 2002) have begun to explore what offenders actually make of the experience of house arrest, and only Ansay (1999) has studied the experience in depth and considered the effects of the sanction on families and intimates. In her unpublished dissertation, Ansay argues that house arrest programs tend to ignore the relationships and responsibilities of clients as family members, and that their use creates undue hardship for intimates who end up sharing the experience of the sentence. She points out that all house arrestees are subject to the same set of program rules and restrictions, yet their lived, domestic worlds are varied and complex (115). The relationship between their official lives and identities as correctional clients and their familial lives and roles as husbands, wives, partners, parents, sons, and daughters must be constantly negotiated in an attempt to satisfy often competing demands.

Building on Ansay's research, the offender narratives presented here reveal how the disciplinary regime of house arrest produces important consequences for those significant others and intimates caught in the collision of these two worlds. These consequences include disruptions to everyday family life and adaptations required in response to the bureaucratically ordered life associated with house arrest. Among other things, intimates must deal with frequent, random phone calls, especially at night; visits by corrections officials; the need to rearrange schedules and activities; and the limits placed on a client's participation in his or her roles as parent, partner, friend, and worker. I focus specifically on the various forms of emotional, mental, and physical labor—what I call "back-up work"—in which family members and others often engage because of their relationship with the offender. First, I show how through this back-up work, individuals who have been convicted of no crime concurrently experience monitoring by the state and become monitors themselves. Second, I show how these effects, changes, and adaptations often produce shared experiences among the clients and others in the home, or what I call "co-experiences," such as stress, tension, and the other consequences of being disciplined and controlled by house arrest. After all, intimates are often woken up by phone calls to the client, they are there when officials visit their home, and their lives are affected by a rigid confinement schedule set by strangers in a state bureaucracy.

Studying House Arrest

During the course of my research in 2001, I visited the house arrest program's office about a dozen times to conduct face-to-face, open-ended interviews with clients. While I waited in another room, program personnel asked clients whether they were interested in participating in a study about house arrest that was being conducted by a researcher from a local university. About one in three declined to participate. If a client agreed to take part, we would be introduced, then we would move to a private office in the facility. Informed consent statements were proffered, and I addressed any concerns or questions about the study before we began. Importantly, I assured all clients that I had nothing to do with the program or the staff and that anything they told me would be kept confidential. Each interview took approximately thirty minutes to conduct. Interviews were taped and later transcribed. I used an interview guide of about a dozen general questions centered on the experience of house arrest. My sample group included fifteen European Americans (twelve males and three females) and eight African Americans (seven males and one female). The mean age was thirty-three, with a range of eighteen to seventy-four.

At the time of my research, the house arrest program had been in operation for more than a decade. The office is located in an isolated industrial area of the county and shares a building with the county Department of Corrections' 172-bed residential program (referred to here as "The Center"). House arrest, as practiced by this community corrections department, is a highly structured program that involves mandatory employment, educational and treatment programs, frequent drug and alcohol testing, and an offender fee payment. Once assigned to house arrest, offenders sign a three-page, seventeen-point contract that outlines all the conditions and behavioral expectations of the program. Clients must develop a daily schedule of approved activities (e.g., work, school, Alcoholics Anonymous meetings, and doctors visits). Weekly face-to-face meetings with a house arrest officer are required to review and update schedules, to verify compliance through testing for drug or alcohol use, and to turn over paycheck stubs and signed verification of attendance at required treatment programs. House arrest officers meet with family or friends, referred to as "collateral contacts," who agree to serve as a secondary means of contacting offenders; the officers also make unannounced visits to places of employment and residence. In addition, a computerized Mitsubishi Electronic Monitoring System (MEMS) device is installed in the offender's home. The device verifies compliance with the house arrest contract by recording the offender's voice, taking his or her picture, and collecting breath samples for analysis. The house arrest officer assigned to each case determines the appropriate number of calls for specific blocks of time, and the system randomly calls the offender within those blocks.

When a call is made, a computer-simulated human voice tells the person answering the phone that the call is from the house arrest office, and a short pause gives the offender time to get to the phone in case someone else has answered. The system then instructs the offender to take his or her own photograph and to submit a breath sample through a straw inserted into the home monitoring unit. The photograph is displayed on a computer screen in the house arrest office next to a reference photo previously entered into the system; this allows staff to verify the identity of the person answering the call. The black and white photographs have a sort of grainy, fish-eye effect and, because they are often taken at night, frequently show clients in a disheveled, sleepy state. The results of the alcohol breath test are recorded in the computer and displayed on screen with the photo of the offender, his or her name, and the date and time of the call. If the client does not answer the phone, the computer immediately places a second call. If the second call results in a violation, an alarm alerts staff at the house arrest office.

Many of the clients told me that there is little leeway for those violating the conditions of their house arrest contract. If clients do not respond to phone calls, they have a two-hour window to either call the house arrest office or show up to the office in person. If they do not contact the office within this time frame, their house arrest officer deems them "violated," meaning that they have broken their house arrest contract. Likewise, having a "hot UA" (a positive urine analysis) results in an infraction. Program staff frequently call on local law enforcement to conduct residence checks, to look for clients suspected of being AWOL, to provide arrest and detention services, to investigate allegations of abuse in the home, and to verify whether or not an offender is driving on a suspended license. The program requires offenders to pay a daily monitoring fee and all fees associated with the program, including drug testing. All of the clients with whom I spoke were court ordered to maintain full-time employment.

In the year 2000, 1,048 adult clients participated in this midwestern county's house arrest program, with about eighty to one hundred individuals monitored at any given time. The typical house arrest sentence lasted between thirty and ninety days. Males accounted for 81 percent of the cases. The majority (68 percent) of all participants were sentenced directly to the house arrest program. Other participants were placed on house arrest as a condition of a bond, pending a probation violation hearing, as an internal sanction of the Intensive Supervision Probation program, or as part of a conditional release agreement from a residential/work release program. Felony offenders accounted for approximately 34 percent of the 1,048 adult clients ($n = 361$). DUI cases made up 30 percent of felony offenses, burglary and theft 19 percent, and drug possession 18 percent. Of the misdemeanor cases served ($n = 687$), 50 percent were DUI, 18 percent were theft or larceny, and 16 percent were drug possession. Clients were charged twelve dollars per day for house arrest monitoring and seventeen dollars per drug test. The program collected more than $211,000 in fees from clients in 2000.

"Where Are You and What Are You Doing?"

As I indicated above, "back-up work" refers to forms of emotional, mental, and physical labor in which family members and other people often engage because of their relationship with the offender on house arrest. Clients reported that intimates wake them up when surveillance calls come; drive them to and from work and other places when their license is suspended; act as their emergency, or "collateral," contact for corrections officials; worry about them; and berate them to "stay on the right track." From the perspective of officials, clients, and even significant others, these actions may be considered a positive contribution since this kind of "support" improves completion rates and helps keep clients out of jail, a result that is seemingly in the best interest of all concerned. And yet, even if intimates gladly offer this assistance, this back-up work is still work—emotional, mental, and physical labor—and is therefore a collateral consequence imposed on individuals simply because of their relationship and proximity to the offender. Moreover, through their actions and behaviors in support of those on house arrest, these significant others may end up functioning as ancillary "watchers," policing the offender's behavior and prodding him or her to stay in compliance with program demands. In this way, intimates are indirectly turned into surrogate agents of the state (Donzelot 1979) as the surveillance regime of house arrest intrudes into their now "deprivatized" (Gubrium and Holstein 1990) domestic lives.

A number of interviewees indicated that family members watch over them and help them stay in compliance with program rules and procedures. Efforts included answering the telephone, responding to the needs of the interviewee, and even assuming responsibility for the interviewee's behavior.

Answering Phone Calls

Frequent telephone calls are a constant interruption in the lives of those living under house arrest, as well as in the lives of those with whom they live and the lives of their emergency contacts. Jeff, the twenty-four-year-old plastics fabricator I quoted above, described how his father is woken up in the middle of the night by the phone calls and is often put in the position of having to "make sure that I am up and I am on the phone so I don't get in trouble." When I asked Jeff what he thought of house arrest, he discussed these interruptions in his father's life: "It's kinda irritating because there's other people, like my father, he works, so it's kind of irritating for him to be sleeping at night and then his phone rings and then I have to get it. I don't think [the program officers] have any consideration if you do stay with somebody else, and there's other people living in that household, too, that work, too. I don't think there's much consideration about that."

Given his erratic and disturbed sleep pattern, Jeff told me that "there's times when I have to have someone yell at me" at two thirty or three o'clock in the morning to get up and answer the phone on time. When I suggested that family members might end up watching over arrestees, Jeff said, "Right. Feels like you got a babysitter there; not just a machine but you also have your family, too." Likewise, when I asked twenty-year-old Justin, a European American landscape worker serving sixty days on house arrest, whether his parents are involved in making sure he gets the phone, he responded affirmatively: "Very much so. They're almost as controlling as house arrest is to me."

Two women I interviewed suggested that the involvement of others might extend beyond the immediate household to include kin within the larger, familial network. Barbara is a thirty-six-year-old European American mother of two children who is employed as a waitress. She described a time when she was having technical problems with the MEMS machine; because the house arrest officer could not reach her, Barbara's aunt was called: "So they called my aunt, who lives, like, thirty minutes from me, and made her come out to our house at ten o'clock at night. [She is] my emergency contact. So she came out and said, 'They are having a problem getting a hold of you. You need to call them as soon as you can.'" Later in the interview, Barbara added, "And she's very, my aunt's very good about it and very supportive because everybody knows the alternative is being in jail, so at least I'm home, you know. But it's, it just spills over into everybody in the family."

Julie, a European American in her thirties who is mother to three children, was a house painter and now manages a fast food outlet. Similar to what Barbara said, Julie told me about how members of her family became involved one night when she forgot to bring the phone to bed with her: "I used to sleep with the cordless right here at my ear, so that I would hear it. One night I forgot to bring the phone to bed and it was in the other room and I almost freaked. [The house arrest officer] ended up calling my cell phone and then they called my mom; my mom called me just as I was getting the message off of my cell: 'Where are you and what are you doing?' I'm like, 'I forgot and left the phone in the other room.'" Barbara and Julie's narratives illustrate that the involvement of others may extend beyond the immediate household and may also include other kin within the larger familial network.

Taking Care of Other Needs

In addition to answering phone calls, family members also fulfill other obligations of daily life that the constraints of house arrest (or other conditions associated with the arrestee's sentence) prohibit the clients from performing themselves. For example, because Jeff had his license suspended, his father has to drive him to and from work every day. Although this allows his father to monitor Jeff and Jeff's schedule, it is nonetheless an additional demand on the father's time and energy. Barbara pointed out that others must do her grocery shopping; she indicated that this is not only a burden on others, but it infantilizes her as well: "When you're in your middle thirties, it's kind of strange having other people taking care of you again. Basically, you know, I can't even go to the grocery store. You know, I have to write a list and send somebody else. . . . My kids have probably more freedom than what I do right now. . . . You have to depend on other people to take care of your needs basically."

Assuming Responsibility

Beyond these concrete actions, other evidence suggests that family members take on the psychological burden of responsibility for compliance. Barbara, who lives with her eighty-three-year-old mother-in-law, told me that the older woman "feels a sense of responsibility to kind of keep an eye on me and that kind of thing. And even though she doesn't have that legal responsibility, that's something that she feels personally, you know." Dusty is a European American male in his late twenties who lives with his brother and another roommate. He works at a car wash and is trying to finish a computer degree. He has been twice convicted of drug offenses and has served more than sixty days on house arrest. I commented that I had spoken to several people who said that their family members also watch them to make sure they stay on the program. Dusty replied, "Oh, as far as them watching me? Yeah, ah, I think my brother who I'm living with thinks, you know, this is my final draw, and he knows when things come down like this. I'm pretty responsible, so he feels pretty strong that I'll accomplish it pretty good."

Blurring the Boundary between Public and Private

House arrest means that many individuals are aware of the client's situation. Because of the way house arrest touches everyday lives, it cannot be concealed (as might be possible with a prior jail sentence or a fine following a conviction for a crime or misdemeanor). For example, I spoke with Barbara specifically about the private versus public nature of house arrest. She talked about how her employer knew what was going on, as did many other family members:

> *Barbara:* You have to let almost everybody know that you're on it. You have to let your employer know, and of course all your family members know. Generally the neighbors will find out, you know, and things like that. Because of your inability to go about your life freely. You know, and they, um, they'll call your work and make sure that that's actually where you work.
>
> *Staples:* So your employer knows about it?
>
> *Barbara:* Oh, yeah.
>
> *Staples:* And so there's a lot of the accountability of jail, but . . .
>
> *Barbara:* It's in a community. Yeah, and it makes, um, a lot of people, that maybe you don't know very well, kind of responsible for you. You know, my employer has the responsibility of, accounting for me, because they make a copy of my work schedule and they call her and things like that.

Julie, the woman employed as a fast food manager who had been convicted on drug charges and was serving her second time on house arrest, also commented on how others are aware of her situation. In contrast to Barbara, Julie appeared to believe that this knowledge helps protect—rather than merely infantilize—her. Speaking affirmatively, she likened her "support group" to a "big circle":

Staples: Tell me what it is like for you living under house arrest.

Julie: Yes, very nice. Um, I was able to be at home with the kids. . . . You learn to be accountable for yourself. Make sure other people know. And I think a lot that letting the other people know, so that it's out there, you're used to letting people know where you're at. So the people that, you know, like I have children. The school knows where I'm at all the time. Or say, like, my parents know where I'm at all the time. And my good friends that may help me out with my kids know where I'm at all the time. You know, it's like a big circle. Like in here [The Center], you have a little circle. And out there, you're on your own circle. So you're, the accountability does really carry over a lot.

Staples: Do you mean that all those people would normally know where you are? But with house arrest, it adds another group that knows what you're doing?

Julie: Like the house arrest people, exactly, 'cause you're, like, on the accountability thing. You've got to let all these people here know where you're at—the house arrest people. And like this one, everybody's got to know where you're at, too, for the first two weeks. And it conditions you to be used to telling your people on the street where you're at.

Staples: Did those people know that you were on house arrest?

Julie: Yeah, everybody that I associate with, everybody that I talk to knows what's going on with me. I'm not ashamed to admit what I've done 'cause I'm paying for it. I took accountability for what I did and the responsibility for what I did, and I'm trying to put it all behind me and move on, and they are trying to help me. They are trying to help me put it all behind me and making sure that I stay on the right track. I've got an excellent support group. A lot of people don't have that, but I'm very fortunate that I do.

Later in the conversation, even as she returned to discuss how house arrest interrupts the lives of those closest to her, Julie continued to be positive about the involvement of so many people in her life:

Staples: Are the people in the house affected by you being on house arrest?

Julie: Well, my mom lives at a different house. They had two phones to get hold of me at, at my house . . . and I also left them [my mother's phone number] as an emergency number. That has an answering machine on it, my mom's number. Just in case my phone, I wasn't able to get to it and, all they have to do is call my mom's house. . . . But see, and that's good because, like, they'd have, like, somebody else that they could call. That support group that calls me and says, "What are you doing?" People are bugging me in the middle of the night, "You're not being accountable, you're not being responsible." A big old slap in the face saying, "Wake up, hello." And you know, it helps to have people that do that.

Accepting Stress

For many clients, the generally strict, "no second chances" stance of the program, which was backed up by the very real threat of jail time if they "messed up," was a constant source of stress and anxiety not only for the clients but also for those with whom they shared their lives (Holman and Quinn 1992). As Jesse, a European American window salesman in his early thirties with a pregnant fiancée and two children at home, put it, "It's nerve wracking, though, 'cause every day, basically, they just hold it over your head." When combined with the regime of weekly appointments, possible home and work visits, drug testing, and random phone calls, it is little wonder that nearly all the clients with whom I spoke characterized house arrest as a stressful experience:

> *Mark:* It's just really stressful.
> *Barbara:* Ah, this time, this time around it's more stressful than the first time.
> *Jesse:* I don't think of myself as being a high-anxiety or stressful person at all, but this last three weeks, I mean, I've been just, my stress level was just out the roof.
> *Ronald:* I was very anxious the whole time.
> *Charles:* If you don't know exactly how this thing's going to play out, then that puts a little stress in your life.
> *Paul:* I was kinda panicking.

Given the levels of stress and anxiety reported by many of the clients, it is not surprising that their emotional states and the conditions of their house arrest have a significant impact on the people with whom they live. This results in both strain on their relationships and stressful co-experiences for these significant others. Intimates were said to be bothered by, and anxious about, the intrusion of the monitoring technology into their homes; concerned about clients getting the phone calls and passing their drugs tests; and worried about clients completing the program without getting sent to jail. For intimates, a sentence to house arrest is a constant reminder of their familial troubles and the incursion of the justice system into their household.

Jesse has been twice convicted for DUI and at the time we spoke had been on house arrest "a little over twenty-one days." He described his very hectic life and mentioned that he was going to try to negotiate with his house arrest officer for more time to be at work. Even though he was working the maximum allowed fifty hours per week, he was falling behind and not making his quota of sales. Jesse also mentioned that the intrusion of phone calls was stressful for his fiancée. He explained as well that his hectic life means that he is frequently returning home minutes after a call is expected and that, as a result, his fiancée is constantly worried that he will miss a call:

> *Staples:* Fifty hours a week and you are falling behind?
> *Jesse:* I can only take, like, a five o'clock or eight o'clock appointment, or two o'clock, I've got kids and day cares, and picking people up from work, I did just have a car break down, uh, last week, so now we got just one car, trying to get somebody to, 'cause I'm on house arrest I can't do that, um. My fiancée is also pregnant, too; she isn't real thrilled when she wakes up at 2:30 AM from a phone call.
> *Staples:* And you said also that it's affecting your family, your fiancée, in the sense there is a spillover effect with the phone calls. Do they get kinda caught up in the whole anxiety of it?
> *Jesse:* Ah, she does because so many times I've been pushing that, I need to be home at 1:30 or something, or whatever time it is, and I'm getting in the door at 1:31 and I'm flying to make it work.
> *Staples:* So she knows your schedule, she knows that they are going to call, and she's waiting for you to come in . . .
> *Jesse:* Right. She has gotten phone calls before, you know, where she sees it on the caller ID, she can't answer the phone 'cause I'm not there yet . . . I may get the second call 'cause I'm ten or fifteen minutes late, and she is just expecting them to come pick me up any day and come put me in jail. Which, in return, if they put me in jail for this amount of time then I'm gonna lose my house, I'm gonna lose my job, cars.

Jesse is desperately trying to balance the demands of house arrest and his role in financially supporting his family. Meanwhile, his fiancée is co-experiencing the intruding phone calls, worrying about whether Jesse will make it home on time for a call, and living on the edge as to whether he will have to go to jail.

Thirty-three-year-old Rita is an African American woman with a newborn child who is living with her mother-in-law and her mother-in-law's male companion. Rita works as a housekeeper at a motel and is aided by the government's Women, Infants, and Children (WIC) program, which helps low-income women with food assistance. When we spoke, Rita had been on house arrest for two weeks following a sentence to the residential treatment center for forging a check. Rita was one of the few people with whom I spoke who found house arrest to be less attractive than the alternative option of incarceration. In fact, given her difficulties, she told me that it would have been easier for her, despite the child, to just do another thirty days in the residential treatment center than to do the same time on house arrest.

Asked to describe her experience, Rita detailed the ways that household members became involved in coming to her aid and enforcing her compliance with the house arrest program. Her discussion revolved around the concrete manifestations of stress this caused other family members—namely, having to drive her to appointments and leave the telephone free for calls to come through. Rita also pointed to the ways in which these obligations might spill over into other sets of interpersonal relationships. For example, in the following discussion, Rita explains that not only does her mother-in-law get drawn into the conditions of her house arrest, but also her mother-in-law's male companion resents those obligations, thus causing trouble within that relationship.

> *Staples:* Describe what it's like living under house arrest.
> *Rita:* It's really *hard!* For one, they call you, like, every hour on the hour, and they expect you [to answer]. You know, sometimes the machine messes up the phones, the phone line, and you don't get no phone call, in four hours you gotta come back all the way out here, and sometimes you don't have transportation to come out here when they want you to come. My mother-in-law works, you know, and it's hard for her to keep bringing me out here when they want me to come out here . . .
> *Staples:* So you don't have a car?
> *Rita:* Not me, no. So [my mother-in-law] does. And to me it's hard, I can't, I can't do it. For real. You gotta come on out here, see 'em

when *they* want, it could be ten o'clock at night, two o'clock [in the morning] they want you to come all the way out here.

Staples: Are other people in your house affected by it?

Rita: Yeah, because the one, the phone keep ringing and then, for another, ah, they have to keep bringing me out here. My mother-in-law has to get her boyfriend to bring me out here, he's old, and he gets upset, and he takes it out on her, and you know, I ask her, and she asks him, so it's a little confusing.

Staples: It's hard, then. Tension in the family?

Rita: Yeah. And then with that one [phone] line thing, you know, they act like she can't be on her own phone, that's her problem. . . . And, if they can't get through they think you got somebody holding the line for you so they ain't get through. But she be, they have to use that phone, I can't stop them from using their own phone.

Staples: So you are living with your in-laws. How many other people in the house?

Rita: Just me, her, and her boyfriend. They keep saying, "Why do they keep calling you back-to-back like that?" and stuff like that, they gettin' upset with me, I don't want them gettin' upset with me.

For Frank, a married forty-five-year-old African American who is self-employed at odd jobs, the restrictions of house arrest meant that *he* could not help his wife and other family members by taking them to work and the like. The phone calls produced co-experiences of stress and anxiety for his wife, who also worked to help him get the calls and stay in compliance.

Convicted of a DUI and on house arrest for only about a week, Frank was very upset during most of our interview about the treatment he received from the court and the house arrest program. I asked Frank how his wife was affected by his house arrest:

Frank: My wife, she'll pick up the phone, "It's for you," 'cause she's hearing them in the background, the computer click off and she say, "Go on in there [to the phone]."

Staples: So, it's affecting her?

Frank: Yeah, it's affecting her, too, because we ain't use to the phone ringing like it does. She just wants to make sure that I get the calls 'cause, it's like, we both want to get through with this. But she, you know, the phone rings and either it's her sister or something and we're both just sitting there [shows tensed expression] you know,

she just had a blow-a-thing through her heart. Doctor took her off
that same evening I come and got it [the MEMS]. I can't take her
to work like I normally do [or] pick her up.

The Special Stresses of Seeing a Child under House Arrest

The stress of living under these controlled conditions seems to be exacer-
bated for parents who live with a son or daughter under house arrest. The
stress parents face can be attributed, at least in part, to the fact that the conditions of house arrest serve as an emotionally laden reminder of their offspring's troubles and possibly what parents view as their own shortcomings.
One can imagine these parents and family members performing various
forms of "emotion work," struggling to bring their feelings of disappointment
and failure in their sons or daughters into line with the normative "feeling
rules" for the unwaveringly supportive parent (Hochschild 1983).

For example, Derek is a twenty-one-year-old European American who
works as a carpet layer. He lives with his father now but previously lived with
his mother. He has been on house arrest three different times for a total of
five months. When I asked him whether his parents were affected by the
house arrest, he responded,

> Hmm. In a way, you know, it's a disappointment. She don't want to see her
> kids do wrong. It's a thing that all parents go through. They don't want to
> see their kids in jail; they'd rather see them on house arrest than in jail,
> but they really don't want to see them on neither. [They] like to see them
> stay out of trouble, so I think for her it was disappointment more than
> anything.

Patrick, a twenty-year-old European American, was serving sixty days
of house arrest. When I asked about his family members' involvement, he
said, "Yeah, they do [get involved]. Like, yeah, I look at my dad and my little
brothers, and they look out for me, you know. My dad acts like he doesn't
care but, like, he's like, 'You better be home or you're screwed.'" When I
asked twenty-year-old Justin whether his parents are anxious to make sure
he gets the phone, he responded affirmatively: "At least my mom is, uh, she's
always nervous. My family's been very, very supportive. They've been that
way throughout my entire life."

Mark is an African American male in his early twenties who attends a
local community college. He was convicted of both driving while intoxicated
and manslaughter following a car wreck that killed one of his passengers.

Mark is serving twenty-one days on house arrest following a stay in the residential treatment center. He is living with his parents in a well-to-do suburb. When I asked Mark if he thought his parents were affected by his house arrest, he told me,

> My mom, she's affected because it's still a stress on her, because she worries about me so much, and then she's like, "Oh my God, the phone, the phone, the phone." And I'm like, "The phone probably isn't ringing," and she's saying "The phone." . . . It's always her protection thing. It's just how she is. Yeah, it worries her, it will be a stress off her when I get off of [house arrest], because it really is a stress, the whole situation has been stressful.

Finally, Duane is a thirty-six-year-old African American who works as a night grocer. At the time we spoke, he had fulfilled two weeks of a thirty-day sentence to house arrest. Duane has a wife and three children, but he is staying with his mother as he transitions from jail through house arrest to his own home.

> *Staples:* You mentioned your family. Do you think other people are affected by it?
> *Duane:* Yeah, um . . . I'm having to stay with my mom at this time 'cause I'm in the process of getting, you know, my place. I've gotten it and everything, but I can't move in there. Cause, since I've gotten out [of jail] I, you know, got "okayed" to be there in my mom's house. Yes, she says she's affected by the phone calls and all through the night and, ah, just worrying about her son, if I'm going to be okay, you know. Ah, gotta do this thing, you know, like a setback.
> *Staples:* Anybody else?
> *Duane:* My wife . . . wife and kids, and like I said, they're also worried about me, you know, I've been away from them long enough, you know, it's time for me to get my life back into order. You know, get things straight in my family.

Conclusion

In exploring some of the collateral consequences associated with a sentence of house arrest, I have attempted to show how this form of punishment is made meaningful in the everyday lives and experiences of the clients interviewed, as well those sharing their domestic worlds. From these offender narratives, I identified a general type of collateral consequence for the intimates, family members, and friends of these house arrest clients: back-up work, or the forms of emotional, mental, and physical labor in which family members and others often engage because of their relationship with the offender on house arrest.

Back-up work and other collateral consequences result from the imposition of a state regime of accountability into the social space of the household, where family members and intimates share a complex web of affiliation and emotional ties with the offender. This regime may be seen as a "disciplinary technology" (Foucault 1979, 26) intent on the production of "docile bodies" (131), both through "hierarchical observations" (170) designed to instill the gaze of authorities and produce self-control and through "normalizing judgments" (183) that set the behavioral standards to be upheld. Since disciplinary power appears multi-directional, fragmented, capillary, and productive, it links up and colonizes the family itself. Much as Donzelot (1979) describes the transformation of mothers into agents of the state in early-twentieth-century France, in the early-twenty-first-century postmodern United States we see how intimates, through their efforts at supporting those on house arrest, get caught in the role of ancillary "watchers" for the program. A kind of collusion is created between the family goal of getting the offender through his or her troubles and punishment and the official goal of ensuring program compliance.

The exercise of disciplinary power may also generate tensions and resistance that are reflected in the contradictory emotions and experiences of clients and those who share their domestic worlds. While many clients report viewing back-up work as supportive, some perceive it as controlling and infantilizing. While some family members exercise informal social control over their children, seemingly in the interest of the state, they also resist aspects of the agency's intrusion into their lives. "They'll come in, walk around the house, and my Dad wasn't very big about that," Jeff told me. "He was like, 'They don't need to walk around in my house.' He's like, 'They can come in through the front door, they can see the living room, you can let them come in the kitchen, they can see the phone in the kitchen, that's all they need to see.' "

Proponents of intermediate sanctions like house arrest have argued that these new forms of punishment, in addition to costing less than incarceration and providing more supervision than traditional probation, can encourage and strengthen bonds to adult roles and attachments to work and family, particularly when coupled with rehabilitative strategies such as substance abuse treatment and education and employment programs (Jones 1990;

Morris and Torny 1990; Petersilia and Turner 1990; Renzema 1992; Smith and Akers 1993). Yet it seems that none of these advocates has anticipated the collateral consequences that are frequently associated with a sentence to house arrest. Only by examining the actual lived experiences of those sentenced to house arrest are we able to truly appreciate the extent and complexity of these ancillary effects.

Notes

1. The names used in this chapter are fictitious. The research protocol was conducted within the ethical and procedural guidelines set out by the Human Subjects Committee of the University of Kansas, the American Correctional Association, and the American Sociological Association. Ellipsis dots in quotations throughout the chapter indicate an editorial omission.
2. This approach is consistent with the "law in everyday life perspective" (Sarat 1998; Garth and Sarat 1998; Ewick and Silbey 1998) that considers law a social process and seeks to investigate how it actually operates in routine, everyday ways.

References

Ansay, Sylvia J. 1999. When Home Is a Prison Cell: The Social Construction of Compliance in House Arrest. PhD diss., University of Florida.

Courtright, Kevin E., Bruce L. Berg, and Robert J. Mutchnick. 1997a. The Cost Effectiveness of Using House Arrest with Electronic Monitoring for Drunk Drivers. *Federal Probation* 61: 19–22.

———. 1997b. Effects of House Arrest with Electronic Monitoring on DUI Offenders. *Journal of Offender Rehabilitation* 24: 35–51.

———. 2000. Rehabilitation in the New Machine? Exploring Drug and Alcohol Use and Variables Related to Success among DUI Offenders under Electronic Monitoring—Some Preliminary Outcomes. *International Journal of Offender Therapy and Comparative Criminology* 44: 293–311.

Donzelot, Jacques. 1979. *The Policing of Families*. Trans. Robert Hurley. Repr., Baltimore: Johns Hopkins University Press, 1997.

Ewick, Patricia, and Susan S. Silbey. 1998. *The Common Place of Law: Stories from Everyday Life*. Chicago: University of Chicago Press.

Feeley, Malcolm, and Jonathan Simon. 1992. The New Penology: Notes on the Emerging Strategy of Corrections and Its Implications. *Criminology* 30: 449–74.

Foucault, Michel. 1979. *Discipline and Punish: The Birth of the Prison*. Translated by Alan Sheridan. Repr., New York: Vintage Books, 1995.

Gainey, Randy R., and Brian K. Payne. 2000. Understanding the Experience of House Arrest with Electronic Monitoring: An Analysis of Quantitative and Qualitative Data. *International Journal of Offender Therapy and Comparative Criminology* 44: 84–96.

Garth, Byrant G., and Austin Sarat, eds. 1998. *How Does Law Matter?* Evanston, IL: Northwestern University Press.

Glaser, Daniel, and Ronald Watts. 1992. Electronic Monitoring of Drug Offenders on Probation. *Judicature* 76: 112–17.

Gubrium, Jaber F., and James A. Holstein. 1990. *What Is Family?* Mountain View, CA: Mayfield.

Harrison, Paige M., and Jennifer C. Karberg. 2003. Prison and Jail Inmates at Midyear 2002. *Bureau of Justice Statistics Bulletin*, U.S. Department of Justice, Office of Justice Programs (April).

Hochschild, Arlie Russell. 1983. *The Managed Heart: Commercialization of Human Feeling*. Berkeley: University of California Press.

Holman, John E., and James F. Quinn. 1992. Dysphoria and Electronically Monitored Home Confinement. *Deviant Behavior* 13: 21–32.

Jolin, Annette, and Brian Stipak. 1992. Drug Treatment and Electronically Monitored Home Confinement: An Evaluation of a Community-Based Sentencing Option. *Crime and Delinquency* 39: 158–70.

Jones, Mark, and Darrell Ross. 1997. Electronic House Arrest and Boot Camp in North Carolina: Comparing Recidivism. *Criminal Justice Policy Review* 8: 383–403.

Jones, Peter. 1990. Community Corrections in Kansas: Extending Community-Based Corrections or Widening the Net? *Journal of Research in Crime and Delinquency* 27: 79–101.

Klein-Saffran, Jody. 1993. Electronic Monitoring versus Halfway Houses: A Study of Federal Offenders. PhD diss., University of Maryland.

Lilly, J. Robert, Richard A. Ball, David G. Curry, and John McMullen. 1993. Electronic Monitoring of the Drunk Driver: A Seven-Year Study of the Home Confinement Alternative. *Crime and Delinquency* 39: 462–84.

Maidment, MaDonna R. 2002. Toward a "Woman-Centered" Approach to Community-Based Corrections: A Gendered Analysis of Electronic Monitoring (EM) in Eastern Canada. *Women and Criminal Justice* 13: 47–68.

Mauer, Marc, and Meda Chesney-Lind, eds. 2002. *Invisible Punishment: The Collateral Consequences of Mass Imprisonment*. New York: New Press.

Maxfield, Michael G., and Terry L. Baumer. 1990. Home Detention with Electronic Monitoring: Comparing Pretrial and Postconviction Programs. *Crime and Delinquency* 36: 521–36.

Mele, Christopher, and Teresa Miller, eds. 2005. *Civil Penalties, Social Consequences*. New York: Routledge.

Morris, Norval, and Michael Tonry. 1990. *Between Prison and Probation: Intermediate Punishments in a Rational Sentencing System*. New York: Oxford University Press.

Newman, Graeme. 1999. *The Global Report on Crime and Justice*. Oxford: Oxford University Press.

Payne, Brian K., and Randy R. Gainey. 1998. A Qualitative Assessment of the Pains Experienced on Electronic Monitoring. *International Journal of Offender Therapy and Comparative Criminology* 42: 149–63.

Petersilia, Joan M., and Susan Turner. 1990. Comparing Intensive and Regular

Supervision for High-Risk Probationer: Early Results from an Experiment in California. *Crime and Delinquency* 36: 87–111.

Renzema, Marc. 1992. Home Confinement Programs: Development, Implementation, and Impact. In *Smart Sentencing: The Emergence of Intermediate Sanctions*, edited by James M. Byrne, Arthur J. Lurigio, and Joan Petersilia. Newbury Park, CA: Sage.

Sandhu, Harjit S., Richard A. Dodder, and Minu Mathur. 1993. House Arrest: Success and Failure Rates in Residential and Nonresidential Community-Based Programs. *Journal of Offender Rehabilitation* 19: 131–44.

Sarat, Austin. 1998. *Crossing Boundaries: Traditions and Transformations in Law and Society Research*. Evanston, IL: Northwestern University Press.

Smith, Linda, and Ronald Akers. 1993. A Comparison of Recidivism in Florida's Community Control and Prisons: A Five-Year Survival Analysis. *Journal of Research in Crime and Delinquency* 30: 267–92.

Staples, William G. 1994. Small Acts of Cunning: Disciplinary Practices in Contemporary Life. *Sociological Quarterly* 35: 645–64.

———. 2000. *Everyday Surveillance: Vigilance and Visibility in Postmodern Life*. Lanham, MD: Rowman and Littlefield.

Ulmer, Jeffery T. 2001. Intermediate Sanctions: A Comparative Analysis of the Probability and Severity of Recidivism. *Sociological Inquiry* 71: 164–93.

3

Bring It On Home

Home Drug Testing and the Relocation of the War on Drugs

Dawn Moore and Kevin D. Haggerty

The award-winning movie *American Beauty* provides a popular depiction of what we suggest is an extension of anti-drug initiatives in which drug testing, coterminous with a change in the anti-drug discourse, is introduced into the homes of white middle-class America. The story unfolds in a stereotypical, middle-class suburb. In one scene an attractive, white, teenage boy sells marijuana to his middle-aged neighbor. The neighbor asks about a container of yellow liquid and the boy responds that it is urine. His parents, he explains, drug test him.

This article explores this most recent extension of America's anti-drug initiatives into a new and relatively untouched space, the realm of middle-class domesticity. Widely proclaimed failures of the "war on drugs" have prompted a renewed emphasis on attempts to eradicate the demand for drugs. In the process, the metaphor of drug use as a "disease" has been revived. This trope works in the context of a distinctive constellation of actors, institutions, and interests to advance home drug testing as a potential solution to one manifestation of America's drug problem. Parental drug testing of teenagers advances anti-drug initiatives into the home and into a child's body by effectively deputizing parents, making them unique articulations of private police. We argue that the use of such tests is characteristic of wider trends in neoliberal approaches to governing crime. Home drug testing is part of a turn to technology in governmental strategies which suggests that

Excerpted from Dawn Moore and Kevin D. Haggerty, "Bring It On Home: Home Drug Testing and the Relocation of the War on Drugs" (© *Social and Legal Studies*, 2001), by permission of Sage Publications Ltd.

analysts must pay greater attention to the minutiae of such tools and the social factors that help to position them as potential solutions to crime problems. However, the drug testing example indicates that rather than being embraced exclusively due to their demonstrated abilities to reduce crime risks, governmental technologies can be adopted for a host of less rational reasons. In the process, they can also prompt some highly distinctive forms of resistance.

We draw from various research sources, including approximately 50 websites dealing with drug testing, numerous hard-copy pamphlets and informational packages pertaining to such tests, and advertisements in specialty magazines aimed at drug users. Telephone interviews were conducted with five representatives of companies that market home drug tests. The minutes of hearings into the regulation of home tests by the US Food and Drug Administration provided valuable insights into who originally advocated on behalf of these tests, and the types of problems they thought these technologies might solve (Food and Drug Administration, 1997).

The Failed "War" on Drugs and the Revitalization of the Drug Use "Disease"

It has only been over the last century that drug use has been problematized in Europe and North America. During this time, the discourse surrounding opiates, and eventually a cornucopia of psychoactive substances, has oscillated between notions of criminality and notions of disease. The degree of purchase each of these binaries has held at a given point has contributed to how officials have responded to the "drug problem." Criminality and disease have acted as useful tropes, repeatedly invoked in the practice of governing populations or behaviors. The criminalization of drug use has revealed itself time and time again as a means of controlling, isolating, and excluding from mainstream society "problematic" minority populations (Giffen, Endicott, and Lambert, 1991; Tonry, 1995). The notion of disease, in contrast, tends to work with techniques of inclusion, subjecting a population to a scrutiny of its morals, normalizing some behaviours and pathologizing others (Peele, 1995). Each of these tropes is well suited to specific social contexts. Criminalization has served as an effective technique of control over specific populations in social climates where concerns over immigration and xenophobia have run high (Giffen, Endicott, and Lambert, 1991). Disease, on the other hand, is invoked when governance is directed at more privileged populations. Looking at the governance of drug use over the last century, we see that while both tropes have always coexisted, one is typically privileged as the appropriate response to the inevitable failure of the other strategy. Thus, the treatment movement in the 1970s was largely driven by concerns over the failure of heavy-handed drug control strategies in the 1960s to effectively control drug use (White, 1998). Likewise, the war on drugs in the 1980s and 1990s was a response to the inability of the 1970s treatment movement to significantly decrease the number of drug users.

This most recent war on drugs has also failed. Almost 20 years after its official declaration, commentators of all political stripes now routinely acknowledge that this campaign has not come close to meeting its proclaimed goal of eliminating the drug supply through the criminalization of certain populations (Chambliss, 1995; Douglas, 1995; Goode, 1993). . . . This is not to say that the war on drugs has been inconsequential. The war on drugs has helped to marginalize and criminalize a generation of ethnic minorities (Miller, 1996), reinforced a conservative crime-control agenda, increased law enforcement budgets, and expanded the network of treatment and social work professionals. Such developments have resulted from efforts by disparate individuals and organizations to capitalize on the opportunities offered to them by the drug war. Failure, however, can also provide its own possibilities, and it is partially the recognized failure of the drug war that has opened up a social space for home drug testing. For example, an Internet website that sells such tests claims: "The sad truth is we're losing the War on Drugs, and our children are the casualties of that war . . . That's why I created the Parent's Alert Home Drug Testing Service." Another company proclaims that "We are *not* winning the war on drug and alcohol abuse . . . Screening of employees and others for drug or alcohol abuse is becoming commonplace and necessary" (original emphasis).

The failure of the drug war is also acknowledged by individuals at the forefront of the state's anti-drug efforts. In keeping with the tendency to oscillate between criminality and disease, leading public figures have started to adopt a discourse that downplays the war rhetoric in lieu of approaching drug use as a disease. . . .

The disease metaphor helps shape American anti-drug efforts. However, some caution should be taken against the impression that this metaphor alone can "determine" the types of solutions advanced on the policy front in any straightforward fashion. A metaphor's power is tempered by the unique social, cultural, and technological environment in which it is invoked. The renewal of the disease metaphor, after an approximate 20-year hiatus in which the discourse was dominated by talk of a war on drugs, demonstrates how the *same* metaphor can be aligned with novel policy initiatives and technological solutions. Rather than there being a single cause for the appeal of home drug tests, it is better to consider the unique combination of factors which helps advance home drug testing as an attractive technology of governance directed at a particular segment of American society. The remainder of this article analyzes the contemporary context in which the disease metaphor now operates in relation to home drug testing.

Shifting Metaphors

. . . Efforts to reframe anti-drug efforts in the language of disease offer distinct attractions and possibilities. The disease metaphor promises to renew flagging public support for anti-drug initiatives. The disease frame also suggests new policy targets and tactics. For example, talk of disease breaks down the us/them dualism intrinsic to the trope of criminality that gives rise to such wars. While the racialized other is the target of criminalization through wars, disease—with cancer being the classic example—affects everyone. And while diseases have particular demographic profiles, they are not intrinsic to poor, ethnic, and otherwise marginalized populations. As disease is effectively everywhere, drug use, by analogy, becomes everyone's problem. At the same time, talk of disease does not imply a homogeneity of treatment of afflicted or at-risk individuals. Those with the financial means can receive better private care and more ready access to early detection technologies and other preventative measures. The disease metaphor also encourages the embrace of diagnostic technologies into anti-drug campaigns. Early detection has become the mantra of the medical profession, and such detection is routinely aided by technological tests and screening systems. If drugs equal disease, the "best defense" against drug use is easily portrayed as involving early detection through drug screening technologies. . . .

Domestic Governance

Parents can now purchase a variety of "kits" that test for drugs in urine or hair samples, and only very recently, in samples of breath and nail clippings. Home tests can provide results in as little as five minutes, although some require that a sample be sent to a laboratory for analysis. The simplicity of these tests makes them attractive to parents who do not have the clinical skills, facilities, and credentials to test samples of extracted blood (Nickell and Fischer, 1999; Saferstein, 1995; Zonderman, 1999). New tests can also track the presence of a substance in the body through a longer time period than is possible with blood tests. The presence of trace amounts of a drug in the urine, for example, is detectable anywhere from 12 to 96 hours after it exits the bloodstream (Greenblatt, 1993), while traces of marijuana can be detected in hair samples up to two months after drug use.

The extent of home drug testing in America is difficult to gauge. There are no national statistics on such tests, and home tests are frequently a subcomponent of corporations that market drug tests to industry and government. This makes it difficult to disaggregate the specific number of home tests. The testing industry is also highly competitive, a fact which fosters a degree of secrecy. Industry representatives who are otherwise very forthcoming generally have refused to provide precise sales figures for their tests. Nonetheless, one gains the impression that this is a small but growing sector. One company spokesperson suggested that home test kits might come close to representing 10 percent of their $20 million testing business. Another representative claimed sales of approximately 3,000 units a month, a figure that was rising steadily. Only six weeks after introducing its home drug test nationally, ChemTrac Inc. had shipped more than 10,000 units to American drug stores. Recent decisions by major American retailers, such as Walgreens, to stock home test kits will likely result in increased sales.

It is tempting to approach the development of these tests as an intensified form of social control. However, the undifferentiated notion of "social control" often brings with it an image of subjects being forced to yield to an external power. In contrast, we suggest that home drug tests exemplify some of the dominant tendencies in neoliberal approaches to governing deviance. In his later work, Michel Foucault (1991) introduced the notion of "governmentality," which amounts to an interrogation of how the practical art of government is envisioned and executed. Governance involves rational policies and practices that act on conduct to direct behavior towards desired ends. These techniques differ by virtue of how individuals are acted upon and the role played by individuals in their own subjectification. Neoliberal strategies of governance ideally minimize repression in favor of techniques that work *with* a subject's limited freedom of choice and action. They structure the context of decision making, creating an environment where individuals freely choose to act in the manner desired by governing authorities. Rather than working against a subject's will, forcing him or her to yield to sovereign power, the will becomes the target of subtle strategies that seek to have individuals behave voluntarily in a certain manner.

In the case of home drug tests, this involves efforts to operate on an adolescent's will by making individual behavior more visible. The ultimate aim of these tests is not so much to detect past drug use or current intoxication as it is to create an environment where youths choose "freely," in light of this newly intensified surveillance regime, not to use drugs. As such, the tests are a technology that governs the behavior of the tested subject from a distance by structuring his or her choices about drug use. However, because these tests presuppose and target the free will of the tested subjects, they also leave opportunities for subjects to subvert the aims of governance, a tendency we discuss below.

Echoing the earlier work of Stanley Cohen (1985), Nikolas Rose (2000) has recently suggested that we can divide strategies of crime control into those that seek to govern by situating individuals in circuits of inclusion versus those that operate on pathologies through a series of exclusions. Such a binary helps to situate home testing in relation to other anti-drug strategies. In keeping with the disease trope, home drug testing is a strategy of inclusion, situating the detection and punishment of criminal behaviors in the compassionate embrace of the family. In contrast, the state's anti-drug policies constitute a strategy of exclusion, which follows the trope of criminality, to remove individuals from their usual social settings, subjecting them to more intensive forms of repression.

A characteristic feature of inclusive neoliberal strategies of crime control is the minimal role played by the state. The state increasingly has withdrawn from direct efforts to guarantee security in lieu of seeking to facilitate the development of private networks of security, expertise, and technology. In the context of home drug tests, the state's facilitative role has involved loosening the FDA regulations so that drug tests can be sold legally over the counter. This was done in response to the lobbying efforts of major pharmaceutical, chemical, and drug testing companies (Food and Drug Administration, 1997).

The ultimate target of such tests is the responsibilized individual. No longer able to rely on the state as a source of security, individuals under neoliberal regimes are constituted as their own personal security manager. O'Malley (1996) has characterized this as a form of prudentialism which can manifest itself in the purchase of private health care, insurance, and various tools that ostensibly reduce the risk of criminal victimization. Governmental experts, both public and increasingly private, offer advice, strategies, and technologies designed to enhance the security of the individual and his or her family. Home drug tests are one in an expanding array of such security-enhancing tools.

Familial Circumstances

Home drug tests are being marketed primarily to the middle-class, white, suburban family. As Garland (2000) has pointed out, the specific dynamics of contemporary middle-class professional families provides a fertile bed for the growth of fears about crime and victimization. Able to spend less and less time in the direct supervision of their children, such parents are now turning to technological forms of scrutiny to satiate a desire to know the specific risks a child might face. Some of the tools being employed towards that end include Internet-connected cameras in daycares (and now high schools), devices to monitor adolescent Internet use, and, most recently, teen drug tests. Such a longing is apparent also in the remarks of David Evans of the National On-Site Testing Association to the Food and Drug Administration hearings on the regulation of home tests. There he observed, "You know, if my kid was on Sudafed, I'd want to know that. If a drug test would show that to me, I'd like to know that. Prescription drugs can be abused, non-prescription drugs can be abused. Most kids are using marijuana and cocaine. . . . I'd like to know everything my kids are doing. Any drug that goes in their body, I'd like to know about it."

Again, drawing on the disease trope, there is a supposition here that "exposure" to drugs is a grave concern. Following the popular logic, just as exposure to a disease increases one's chances of contracting the illness, exposure to drugs increases the risk that a youth will develop a dependence disorder. This is especially distressing given the attention now focused on the long-standing fact that adolescent drug use and experimentation is relatively common. Early interventions such as drug testing are indicated in the same way that we are encouraged to get flu shots every fall in anticipation of the high rate of exposure to the virus that we all experience through the winter.

While the family has long been a site of surveillance and control, home drug tests intimately connect the home with broader programs of governance. As Foucault (1991: 100) observes, the family has become "the privileged instrument for the government of the population." As the material embodiment of social and scientific expertise, drug tests are yet another vehicle that allows the family to be penetrated by a profusion of expert governmental knowledges. The tests contribute to the ongoing historical transformation of parenting as a role where a general competency was assumed, to a series of activities that depend on an array of expert advice, techniques, and technologies. Rather than being something that simply *is* by virtue of kinship and living arrangements, the family is understood as a series of processes to be effectively governed.

The discourse surrounding home testing that can be found in pamphlets and informational packages, and on talk shows and various websites, situates drug tests as one component in a larger effort to rationally govern the white, middle-class family, an institution that has, up until recently, enjoyed an acclaimed capability to regulate itself. Such sources offer advice on the minutiae of family management so as to increase the probability of raising drug-free children. One website, for example, encourages parents to use drug testing as part of an explicit "drug policy." Such a policy could include working in partnership with parental support groups, communicating the risks of drug use to youths, and using a written contract to detail the implications of straying from that policy. Parents are encouraged to "Explain to your child that you trust them, but recognize the outside pressures and outside conflicts they face." Another website that sells a hair test kit includes a link to "A Parent's Guide to Prevention" produced by the US Department of Education. This guide reflects back on potential customers a middle-class view of the family, including bromides on the necessity of communicating to children the family's values, the need for parents to watch for conflicts between their own words and deeds, and the importance of establishing and enforcing strong rules. Some drug test websites contain hyperlinks to information about the prevalence and effects of drug use. Such informational sources are usually characterized by a singular emphasis on the harms of drug use and are devoid of any moderating voices that might downplay the risks of recreational drug use or emphasize the dangers of overreacting to such behavior.

The fact that all drug testing companies promise anonymous results speaks to the distinctive fears that these tests seek to allay. In exchange for becoming deputized agents in the anti-drug campaign, white, middle-class parents can divert their child from the state's official system of drug regulation. State-based anti-drug initiatives are actually one of the main risks faced by middle-class families of teens who use recreational drugs. This is apparent in a drug testing website that depicts a white, teenage boy staring plaintively at the viewer from behind prison bars. The caption over the photograph reads, "Drug Testing would have been a better way for my parents to find out I was doing drugs." It sends the clear message that while poor, minority parents continue to witness their children repeatedly coming into conflict with the law, white, middle-class parents should not, and need not, rely on the state to monitor and respond to their child's drug use. Furthermore, it implies that the state's strategy in the war on drugs—criminalization—is not the most effective, desirable, or appropriate way to govern this population of offenders. This is in line with more general trends in late-modern forms of governance, where responsible individuals are encouraged to manage their own affairs with a minimal reliance on the state (O'Malley, 1996). Instead, parents can obtain the necessary evidence themselves, and respond in ways that are free from the dangers posed to both the family and child by the official criminal justice system. . . . Such a development represents a historical reversal in the audience for credentials. Historically, the rise of personal markers such as degrees, passports, and criminal records were designed to give unknown strangers some indication of a person's reputation (Nock, 1993). In contrast, home drug tests bring the gaze home. They are a standardized means to establish an adolescent's reputation for those individuals who would ostensibly be most intimately aware of the child's character—his or her parents. These tools stand in the place of a host of more traditional paternalistic ways to establish a child's reputation, freeing parents from the need to listen in on their children's phone calls, search their children's rooms, or piece together the various bits of evidence pertaining to their children's drug use, such as withdrawn behavior, constant need for money, general malaise, and weight loss.

The search for chemical deviance implies that parents can assemble genitive evidence through a very septic and narrowly focused examination. Drug tests consider only one product of the body in isolation. For the most part, tests like EMIT (Enzyme-Mediated Immunoassay) are only able to detect the presence of one particular drug enzyme in urine or liquefied hair. This is done by introducing the enzyme's antibody into the test substance and monitoring the solution for a reaction (Hanson, 1993; Zonderman, 1999). Only a limited range of chemicals are scrutinized, which represents a profound narrowing of the gaze. It lacks the panoptic dimension whereby a single watcher invisibly scrutinizes the many. Instead, the tests provide harried middle-class parents with the semblance of some supervisory role in their child's life. This despite the fact that parents who rely on the tests need not actually even engage with the child, to look him or her in the eyes (both figuratively and *very* literally), to monitor their behavior. Instead, they can stare detachedly at the rational products of science.

Home drug tests extend governmental strategies by helping to transcend two privacy constraints that have traditionally hindered anti-drug initiatives. First, the difficulty in definitively determining whether a person uses drugs, outside of those instances where they are obviously inebriated or incapacitated, has long been a problem for anti-drug efforts. Home tests address this problem by penetrating the bodily integrity of tested subjects, forcing their ostensibly private bodily substances to yield to chemical scrutiny. Residing in the legal gray area of adolescence, tested subjects cannot even marshal the limited privacy rights accorded to adults to resist such bodily intrusions. Second, drug tests infiltrate the privacy of the home, which has long been recognized as hindering policing efforts (Reiss, 1987). As an advertisement for the "Drug Test" company observes, "The War on Drugs has been fought in the growing fields, the borders, streets and schools. ONLY NOW is there a way to bring it where it matters most—AT HOME" (original emphasis). While middle-class parents would ostensibly oppose the physical intrusion of state agents into their homes, they appear willing to open the door to anti-drug initiatives, on the condition that they maintain exclusive authority over the results of such tests. This incorporation of middle-class parents into anti-drug efforts indicates that privatization, especially in the realm of criminal justice, occurs not just by making private that which was once public, as in the development of private police forces, but also by encouraging that exemplar of the private realm—the family—to take up crusades that were originally concerns of the state.

Private Commodities

. . . Earlier we noted the general bifurcation in strategies of criminal justice governance between inclusionary and exclusionary approaches. Ewick's (1993) work on the institutionalization of deviants points out how a class hierarchy can be overlaid on these two extremes. She details how a class-based two-tier system works to exert different modes of control over different social groups. While the lower classes continue to be directed towards prisons, the exemplar of exclusionary institutions, private organizations now use therapeutic approaches to govern the criminal behavior of the middle classes who are able to pay for their services. Private drug testing establishes a similar cleavage in campaigns against drug use. Home drug tests are not concerned with the generalized betterment of all sectors of society, but are specialist tools available to more affluent parents. While some of the kits sell for $5 or $10, most cost $50 to $60. These costs are amplified by the fact that tests are not reusable and many can only trace one substance. A parent who wished to place his or her child on a periodic drug test regime (testing once a month for marijuana, cocaine, and heroin) could easily spend $500 a year or more on such an endeavor.

The spokesperson for a company that sells a hair test kit accentuated the narrow class-based market for these commodities when he noted that the specific demographics for his products were "upscale, suburban, newspaper-reader, soccer-moms. Less of the inner-city types." The racial division embedded in that sociodemographic characterization should be self-evident. This implicit racial targeting is reinforced by the fact that outside of the prominent display of Oprah Winfrey, who has endorsed one particular home drug test, the packaging and advertisements for these products depict almost no people of color.

Middle-class parents who have assumed the responsibility for governing their children's drug use, and who have the resources to purchase the tests, work to keep their children out of the "hard end" of the system, governing their drug use through an inclusive paternalistic model. The poor and racialized, however, continue to have their illicit drug use regulated through the coercive state-based war on drugs. Indeed, the US "war on drugs" has become a de facto undeclared war on young African American and Hispanic men. According to the US Sentencing Project, on any given day nearly one-third of all African American men between the ages of 20 and 29 years are under criminal justice supervision, meaning that they are either in prison, on probation, or on parole (Mauer and Huling, 1995). Drug offenders account for the majority of this population (Tonry, 1995). This racialization of the drug war becomes entrenched in policies such as California's "three strikes" provisions and the federal law which now requires judges, in sentencing drug offenders, to treat 1 g of crack as the equal of 100 g of cocaine. Since more than 90 percent of crack defendants are African American, as opposed to only 20 percent of those accused of possession of powder cocaine, the law further increases the disproportionate number of African Americans in the prison system (Lemann, 1998: 25).

Authors writing about neoliberal forms of governance have accentuated the calculative attitude that responsibilized individuals are encouraged to adopt in making decisions about how to enhance their security. . . .

Parental fear underpins the attraction of home drug tests. At the most general level, the testing industry benefits from the angst generated by the ongoing moral panic surrounding illicit drug use. Individual companies also employ a range of subtle and not-so-subtle efforts to capitalize on, and augment, parental fear. For example, most of the drug testing promotional literature employs the common strategy of invoking "shocking numbers" (Best, 1989; Orcutt and Turner, 1993) to dramatize the prevalence and dangers of drugs. These figures are typically unreferenced, or consist of sweeping generalizations, such as "Drug use among our teens is at its highest level in nine years." Other companies hone in more specifically on the fears of that class of individual who can afford their kits, as is apparent in the "informational" component of the website for the "Drug Test" company that claims that "heroin, PCP and others with high death rates are gaining in popularity; *particularly among more affluent sectors*" (emphasis added). Speaking to the FDA, the representative from ChemTrak made a similar point, suggesting that "Unfortunately, good children from good homes who live in nice neighborhoods use drugs. The problem is not one limited to the inner city. Sixty percent of the problem occurs in suburbs, many of them affluent suburbs." More disturbingly, Hanson (1993: 128) reports that the National Drug Awareness and Detection Agency of Houston randomly sends postcards to families that state, "We have been informed that your children may be using ILLEGAL DRUGS . . . Please call us IMMEDIATELY" (original emphasis). Those who call the number on the card are given a lengthy presentation about the dangers of drugs. They are then urged to send $99.95 to purchase a kit that claims to detect drug use by measuring the pupil of a suspect's eye with a "pupilometer."

Dialectics of Observation and Resistance

Governance seeks to shape the behavior of subjects in the directions desired by authorities. The success of a particular governmental technique, however, is not preordained. The targets of governmental strategies can at times resent or resist efforts to modify their behavior. Constituted as relatively autonomous agents, tested subjects can employ their limited scope for agency to subvert governmental ambitions. Privileged adolescents increasingly have at their disposal a range of commodities which purport to beat drug tests. Predictably, such counter technologies and tactics have sparked further refinements to monitoring regimes and testing procures, resulting in an escalating dialectic of observation and resistance.

The notion of resisting surveillance brings to mind someone standing outside of the gaze, finding cracks and fissures where surveillance does not penetrate. Resisting surveillance, however, can also involve strategies that work creatively within the field of visibility through imaginative engagements with the particularities of an observational regime (De Certeau, 1984). These involve various techniques that use simulations to stand in for or (mis)represent assorted originals (Baudrillard, 1983; Bogard, 1996). Such simulations depend on an intimate familiarity with the minutiae of the tools and procedures of a particular surveillance regime: how it operates, what it scrutinizes, and how.

Various techniques are available to beat drug tests, and these differ in their specifics and efficacy according to what drug is being tested for, the type of sample collected, and the manner through which this is done. Urine tests appear to offer the greatest range for evasion. If one knows when a urine sample is going to be collected, for example, a clean test can be produced by simply abstaining from drug use for a limited period of time prior to the test, often as little as three days. Urine tests can also be defeated through dilution, which can involve adding water to the sample or drinking copious amounts of water prior to the test.

One of the most straightforward simulations employed to defeat a drug test involves replacing a tainted sample with a clean one. Recall the scene in the movie *American Beauty* mentioned above, where the youth relates that his parents test him for drugs. He then proceeds to explain that this does not pose a problem, as he substitutes someone else's clean urine for his own. Drug users can acquire untainted samples from friends who sell or donate their urine. Individuals can also purchase urine in "natural" or dehydrated form through mail order and Internet-based companies.

Drug users now also have at their disposal a host of purifying commodities sold through specialty drug magazines or over the Internet. With corporate names like "Urine Luck," "Clear," and "Detoxify," these products subvert drug tests by chemically masking the tested-for markers of drug use. Some of these products are added to the sample itself, while others are ingested by the test subject prior to the test. . . . Adolescents who might want more information on which techniques work and which are spurious can call the 24-hour telephone hotline run by the drug magazine *High Times* that is dedicated exclusively to disseminating information on how to beat drug tests.

Perhaps the most surreal example on this hyperreal continuum of countersurveillance fakes is the "Whizzinator 2000." This amounts to a (limitedly) operational plastic prosthetic penis that is sold in a variety of "natural, lifelike skin tones." Worn under a man's underwear, the prosthesis ostensibly allows him to "urinate" toxin-free urine that can be purchased with the "Whizzinator" or acquired elsewhere. He can thereby defeat the visual and chemical scrutiny of even the most conscientious parent or technician.

Not surprisingly, the development of such tools and techniques has introduced an escalating dialectic into drug monitoring regimes, as avoidance techniques are countered by more restrictive and intrusive testing procedures. Testing companies have capitalized on this trend by selling new tests that detect sample alteration. One such product claims to detect various techniques and products that can be used to beat drug tests including excessive fluid consumption, Klear, Urinaid, Instant Clean, bleach, vinegar, eyewash products, sodium bicarbonate, drain cleaners, soft drinks (and other urine look-alikes), and hydrogen peroxide.

Although one might presume that the companies that market these technologies would be aligned with a specific political agenda, with pro-drug organizations selling drug evasion tools and anti-drug advocates selling drug testing tools, this is not necessarily the case. Instead, the greater allegiance at times appears to be to the quest for profit. For example, the web page for TriCorp labs markets a series of drug tests, and also includes a hyperlink labeled "Need Help Passing a Drug Test?" This connects viewers with a site that markets various technologies designed to *beat* drug tests! A website for the company "Urine Luck," whose company spokesperson is drug comedian Tommy Chong, sells a variety of flushing capsules, detoxifying drinks, and urine additives that purport to beat drug tests. It also sells its own home tests for detecting THC, cocaine, opiates, amphetamines, and barbiturates. Both the testing of potential drug users and attempts to beat these tests ultimately benefit the same industry, and at times may benefit the same companies.

Conclusion: Towards an Ambiguous Result

The American campaign against illicit drug use is expanding its vocabulary beyond the "war" metaphor to reinvoke the image of drug use as a disease. Such terminological oscillations warrant critical attention because new public policy discourses can bring in their wake new problematizations and an attendant set of self-evident solutions. However, we should be cautious not to overstate the role that new metaphors can play in bringing about such transformations. It is not exclusively the discourse that prompts change, but how metaphors resonate with a broader social situation that makes particular governmental strategies thinkable and actionable.

Previous manifestations of the disease metaphor in campaigns against illicit drugs did not lead, indeed could not have led, to the embrace of home drug tests. At the most obvious level, this is because these technologies did not then exist. The advent of such tests produces new possibilities for governing children and families. However, this is not a technologically determinist result, as the mere availability of such tests cannot explain their use. As we have demonstrated, the embrace of home testing can be partially attributed to how private interests have expounded their benefits to a particular class and race of parents. Encouraged to be obsessed about adolescent drug use, responsibilized parents are also persuaded through efforts that capitalize on such fears to employ a host of private commodities to ensure the security of their families.

Part of the parental appeal of drug tests derives from their promise of scientific certainty in determining whether their child is using drugs. Scientific certainty notwithstanding, parents can still find themselves in a remarkably ambiguous situation should their child test positive. Much in the same way that youths now attempt to explain away the non-scientific markers of drug use, they will undoubtedly attempt to explain away positive test results. Parents must then decide whether to trust their own progeny or to trust the systems of abstract knowledge embedded in the test itself. Those who accept a positive test as definitive proof of drug use must then decide how to proceed. The tests themselves, however, offer little guidance for what a parent should do in the event that their child tests positive. Given that such tests hold out the promise of keeping white, middle-class children out of the official criminal justice system, parents would be loathe to turn their drug-using child over to the authorities. As yet, however, there are few formal arrangements for a seamless transition from positive test to institutional response. If home-based drug tests become more popular we can anticipate the increasing establishment of a host of drug "treatment" policies and techniques designed for youths who have tested positive. Such a development would continue the bifurcation between the white, middle-class inclusionary treatment and lower-class racialized exclusionary repression of illegal drug use. However, the efficacy or ethics of such efforts would remain an open question. This is because contrary to the emerging discourse, the drug habits of recreational users—the population most likely to be caught by such tests—are *not* a disease. Notwithstanding recurring moral panics about drug use, there is little evidence that casual use of drugs leads inextricably to addiction and even less evidence to indicate that addiction is itself a disease in the original biological sense of the term. Lacking any precise scientific and biological meaning, the disease trope invokes powerful imagery of teens requiring treatment, irrespective of the lack of a clinical diagnosis of a medically accepted syndrome.

The advent of home drug testing indicates that anti-drug campaigns are far from over. The United States continues to refuse to adopt harm reduction and decriminalization initiatives. If the focus on eradicating drug demand through the private mobilization of families effectively replaced the supply-side, criminal justice responses to the "drug problem," then techniques like home drug testing might be considered tools of decriminalization. If this was the case, at least it could be said that criminal sanctions were no longer the derivative harms of anti-drug initiatives. This, however, is not the case. The war on drugs continues, having become very much like a disease itself, a cancer that increases in size and works its way further and further into the American social body.

Note

The authors would like to thank the following individuals for the valuable comments on earlier versions of this article: Catherine Carstairs, Aaron Doyle, Kelly Hannah-Moffat, Pat O'Malley, James Sheptycki, Mariana Valverde, Robin Room, and two anonymous reviewers.

References

Baudrillard, Jean. 1983. *Simulations*. New York: Semiotext(e).

Best, Joel. 1989. Dark Figures and Child Victims: Statistical Claims About Missing

Children. In *Images of Issues: Typifying Contemporary Social Problems*, edited by Joel Best, 21–37. New York: Aldine de Gruyter.

. . .

Bogard, William. 1996. *The Simulation of Surveillance: Hypercontrol in Telematic Societies*. Cambridge, UK: Cambridge University Press.

. . .

Chambliss, William. 1995. Another Lost War: The Costs and Consequences of Drug Prohibition. *Social Justice* 22: 101–24.

Cohen, Stanley. 1985. *Visions of Social Control: Crime Punishment and Classification*. Cambridge, UK: Polity Press.

. . .

De Certeau, Michel. 1984. *The Practice of Everyday Life*. Berkeley: University of California Press.

Douglas, Joseph D., Jr. 1995. Why Is the War on Drugs Going Nowhere? *Conservative Review* 6: 15–21.

. . .

Ewick, Patricia. 1993. Corporate Cures: The Commodification of Social Control. *Studies in Law, Politics and Society* 13: 137–57.

Food and Drug Administration. 1997. Clinical Chemistry and Clinical Toxicology Devices Panel of the Medical Devices Advisory Committee. Bethesda, MD: US Food and Drug Administration.

Foucault, Michel. 1991. Governmentality. In *The Foucault Effect: Studies in Governmentality*, edited by Graham Burchell, Colin Gordon, and Peter Miller, 87–104. Chicago: University of Chicago Press.

Garland, David. 2000. The Culture of High Crime Societies: Some Preconditions of Recent "Law and Order" Policies. *British Journal of Criminology* 40: 347–75.

Giffen, P. J., Shirley Endicott, and Sylvia Lambert. 1991. *Panic and Indifference: The Politics of Canada's Drug Laws: A Study in the Sociology of Law*. Ottawa: Canadian Centre on Substance Abuse.

Goode, Erich. 1993. *Drugs in American Society*. New York: Knopf.

Greenblatt, D. J. 1993. Basic Pharmacokenetic Principles and Their Application to Psychotropic Drugs. *Journal of Clinical Psychiatry* 54: 8–13.

Hanson, F. Allan. 1993. *Testing Testing: Social Consequences of the Examined Life*. Berkeley: University of California Press.

Lemann, Nicholas. 1998. Justice for Blacks? *New York Review of Books*, March 5.

Mauer, Marc, and Tracy Huling. 1995. Young Black Americans and the Criminal Justice System: Five Years Later. Washington, DC: The Sentencing Project.

Miller, Jerome G. 1996. *Search and Destroy: African-American Males in the Criminal Justice System*. New York: Cambridge University Press.

Nickell, Joe, and John F. Fischer. 1999. *Crime Science: Methods for Forensic Detection*. Lexington: University of Kentucky Press.

Nock, Steven L. 1993. *The Costs of Privacy: Surveillance and Reputation in America*. New York: Aldine de Gruyter.

O'Malley, Pat. 1996. Risk and Responsibility. In *Foucault and Political Reason: Liberalism, Neo-Liberalism and Rationalities of Government*, edited by Andrew

Barry, Thomas Osborne, and Nikolas Rose, 189–207. Chicago: University of Chicago Press.

Orcutt, James D., and J. Blake Turner. 1993. Shocking Numbers and Graphic Accounts: Quantified Images of Drug Problems in the Print Media. *Social Problems* 40: 190–206.

Peele, Stanton. 1995. *Diseasing America: How We Allowed Recovery Zealots and the Treatment Industry to Convince Us We Are Out of Control.* San Francisco: Jossey-Bass.

Reiss, Albert. 1987. The Legitimacy of Intrusion into Private Space. In *Private Policing,* edited by Clifford Shearing and Phillip Stenning, 19–44. Thousand Oaks, CA: Sage.

. . .

Rose, Nikolas. 2000. Government and Control. *British Journal of Criminology* 40: 321–39.

Saferstein, Richard. 1995. *Criminalistics: An Introduction to Forensic Science.* Englewood Cliffs, NJ: Prentice Hall.

Sontag, Susan. 1977. *Illness as Metaphor.* New York: Farrar, Straus & Giroux.

. . .

Tonry, Michael. 1995. *Malign Neglect: Race, Crime and Punishment in America.* Oxford: Oxford University Press.

White, William. 1998. *Slaying the Dragon: The History of Addiction Treatment and Recovery in America.* Bloomington, IN: Lighthouse Institute.

Zonderman, Jon. 1999. *Beyond the Crime Lab: The New Science of Investigation.* New York: Wiley.

Part II

We're Watching You, We're Watching Each Other

The essays in this section explore how members of the public monitor the behavior of families in order to hold those families accountable to social norms of what it means to be a family and to individual ideas of appropriate parenting. As in the previous section, some chapters explore the new surveillance technologies (e.g., the Internet) and others focus on more conventional monitoring approaches (e.g., observation and gossip). Issues of race/ethnicity, social class, and gender become central in both forms of monitoring as members of the public make assumptions about family boundaries and appropriate behaviors on the basis of these social locations.

4

Interracial Surveillance
and Biological Privilege

Adoptive Families in the Public Eye

Heather Jacobson

You go in the grocery store and people look. . . . You just accept
it. Yeah, people just stare at you. But [my children are] both
so beautiful and [people] go, "Oh, she's so cute and pretty!"

—Eloise Nolan, white mother of Tara and
Lani, both adopted from China

We wanted her to look like ours (I don't know how
to say that without being, you know), so it's not as obvious
when we're out with her.

—Jean Kerne, white mother of Lucy,
adopted from Russia

Contemporary families in the United States are characterized by a range of
configurations and kinship relations.[1] Relatively high rates of divorce, remarriage, nonmarital unions, single parenthood, and cohabitation coupled with
broader social acceptance of interracial marriage, adoption, and same-sex
relationships mean there are many ways to "do family" (Nelson 2006) in the
contemporary United States. Paradoxically, despite this family diversity, in
mainstream cultural representations and public discourse an idealized and
static image of "the family" is often posited—a nuclear unit of heterosexual,
married parents and their biological children (Coontz 1992; Hansen 2005;

Another version of this chapter appears as chapter 5 in Heather Jacobson, *Culture
Keeping: White Mothers, International Adoption, and the Negotiation of Family
Difference* (Vanderbilt University Press, 2008).

Smith 1993; Wegar 1997). This family is often white and middle class (Collins 1994; Garey and Hansen 1998); it is almost always monoracial. When other types of families are invoked, they are often referenced against this "traditional family" and found to be lacking. In this way, although not everyone "participates in identical sorts of kinship relations [or] subscribes to one universally agreed upon definition of the family" (Weston 1991, 22), a particular ideological understanding of the "American Family" as monoracial, heterosexual, biogenetically formed, middle class, and nuclear is privileged in the United States.

How does this ideological privileging shape our experiences living in diverse family forms? Dorothy Smith (1993) calls the idealized family the "Standard North American Family" (SNAF) and argues that this "ideological code," which includes a gendered division of labor (with a breadwinning father and a stay-at-home mother), infiltrates public policy and political practice. Laws governing marriage and adoption, for example, have historically benefited white, monoracial, heterosexual families. Many institutions, such as schools and the workplace, are organized around the notion of the SNAF, which assumes a dichotomy between "worker" and "parent." Primary school hours and the lack of parental leave policies in many workplaces, for example, often make it challenging for families to manage the demands of child care and employment.

This chapter examines interactions with strangers in public places, another way in which the hegemonic American Family shapes lived experiences in diverse family forms. When in public, families are on display. When they challenge conventional norms, families are especially open to unsolicited attention from strangers—to questions, stares, even violence; when they appear congruent with those norms, families receive less intrusive attention. In either case, monitoring occurs. And this monitoring is especially acute when adults are in public with young children (see Blackford, Chapter 5). In the surveillance of family form and behavior, we see how parents are held accountable for their ability to comply with prevailing norms concerning the shape, behavior, and membership of a family.

Norms about the family are variable; they are neither static nor identical across communities. However, I argue in this chapter that contemporary U.S. families who do not match the hegemonic American Family along the lines of monoraciality and biological kinship often experience a heightened surveillance that results in messages about their failure to meet those particular family norms. International adoptive families are one such group that experiences this type of surveillance.

International adoption is a growing phenomenon in the United States.

The decade from 1995 to 2005 saw a 150 percent increase in the number of international adoptions into the United States, from 8,987 to 22,728 (U.S. Department of State 2009). This phenomenal growth has been attributed, in part, to the opening of China and Russia for international adoption placements (Simon and Altstein 2000; Pertman 2000). During this time period, China and Russia accounted for roughly half of all international adoptions and were the top two countries from which children were adopted into the United States.[2] This decade of growth is particularly interesting because of the resulting racial makeup of these two sets of newly formed families. Data from the 2000 Census indicate that the majority of international adoptive parents are white (Ishizawa et al. 2006). Indeed, the majority of formal adoptive parents in the United States have always been white (Vonk 2001; Zelizer 1985).[3] As such, the increase in adoptions from China and Russia presents a situation in which the two most popular international adoption programs from 1995 to 2005 were split over race: children from China largely helped to form interracial families, while those from Russia largely helped to form monoracial ones.[4]

Given the politics of race in the United States, the contentious history of transracial domestic adoption, and the contemporary process of securing an international adoption placement (which requires parents to be explicit about the "type" of child they wish to adopt; see Jacobson 2008 for a broader discussion), race is clearly involved in international adoption. This chapter examines how interpretations of "race" and "the family" result in particular types of public interactions for adoptive families, and how those experiences differ for families raising children adopted from China and from Russia.

This chapter, then, compares the experiences of families who adopt from Russia and those who adopt from China. My analysis is based on the contrasting themes regarding race and biological kinship found between these two groups in their public interactions and interpretations of those experiences. I approach this work from a social-constructionist, symbolic-interactionist perspective. Central to my theoretical framework is the idea that just as we "do gender" (West and Zimmerman 1987), we "do family" (Nelson 2006): we engage in interactional work around the notion of family, and we enact and react to both internally felt and externally applied notions of who makes a family (including varying degrees of institutionalized support for particular types of families), which in turn gives meaning to the concept. Likewise, I approach "race" and "the family" as sociohistorical constructs, composed of varied socially defined, politically charged meanings that have popularly relied on features visible to others (phenotype and assumed familial form). In examining the public interactions of adoptive families, I mean not to reify "race" and "the family" but instead to highlight the powerful ways in which popular understandings of race and the family influence lived experiences.

Methods

In 2002 and 2003, I conducted in-depth interviews with forty mothers and six of their husbands who live in New England and adopted their children internationally from China and Russia. The interviews were tape-recorded and transcribed and included questions on the adoption decision-making process and adoption procedures. Questions focused primarily, however, on the post-adoption experiences of day-to-day life as an international adoptive family, as well as engagement with the "birth culture" of the child. To supplement interview data I also attended community events that were of interest to international adoptive parents, such as adoption agency information sessions, "culture days" for adoptive families, and adoption conferences.

Of the families in my study, 65 percent ($N = 26$) included married heterosexual parents; the remaining families ($N = 14$) covered a variety of familial configurations—divorced, remarried, single, cohabiting, and homosexual. Most participants in my study came to adoption through infertility, which is typical of contemporary adoptive parents, though 25 percent ($N = 10$) did choose adoption as the first route for expanding their families. The women and men who spoke with me adopted their children as infants or toddlers (from the ages of five months to three years). The children, having been in their present families for a minimum of two years, were between the ages of four and twelve when I spoke with their parents. As is typical of international adoptive parents (Ishizawa et al. 2006), all participants in the study except two were white and professional middle-class.[5]

It is important to note that although the majority of families in this study resided in the greater Boston metropolitan region, an area of the country with relative racial, ethnic, and class diversity, they overwhelmingly lived (physically and socially) in predominantly white, middle-class communities. While several China-adoptive families moved to more racially diverse neighborhoods following their adoption of a child of color, the overwhelming majority did not. Few had established friendships with racial- or ethnic-minority adults or deep connections with racial- or ethnic-minority communities, though most commented on their importance. (I discuss this in depth in Jacobson 2008.) Many of the public interactions with strangers that form the data for this chapter took place in predominantly white, middle-class communities and involved other native-born, middle-class whites. As families traversed the city and larger metropolitan landscape, however, they also recounted having the same experiences with African Americans, Asian Americans, immigrants, and people from a variety of class positions.

The Interracial Surveillance of Families with Children from China

Families with children adopted from China draw considerable attention in public spaces. This attention indicates that others are engaged in the surveillance of families to assess the degree to which they fit the ideological normative family mold. Parents in my study spoke of feeling that they were under surveillance when out in public with their Asian children. This surveillance was characterized by a near-constant trickle of inquiries directed at them in public spaces—such as grocery stores, playgrounds, airplanes, and parking lots—about their adoption experiences and their daughters. The questions families received ranged from the innocuous to the offensive. Lorraine Burg described this ongoing attention and the burden she felt it placed on her family:

> Everywhere we go people look twice at us, and it has become sort of the norm. So we're used to it. But people ask questions, you know: "Is she your daughter?" "Is your husband Chinese?" They ask her, you know, other kids say, "That's not your real mother." So all of those things sort of impact us more than any other piece, just because it's so daily and so constant.

It is the interracial aspect of these families and what it signals to others—nonbiological kinship and international adoption—that drives this surveillance. Unlike families (either biological or adopted) in which all members appear to be biologically related because of shared racial classifications, the members of these families feel as if they cannot hide their nonbiological mode of family formation. Others most often read the racial makeup of these families (white parents, Asian children) to represent transracial adoption rather than an alternative route to whites parenting Asian children: Asian-white intimate partnering. The obviousness of their route to family formation stems in part from cultural understandings of biological race and the near invisibility of interracial Asian-white families in mainstream American public consciousness. In short, these Chinese children are assumed to be adopted because cultural understandings of race and the family do not include the possibility of a white woman giving birth to an Asian-looking child. This assumption is particularly poignant when one parent is out alone with his or her child and therefore the racial status of the other assumed parent is unknown to strangers. As Rachel Abramson explained, the fact of adoption cannot be concealed for these families, even as they skirt the possibility of being taken for a member of an Asian-white romantic couple: "I cannot pretend that she's not adopted. Although sometimes I think when I'm just alone they might think my husband's Chinese. [*laughter*] But it is always out there. We are always [being asked], 'Is she your real daughter?' We are always getting these obnoxious questions."

The questions families received focused on clarifying or fixing the nature of the relationship between adult and child: Are they *really* related? Why are they together? Why is this white woman mothering this Asian child in public? I call these types of encounters "interracial surveillance," a phenomenon by which interracial families or multiracial individuals draw public interest and are scrutinized, monitored, or harassed because of embodying multiple racial positions.[6] Interracial surveillance is similar to "border patrolling," which Heather Dalmage (2007, 218) notes is "a form of discrimination faced by those who cross the color line, do not stick with their own, or attempt to claim membership (or are placed by others) in more than one racial group." However, while border patrolling takes many forms and occurs in multiple settings, including private interactions between family members (Dalmage 2000), interracial surveillance as defined here focuses specifically on the monitoring of families and individuals by *strangers* in *public settings*.

The interracial surveillance of international adoptive families has a unique tenor. It is unlike the surveillance of U.S. black-white intimate relations both in what it includes and in what it excludes. Although black-white couples report public interest in and fascination with their relationships, they also detail being ignored or receiving an edgy hostility directed at them via poor service, cold stares, epithets, and violence in public spaces (Azoulay 1997; Childs 2005; Dalmage 2000, 2007; Reddy 1994). Indeed, a desire to circumvent this type of interracial surveillance plays a role in the selection of China for adoption. As others have noted (Dorow 2006; Kim 2008; Rothman 2005), the popularity of international adoption is partially fueled by a desire to avoid the domestic adoption of African American and multiracial black children. There were a variety of reasons participants in my study desired not to adopt across the black-white divide, including familial prejudice and a sensitivity to the contentious debate surrounding the capacity of whites to raise blacks in a racist society. Participants in my study also indicated a strong desire to circumvent the intensely negative interracial surveillance that they felt would result from the adoption of black children.

Parents reported that prior to adoption, they felt comfortable with the level of interracial surveillance they imagined their new white-Asian families would experience. What they experienced post-adoption, however, was an almost constant interest, with strangers wanting to learn intimate details about their families. While some parents came to terms with this very intrusive surveillance, none reported it as a thorough pleasure, and many experienced it as a sort of assault. Although no families in my study were physically attacked (as has occurred in other cases of interracial surveillance), many used the term "assault" to describe their public encounters, even if recalling them with humor. More so than any one interaction in particular, it is the bluntness and the consistency—in both form and occurrence—of these encounters that characterize them as intrusive. Although families in my study rarely, if ever, experienced a directly hateful or racist remark, they were made aware of their non-normative families through the blunt, repetitive questions they received: Where is she from? Are you her mother? How much did she cost? Is she adopted? She's so cute; does she speak Chinese? These seemingly innocuous questions came from people from varying social locations and occurred in all manner of public settings, often multiple times in one outing.

The interracial surveillance experienced by international adoptive families with Asian children can be thought of, in essence, as one of attraction, while that of biological black-white families can largely be seen as one of repulsion.[7] Both, however, serve to make interracial families the "Other" (de Beauvoir 1984; Kristeva 1991) by communicating the idea of familial difference and norm violation. Parallels can be made to Foucault's (1977, 184) "normalizing gaze" characterized by "a surveillance that makes it possible to qualify, to classify and to punish." Interracial families are publicly gazed upon through a normative family lens and held accountable for their apparent differences by unsolicited attention to their non-normative familial form, inscribed on their bodies through "race." They are made to account for their differences by consistently being asked to explain them to others as they go about their daily lives.

Adoptive parents with children from China use a variety of strategies to deal with interracial surveillance. Crafty mothers shut down conversations ("I'm sorry, we have to go"), deflect questions, dodge possible conversations by moving away from people at the grocery store (or state fair, doctor's office, park, etc.), or avert their eyes from interested strangers. At times mothers refuse to answer questions coming at them from strangers. Nancy Thorne laughed as she told of how she tried to avoid answering questions from several women hounding her:

> I remember this one woman chasing us in a grocery store when we were in Capital City. [I said], "I'm not going to talk about this! Leave me alone!" The

second person just wanted to know, like, everything. "Have you ever heard of boundaries? Why am I going to tell you all of this? I'm just now figuring out how to go grocery shopping with a baby! Okay? I haven't figured this all out yet!" [*laughter*]

An important and telling strategy was refusing to "understand" the nature of the question. This was used most often when presented with a direct question, such as "Is she your daughter?" or "Are you her real mother?" In these inquiries about authentic relationships, mothers recognized the real questions being asked: "Is she your *biological* daughter?" "Are you her *biological* mother?" Yet the mothers refused to acknowledge the intent of the question and instead responded in the affirmative: "Yes, she is my daughter," "Yes, I am her real mother," "Yes, they really are sisters." By doing this, the mothers defined adoptive relationships as *real* kinship. Shannon Lynch, who in addition to adopting a child from China is the aunt of an adopted Chinese girl, shared such a story. Her experience illustrates the lengths to which people extend themselves in order to clarify the relationship between Asian child and white adult:

> One time with [my niece], when she was probably three or four, I was in the car with her. It was in the summertime because the windows were open, and there was a car next to me and [the driver] had a convertible. And I just remember this guy yelling over (he was probably in his mid-thirties or something), "Oh, is she adopted?" And I looked at him and I said, "She's my niece." And I closed the window up.

This strategy of offended or witty reply was especially useful when receiving the "blue ribbon" of supermarket surveillance questions: "How much did she cost?" Adoptive parents particularly dislike and even fear this question, because it alludes to the commodification of children and baby-buying (Dorow 2006). Participants' responses to this question included "not nearly enough," "priceless," and "about the same as a C-section." This refusal to "understand" the nature of the question is an act of resistance (Stiers 2007) through which parents reject the definition of nonbiological kinship as second best.

Interracial surveillance often took the form of paying compliments to children about their looks, such as "What a cutie! Does she speak Chinese?" Although mothers did not deny that their daughters were good-looking, and many even gushed unapologetically about their children, they found this continual "positive" attention from strangers, which they believed relied on

Asian fetishization, problematic. Mothers were worried that so much fawn-ing would direct their children to a particular type of self-identification. They didn't want their daughters to understand their value or worthiness only in their ability to be attractive. Holly Pritchard worried about her daughter privileging looks over intelligence and thus would counter those comments with ones that praised her academic ability: "I didn't want her to just estab-lish her self-image as one of being this cute little Asian kid, you know, be-cause she's very bright. And I said, 'Well yes, she's really good in school, too.' You know, I'd use something like that."

Mothers also reported that this focus on appearance from strangers led their children to draw a connection between their bodily features—which physicalize their "Chineseness," and which cannot be altered (at least not without the aid of cosmetic surgery)—and difference. Leanne Becker noted that the consequence of this kind of attention was "a lot like somebody com-ing up to you and saying, 'You stick out like a sore thumb, and I think it's great.'" They didn't want their daughters made to always feel like "a sore thumb," even if that difference was defined positively. Lynn Werden dis-cussed her approach to the flattering compliments paid to her daughter:

> Because in a certain way you don't want all that curiosity and attention
> focused on your family as if you're some amazing beauty or something. So,
> you know, I guess [I respond with] some combination of answering, some
> combination of avoiding, but really trying just to be really matter-of-fact
> and really happy in that, "yes, she's a beautiful child, blah, blah," but just
> trying to normalize it and kind of keep it cloaked in.

Despite the fact that adoptive parents were often irritated by the inter-racial surveillance they experienced, they did note several positive features associated with being a visibly adoptive family. They saw public interactions as opportunities for educating prospective adopters about adoption from China. As Eloise Nolan noted, "People ask, and they don't always ask just to be nosy." Parents understood that people touched by adoption—especially those in the midst of the adoption process—desire to connect with some-one who has been through the experience. Because study participants were aware of this, they reported replying to inquiries with "Why do you ask?" or "Do you know someone who has adopted?"

Participants also temper strong or negative reactions to interracial sur-veillance out of concern for the reputation of international adoption and in-terracial families. As Holly Pritchard explained, she wanted to act as a posi-tive spokesperson for adoptive families:

People are just nosy, but I don't think—I don't believe people are doing it maliciously, and certainly not consciously. They aren't consciously being intrusive. They just don't see that they are being intrusive. And I don't think it helps international adoption, in general, and mixed, multiracial families, in general, to blow them off, because then they're just—then they go home with an attitude of, you know, in the back of their minds it was a negative experience. . . . But generally speaking, I try to handle them in a positive way, because I just think you can cause more damage refusing it. I really don't—I sincerely don't think people are doing it intentionally to put you on the spot.

Through interracial surveillance, adoptive parents thus learn to act as educators and find themselves in the position of promoting international adoption. Though not always pleased, many participants found themselves content to take on this role.

Another form of education is also practiced when basic social norms regarding privacy of families (Fox 1999)—especially those granted to middle-class whites—are transgressed by interracial surveillance. Parents resist interracial surveillance by reminding the offending party of these social norms. That education can be more overt, but it often falls on deaf ears. Often family members attempt to extend lessons on privacy by establishing a balance of power in the information exchange: they demand the same information of the asking party. But as Leanne Becker's story illustrates, the questions—and the sense of entitlement that leads people to believe they have to right to ask the questions and to receive answers—are unidirectional, in that those asking the questions do not expect to be questioned in return:

You know, [strangers] are very well meaning, but they don't expect those same questions to be asked of them. In fact my daughter, my older daughter, once did. Somebody came up to us and said, "Where is she from?" and I said, "Well, she was born in China." [My daughter] said, "And where are you from?" and the woman started laughing like this was a ridiculous question, because of course, to her, it was. [It was as if this woman was saying,] "Why would you ask? I'm white." [*laughter*] "I belong here. You don't."

As many participants noted, most people who ask these questions of adoptive families in public are unaware of how they are received. Therefore, as Leanne's story illustrates, direct resistance to interracial surveillance is often itself misunderstood and ignored or met with baffled silence.

An interesting dynamic of the interracial surveillance experienced by international adoptive families is that it changes over time for individual families. Although families with older children are still the subject of public interest, parents less frequently have to deal with direct intrusive questions such as "How much did she cost?" Mothers attribute this shift in behavior to social norms about interactions with children. Although babies and toddlers in general (not only adopted infants) draw interest and attention, questions about them are addressed to their adult companions. Questions about older children are often directed to the children themselves. Although the comments associated with interracial surveillance from adult strangers diminished for study participants, questions, stares, and comments from other children increased. Charlotte Gordon spoke of the increased interracial surveillance from children in their multiracial neighborhood perplexed by her family's configuration. A playground encounter she recounted was typical of those interactions: "There was a black child once at the playground running off to his friends, who was several years older than my child, and he stopped and he said to us, 'What are you doing together?' And this was clearly just, 'How come you don't match?' "

Despite the decrease in comments from adults as children age, mothers with older children reported that they felt they had to be even more vigilant in tempering their responses to public encounters because their older children were able to comprehend questions and evaluate the ways in which their parents reacted. Mothers reported that they framed their responses to interracial surveillance specifically with their older children in mind, regardless of how complete or appropriate their answer was for the questioning party. They responded "proudly and calmly," because their children were "going to hear what you are saying and how you say it." Vigilance was especially needed when questions had racist or anti-adoption overtones.[8]

An important positive feature of the visibility of adoptive families with children from China is that it allows adoptive families to find each other, to connect, and to seek support through recognition of each other in public spaces. Mitchell Sorokin emphasized the ability to be recognized as an adoptive parent: "When you adopt a Chinese baby, it's pretty obvious. It's not like you're adopting from some other countries [where] you can almost kind of get away with [pretending] they're your biological kids. People know you're an adoptive parent, and you can spot each other in the malls and stuff. You kind of give each other the little wink or something, that kind of thing."

Because of this ability to "spot each other" and connect, parents enjoy the ability to be recognized as adoptive families by each other. Ironically, therefore, adoptive parents themselves engage in the same type of behavior they bemoan in others. Participants recalled public encounters with other parents that resulted in deep and abiding friendships. Interracial surveillance, then, is at the same time welcomed and reviled. Parents almost simultaneously utter, as Charlotte Gordon did, "Sometimes I just can't stand another goddamned idiot comment," and then approach each other when out and about and ask, "Where is she from?" This complicated terrain of adoptive visibility means that although being "put on the spot," as Holly Pritchard describes it, does occur through interracial surveillance, that "spot" can and often does serve as an important site for educating others about adoption, locating friends, and building networks among adoptive families with children from China.

The Quasi-biological Privilege of Families with Children from Russia

Through the 1990s and into the early 2000s, international adoption from Russia ranked second overall in popularity to that from China. (For a thorough comparison of the two, see Jacobson 2008.) Unlike families with children from China, however, those with children from Russia are not visibly marked as adoptive because parents and children share a single racial categorization. Indeed, the fact that children classified as white are available for international adoption in Russia plays a large role in the choice to adopt from that country. Parents who adopted from Russia hoped that a monoracial or ethnically similar adoption would ease the transition into a family and provide a buffer against what they viewed as the stigma of nonbiological kinship. Not only did participants in my study who adopted from Russia hope to match their child racially, they also explicitly did not want a child of color. It was not only a desire for whiteness, therefore, that drew people to Russia, but also a rejection of non-whiteness. Jean Kerne's reflections on the role race played in her choice to adopt from Russia were indicative of many participants: "Quite frankly, we wanted a child that would look most [like us]—we didn't want a darker skin or a Chinese. You know, to be honest we just felt we weren't comfortable with that. We wanted Caucasian and so that—you know, we chose that."

For these parents, adopting a white child meant avoiding the problems they understood to arise from cross-racial placements: prejudice, racism, stigma, and identity issues. As Emma Moore said, "I did think if we adopted from Russia it's probably likely that the child would be Caucasian and that would be one less thing to deal with." A monoracial placement meant that parents would not have to engage in the work of developing strategies to successfully negotiate these additional parenting challenges. White children, they said, could be more easily integrated into a white family. They wanted their children to "blend in" physically with their families and communities in order to avoid the stares, comments, and interest of interracial surveillance that surrounds interracial international adoption. Parents with this perspective felt that dealing with issues of nonbiological kinship and adoption would be enough for them and their child to deal with and that the additional issue of race was best avoided. Therefore, a large reason these parents chose Russia was because the majority of children available, though not all, are classified as white in the U.S. racial schema.[9]

In their post-adoption lives, these families experience little comment from others regarding their family form. Unless they consciously mark themselves, they are, in essence, invisible to strangers as adoptive families or as families with a child who was born in Russia. Because of shared race, participants in the study with children from Russia remarked that they were often mistaken in public as being the biological parents of their adopted children. This assumption was displayed through a profound absence of public acknowledgment of their adoptive status. They did not experience the stares and questions about adoption that are so prevalent among China adopters. This assumption was also displayed through comments regarding physical resemblance between parent and child. Dotty Cohen described how her daughters, adopted from Russia, are viewed when they are out in public: "My daughters walk around and no one looks at them. I mean, they look a little like me—I don't think it's paramount—or a lot like me, but they resemble us enough that people on the street would never say, 'Oh, okay, [that's an adoptive family].'" This imagined biological link was attractive. As Esther Levenson confided, "I think physically we have some—people think we look sort of similar, a little bit, a smidgen. Which is very exciting to hear that, you know?" Part of the excitement for parents is experiencing normative parenting, because discussions about physical resemblance between parent and child play a prominent role in public interactions for many biological parents.

In a society that privileges biological relatedness between parent and child—especially between mother and child—and problematizes other types of parent-child kinship (such as adoptive, foster, or step-parenting), the ability to appear as if one is biologically related to one's child confers special benefits. I call this "biological privilege." This term is popularly used to describe the ability of women to conceive and bear children. I play on that popular usage when I employ the term to describe not the fact of biologically birthing a child but the privilege of appearing *as if* one has done so. Biological privilege is not granted to all mothers who have birthed their children—regardless of visible mothering behavior—but to those who appear phenotypically similar enough to their children to be readily classified as a biological mother. White biological mothers of children of color, for example, are denied this privilege when their relationship to their children is questioned. Thus, biological privilege is explicitly rooted in normative understandings of the family as a racialized unit—of who is and who can be biologically related to others. Interracial surveillance and biological privilege, therefore, are flip sides of the same coin.

Biological privilege is granted to both individuals and to families and translates most directly into a notion of familial privacy—of anonymity in public spaces because one adheres to the norm of biological relatedness in families. Individuals and families that hold biological privilege are granted public support or acceptance for the form their familial relationships take. This can be seen in the public experiences of parents with children adopted from Russia as compared to those with children from China. As a consequence of their ability to appear biologically related to their children, the status of parents with children from Russia is not publicly questioned. White adoptive parents with white children born in Russia are able to freely move in public with their children without comments from or stares by strangers. They do not receive questions regarding how they came to be a family, and their children do not receive special attention. The families in my study who adopted from Russia experienced a type of quasi-biological privilege in that their adoptive status was invisible to strangers.

In theory, parents who adopt monoracially have available to them the choice to divulge or keep hidden their child's adoptive status. Historically, the adoption community supported the idea that parents and children should be matched in such a way that the visible differences between them were minimized—an "as-if" biological principle (Modell 1994). Because of the strong stigma surrounding adoption this was seen to be in the best interest of both parents and children. Today's adoption practices do not allow for the secrecy and sealed records that were so prominent throughout much of the twentieth century (Carp 1998; Pertman 2000; Melosh 2002). Full disclosure of adoption, especially to the adopted child, is now strongly promoted, and anything less would be cause for concern among adoption workers (Melosh 2002). Cautionary tales of the difficulties experienced by adult adoptees discovering their origins late in life frame and propel prescribed disclosure. Parents in my study argued that it would be considered taboo to hide the fact of adoption from their children, as doing so is presumed to be psychologically damaging to them. Parents such as Bonnie Hill argued that an orientation toward concealment would be enough to disqualify one for adoption: "The question about whether or not to talk about [adoption] is not the issue. And I think that you're very well schooled in that by your adoption agency. I think that if you said to an adoption agency that you were not going to talk about it, you would not get approved. Your home study would not get approved.[10] I really—I mean it's very clear this is what you're supposed to do. So I think you're told that."

Given these contemporary notions about how best to treat the issue of adoption, it is not surprising that all the parents in my sample were open with their children about the fact that they were adopted. From an early age, these children had been informed about how they came to be members of their families. Participants with children from Russia were emphatic that adoption be discussed and processed by their children. (This held true for parents with children from China as well.) Even if these families appear to be biological and are treated as such by people who do not know their exact route to family formation, the parents actively pull back that biological scrim *within their homes* in order to fulfill their responsibility to be open and honest.

In *public encounters*, however, adoption disclosure for families with children from Russia varied. Unlike families with children from China, whose adoptive status is seemingly "obvious" to all, those with children from Russia could choose to divulge or not to divulge their adopted status to strangers. Because of shared phenotype, however, these families actually had fewer occasions for naturally bringing up adoption in public encounters. Opportunities for disclosure did arise, however, when comments about physical resemblance were made. Kerry Mead spoke about the variety of approaches she used in such encounters: "It's funny, people sometimes say to her, or to me, 'Oh, she looks just like you,' or something like that, and depending on who it is we might either tell them, or not tell them, 'Oh, thank you.' You know that kind of thing. We get a chuckle out of stuff like that."

The parents in my study with children from Russia were emphatic that adoption should not be hidden out of embarrassment. They often expressed delight when their children openly and enthusiastically shared their adoption stories with strangers. Dennis Fischer shared such an exchange he witnessed when out with his son, Dimitri: "We were at the bowling alley last weekend and, you know, a girl next to us in the next alley had seen that his name was 'Dimitri' and said what a great name that was, and immediately Dimitri said, 'Well, I'm from Russia. I was adopted at [age] two from an orphanage.' So he's very much into telling everybody, you know, the story."

Parents were familiar, however, with the intrusive questions or inappropriate comments that sometimes follow exposure as an adoptive family. Carol Acher articulated this dilemma between disclosure and protection: "We're very open about [adoption], but some people can say things that aren't very smart to say in front of a four-year-old." As a result, the choice that parents with children from Russia face in public encounters is not only between celebrating adoption or privileging biology, but also between protecting familial privacy or exposing themselves to the possibility of intrusive questions or inappropriate comments. In the occasional choice to maintain the scrim of biology, we can see the privilege of privacy granted to families who match the hegemonic family norms of monoraciality and biological kinship.

Quasi-biological privilege protects Russian-adoptive families from interracial surveillance, but this lack of adoptive visibility is not always completely welcome. Parents in my study reported that the absence of a visibly adoptive identity kept others from "truly seeing" their families. The lack of readily accessible public acknowledgment of their families as adoptive translated into a source of isolation. Many parents spoke with envy about the community available to China-adoptive families that arose through spontaneous encounters in public settings (recall Mitchell Sorokin's mention of the wink in the mall that passes between China-adoptive families). Although there are several factors involved in the difference between the two communities, which I explore in depth elsewhere (Jacobson 2008), one important dimension is the lack of visibility that Russian-adoptive families have in public spaces, both to other Russian-adoptive families and to adoptive families with children from other places. Bonnie Hill articulated this dilemma:

> I would go to playgrounds and I would see these *very adopted families*. I mean, it was like, "Oh, okay, [you're adopted]." And there isn't—and, again, I'd go with my son and there would be no identifying mark. But if I had shown up with a South American child, or an Asian child, you know, it would be like having "A" for "Adopted" stamped someplace on your person, whereas that didn't happen. And so I really do feel like—and I never knew what to do. I never knew whether to just go up to this other parent and say, "So, your kid is adopted. So is mine," you know, because it felt like that would be invading their privacy.

Although they enjoyed freedom from interracial surveillance, parents with children adopted from Russia sometimes wished to have their adoptive status visible to other adoptive parents in order to easily interact in public spaces, bond with others over shared experience, and create friendships. However, because they were not marked through racial classification as "very adopted," they did not have access to a visible adoptive status that would allow them to approach people in what they felt to be a natural way (note Bonnie's statement that she "never knew what to do" when she wanted to connect with a stranger over adoption). In this way, the flip side of quasi-biological privilege and the lack of interracial surveillance, overwhelmingly framed by parents as positives, was the impediment to experiencing support from other adoptive families in public settings, feeling connected to the adoption community, and building friendship networks.

Conclusion

The noted differences regarding surveillance among families with children from China and those with children from Russia bring into focus the important ways in which people are always evaluating other families and expecting others to adhere to a specific set of ideals; these differences illustrate as well the ways in which individuals negotiate those expectations. In addition, the differing race-based experiences of the adoptive families in my sample point to the idea that rather than a zero-sum game, with the privileged American Family on one side and everyone else on the other, the idealized family (and its accompanying privileges) can be seen to fall on a continuum with a range of norms regarding culturally appropriate family forms and behavior.[11] This continuum perspective can be seen in the range of responses to families who fall outside of the idealized American Family. Visibly international-adoptive families (or those who disclose their status) are objectified as interesting curiosities by usually well-meaning but prying strangers, but they are not vilified or discredited as are some other "nontraditional" families. This surveillance does not result in structural discrimination or physical intimidation. Rather, interracial surveillance and the loss of biological privilege challenge the privacy and integrity of these families that are afforded to biological, monoracial ones. The loss of privilege experienced by these families is therefore largely symbolic. However, as Goffman's work on stigma (1963) emphasized, the symbolic loss of normativity is not inconsequential. It is deeply experienced and can have material as well as social and psychological impacts.

Comparing the decision making of parents with children from China and Russia makes visible the nuanced and complicated relationships adopters have to both interracial surveillance and biological privilege. While a variety of constraints pushed participants in my study toward and away from certain countries for adoption, the requirements to adopt from China and Russia were quite similar during the time these parents received their children. For some, the decision to pursue China or Russia was idiosyncratic. However, for many it pivoted on issues of race—especially how the racial make-up of their families would potentially influence the tenor of their day-to-day lives in public settings. This speaks to a larger issue in family formation. It shows how our choices of family members—who we choose to adopt, or even, perhaps, with whom we choose to form a committed relationship or to parent—are influenced by anticipated surveillance, by expectations of how strangers in fleeting public encounters will react to our choices. The consistency of surveillance and the degrees to which people go in order to seek information from adoptive families signals not only an interest but also a cultural anxiety related to ambiguous and non-normative family forms.

Yet the post-adoption experiences of interracial surveillance and biological privilege are complex. Interracial surveillance is intrusive and annoying for families with children from China, but at the same time it is welcomed in that it makes possible links between adoptive families. Likewise, quasi-biological privilege is welcomed in that it grants families with children from Russia cursory support and anonymity. Yet their status as adoptive families is not validated by other adoptive families because it goes unacknowledged. This absence of a marked adoptive status that comes through interracial surveillance means those with Russian-born children lack an acceptable public means to create new connections with other adoptive families.

The experiences of adoptive families in public point to a constant surveillance of the family—all families—that makes us accountable to an idealized norm. These norms, of course, do historically shift and change. The focus of negative or positive assessments of families also differs by context. In communities or contexts where interracial or adoptive families are the norm, we could imagine very different types of interactions. For example, participants reported that it was precisely the supportive interactions regarding family form that drew them to adoptive-family organizations. In public interactions, however, the continued dominance of monoraciality and biological kinship in normative ideas about the family heavily shaped the type of interactions they had with strangers. In their experiences we can see the hegemonic American Family continuing to shape family life despite its anachronistic status.

Notes

1. The names used for all participants and their children are pseudonyms.
2. Between 1995 and 2005, China led in numbers of children adopted into the United States, except for the years 1997, 1998, and 1999, when Russia was the leading country. In 2006 Guatemala surpassed Russia as the second most popular country from which U.S. families adopt children, with China remaining the most popular. For a breakdown of all international adoptions to the United States by country of origin, see U.S. Department of State 2009.
3. It is important to distinguish here between formal and informal adoption. While whites compose the majority of formal adoptive parents in the United

States, informal adoptions—often called "kinship adoptions"—have played an important role in the African American family (Kim 2008; Stack 1974).

4. Although both China and Russia are ethnically diverse, the children coming from these two countries are almost exclusively classified in the United States as "Asian" or "white," respectively. Although the majority of children brought into the United States from Russia are considered white, Volkman (2003, 52n) notes, "in their birth country they may be stigmatized as Roma" (or "gypsy").

5. One participant self-identified as both Chinese and white. Based on a combination of income, education, occupation, and self-identification, the parents in another family were identified as working-class.

6. Qualitative differences exist among the terms "multiracial," "interracial," "biracial," "mixed race," and "transracial." "Interracial couple" refers to a couple comprising adults of two different races; a "multiracial" person ("biracial" and "mixed race" having gone out of vogue) would refer to the biological child of their coupling. "Transracial" is commonly used in the context of adoption and refers to a child of one race being adopted by an adult of another race (Dalmage 2007). I use "interracial families" as an umbrella term to encompass families in which two or more members, including children, can be classified as belonging to different races.

7. I thank Kimberly McClain DaCosta for our conversation, which helped me to clarify this point.

8. It could be speculated that participants also experienced a decline in interracial surveillance because of increasing numbers of international adoptive families in their communities. The families in my study had all adopted in the 1990s; many characterized themselves on the "cutting edge" of international adoption. With the increase in popularity of international adoption (as evidenced by the growing numbers), interracial surveillance of adoptive families overall could be in decline. With more adoptive families in the public eye, perhaps people are less likely to see international adoption as unique and worthy of interest. However, my time spent in the field with recent adoptive families contradicts this idea. On adoption websites and at local and national conferences for adoptive families and adoption professionals, the topic of how to handle intrusive questions in public interactions continues to be popular. Interracial surveillance remains an issue for newly formed families just as it was for those who adopted a decade ago. Consequently, I see the age of the child, rather than the increasing popularity of adoption, as having a greater effect on the reduction over time of comments stemming from interracial surveillance.

9. Ironically, one family that chose to adopt from Russia in part to receive a Caucasian child was referred to a nonwhite child, whom they did adopt.

10. The "home study," during which an adoption social worker visits the home and assesses the fitness of the potential adopters as parents, is an important step in the adoption process.

11. I thank Anita Garey for encouraging this line of thought.

References

Azoulay, Katya Gibel. 1997. *Black, Jewish, and Interracial: It's Not the Color of Your Skin but the Race of Your Kin, and Other Myths of Identity*. Durham, NC: Duke University Press.

Carp, E. Wayne. 1998. *Family Matters: Secrecy and Disclosure in the History of Adoption*. Cambridge, MA: Harvard University Press.

Childs, Erica Chito. 2005. *Navigating Interracial Borders: Black-White Couples and Their Social Worlds*. New Brunswick, NJ: Rutgers University Press.

Collins, Patricia Hill. 1994. Shifting the Center: Race, Class, and Feminist Theorizing about Motherhood. In *Mothering: Ideology, Experience and Agency*, edited by Evelyn Nakano Glenn, Grace Chang, and Linda Rennie Forcey. New York: Routledge.

Coontz, Stephanie. 1992. *The Way We Never Were: American Families and the Nostalgia Trap*. New York: Basic Books.

Dalmage, Heather M. 2000. *Tripping on the Color Line: Black-White Multiracial Families in a Racially Divided World*. New Brunswick, NJ: Rutgers University Press.

———. 2007. Interracial Couples, Multiracial People, and the Color Line in Adoption. In *Adoptive Families in a Diverse Society*, edited by Katarina Wegar. New Brunswick, NJ: Rutgers University Press.

de Beauvoir, Simone. 1984. *The Second Sex*. Harmondsworth, UK: Penguin.

Dorow, Sara K. 2006. *Transnational Adoption: A Cultural Economy of Race, Gender, and Kinship*. New York: New York University Press.

Foucault, Michel. 1977. *Discipline and Punish: The Birth of the Prison*. New York: Vintage Books.

Fox, Greer Litton. 1999. Families in the Media: Reflections on the Public Scrutiny of Private Behavior. *Journal of Marriage and the Family* 61: 821–30.

Garey, Anita Ilta, and Karen V. Hansen. 1998. Analyzing Families with a Feminist Sociological Imagination. In *Families in the US: Kinship and Domestic Politics*, edited by Karen V. Hansen and Anita Ilta Garey. Philadelphia: Temple University Press.

Goffman, Erving. 1963. *Stigma: Notes on the Management of a Spoiled Identity*. New York: Simon and Schuster.

Hansen, Karen V. 2005. *Not-So-Nuclear Families: Class, Gender, and Networks of Care*. Piscataway, NJ: Rutgers University Press.

Ishizawa, Hiromi, Catherine Kenney, Kazuyo Kubo, and Gilliam Stevens. 2006. Constructing Interracial Families through Intercountry Adoption. *Social Science Quarterly* 87 (5): 1207–24.

Jacobson, Heather. 2008. *Culture Keeping: White Mothers, International Adoption, and the Negotiation of Family Difference*. Nashville: Vanderbilt University Press.

Kim, Katherine M. Flower. 2008. Out of Sorts: Adoption and (Un)Desirable Children. In *Mapping the Social Landscape: Readings in Sociology*, edited by Susan J. Ferguson. Boston: McGraw Hill.

Kristeva, Julia. 1991. *Strangers to Ourselves*. New York: Columbia University Press.

Melosh, Barbara. 2002. *Strangers and Kin: The American Way of Adoption.* Cambridge, MA: Harvard University Press.

Miller-Loessi, Karen, and Kilic Zeynep. 2001. Unique Diaspora? The Case of Adopted Girls from the People's Republic of China. *Diaspora* 10 (2): 243–60.

Modell, Judith. 1994. *Kinship with Strangers: Adoption and Interpretations of Kinship in American Culture.* Berkeley: University of California Press.

Nelson, Margaret K. 2006. Single Mothers "Do" Family. *Journal of Marriage and Family* 68: 781–95.

Pertman, Adam. 2000. *Adoption Nation: How the Adoption Revolution Is Transforming America.* New York: Basic Books.

Reddy, Maureen T. 1994. *Crossing the Color Line: Race, Parenting, and Culture.* New Brunswick, NJ: Rutgers University Press.

Rothman, Barbara Katz. 2005. *Weaving a Family: Untangling Race and Adoption.* Boston: Beacon Press.

Simon, Rita J., and Howard Altstein. 1992. *Adoption, Race, and Identity: From Infancy through Adolescence.* Westport, CT: Praeger.

Smith, Dorothy. 1993. The Standard North American Family: SNAF as an Ideological Code. *Journal of Family Issues* 14 (1): 50–65.

Stack, Carol B. 1974. *All Our Kin: Strategies for Survival in a Black Community.* New York: Harper and Row.

Stiers, Gretchen A. 2007. From This Day Forward: Commitment, Marriage, and Family in Lesbian and Gay Relationships. In *Shifting the Center: Understanding Contemporary Families*, 3rd ed., edited by Susan J. Ferguson. Boston: McGraw-Hill Higher Education.

U.S. Department of State. 2009. Total Adoptions to the United States. *adoption.state. gov/news/total_chart.html.*

Volkman, Toby Alice. 2005. Embodying Chinese Culture: Transnational Adoption in North America. In *Cultures of Transnational Adoption*, edited by Toby Alice Volkman. Durham, NC: Duke University Press.

Vonk, Elizabeth M. 2001. Cultural Competence for Transracial Adoptive Parents. *Social Work* 46 (3): 246–55.

Wegar, Katarina. 1997. *Adoption, Identity, and Kinship: The Debate over Sealed Birth Records.* New Haven, CT: Yale University Press.

West, Candace, and Don H. Zimmerman. 1987. Doing Gender. *Gender and Society* 1 (2): 125–51.

Weston, Kath. 1991. *Families We Choose: Lesbians, Gays, Kinship.* New York: Columbia University Press.

Zelizer, Viviana A. 1985. *Pricing the Priceless Child: The Changing Social Value of Children.* Princeton, NJ: Princeton University Press.

5

Playground Panopticism

Ring-around-the-Children,
a Pocketful of Women

Holly Blackford

In his essay on panopticism, Michel Foucault (1995) analyzes the architectural structure of the panopticon planned by Jeremy Bentham in 1791. The structure revolutionized the concept of disciplinary power through the technology of surveillance. The panopticon is a windowed, central tower in which a supervisor can survey the people in prison cells or rooms that occupy the periphery. The prisoners, patients, schoolboys, or workers in the cells can be perpetually seen by the supervisor in the tower, while those that are watched cannot actually see the person watching them. With this structure, the very few can hold power over the many because the tower supplies the very *suggestion* of constant surveillance. Those of us who still notice the surveillance equipment that monitors our movements in banks and stores are conscious of how this feels. It makes us think twice about undressing in front of dressing room mirrors. Recently, a mother was charged with child abuse when store cameras filmed her hitting her child in her car. She pled guilty and said that she was overly frustrated by the child, who continually misbehaved in the store. One wonders why surveillance tools cannot enable store managers to send aid to an overburdened mother *in* the store, who perhaps needs help expediting her shopping. But surveillance equipment is designed for punishment, not intervention.

The concept of the panopticon, I was astonished to find, enabled me to interpret the data that I gathered through two years of participant-observation research on two playground settings in the San Francisco Bay Area. One

Excerpted from Holly Blackford, "Playground Panopticism: Ring-around-the-Children, A Pocketful of Women" (© *Childhood*, 2004) by permission of Sage Publications Ltd.

was an outdoor public suburban neighborhood playground, and the other was a commercial playplace situated in a suburban strip mall. The panopticon model taught me the meaning of the term "supervision," identified as the mechanism of safety in the rhetoric of playground safety and design recommendations (Smith 1998; Wellhousen 2002). The suburban playground that I observed operates upon a similar principle of constant surveillance, with the children playing in the center and the parents—usually mothers, the embodiment of the possibility of surveillance—circled around the children on the park benches. When they have done something questionable, children furtively glance in the general direction of the benches. Although children know who their mothers are and prisoners do not know who is watching them, the park benches similarly represent the constant suggestion of being watched, and thus the automation of panopticism. The adults on the benches may not have actually observed a transgression but "mothers have eyes in the back of their heads," the children know, just as they know that "Santa Claus sees you when you're sleeping." Adults want children to believe that they are seen. Although supervision is equated with keeping children safe, panopticism also seeks to produce a certain kind of subjectivity in children, an internalization of discipline through self-monitoring. In this chapter, I also argue that panopticism creates a certain kind of subjectivity in mothers, who initiated me into the multifaceted meanings of supervising children on playgrounds.

Unlike Foucault's panopticism of the prison, the panoptic force of the mothers around the suburban playground becomes a community that gazes at the children only to ultimately gaze at one another, seeing reflected in the children the parenting abilities of one another. Through visiting several playgrounds with my now-four-year-old daughter, I have come to understand that a complex network of female social relations occupies those benches. Elaborate rules of both playground etiquette and social competition occupy the ring of women that can be found at almost any Bay Area suburban playground in the mid-morning or afternoon. Through encoding the principle of surveillance into its physical structure, the panoptic structure of the suburban playground actually objectifies women as mothers and allows mothers to objectify themselves, because they participate in the female community that is watching and measuring the behavior of the children to assess the mother's mothering.

In this chapter I compare the ring of mothers in Bay Area suburban playgrounds, particularly focusing on the one in my neighborhood of two years, to parents and children at McDonald's PlayPlace, where children disappear from their mothers' gazes into networks of tunnels, enclosed slides, and cages of balls. Around the PlayPlace are not benches but cafeteria tables;

both play equipment and parental tables encourage parallel play. Although the McDonald's is located in "suburban sprawl," the children pass one another in tunnels as urban, anonymous subjects, while mothers socialize with one another instead of watching or talking about their children. Whereas mothers of young children perform governance of their children's conduct in the public playgrounds under study, they rarely interfere with their children's behavior in the PlayPlace, having to some extent "let their guard down" and put their trust in commercial standards for safety. This is true to such an extent that McDonald's has a sign saying, "Police will be called for children unattended by parents." The ironic equation of "commercial" with "safe" is not unlike the irony within the American Halloween ritual, when mothers distrust homemade food and authenticate the safety of packaged candy. The vigilance that the mothers exercise in the suburban playground is relaxed in the commercial play zone, furthered by efforts of companies like Chuck E. Cheese's to provide identity bracelets to parents and children upon arrival and ensure that the right children leave with the right parents.

Commercial sectors represent a broader, more dispersed ideal of surveillance. There, the mothers relax their panoptic responsibilities and experience an intriguing moment of freedom from disciplinary concerns. This explains the appeal of the commercial playplace to mothers and children, who seek relief from surveillance regimes. With the price of a Happy Meal, parents purchase an alternative ideology that tells them, "You deserve a break today," which, apparently, the public playground does not afford them. Curiously, the relaxed form of behavior that parents exhibit in commercial playgrounds allows children to create their own rules for play and conduct their own social interactions, largely free from adult interference. We live in an era when children's spaces are increasingly circumscribed, and their activities—even recess (Pelligrini 1995)—increasingly organized by adults (Postman 1994). Although the commercial playplace represents the privatization of public play space, the actual freedom that the children enjoy there parallels the freedom that urban, working-class children exhibited on the streets in the late nineteenth and early twentieth centuries (Nasaw 1985). Before middle-class social reformers—the ancestors of the suburban mothers I observed—succeeded in developing public playgrounds to get children off the street, working-class children set their own rules for governance and play, with minimal adult interference. Though by no means a public street, the PlayPlace structure serves to symbolize the pipes and ducts under a street, enabling the children to disappear in a way middle-class mothers would not allow in a semi-urban park. The families using the McDonald's PlayPlace, located in the midst of discount outlets, represent a more mixed socioeconomic group than the middle-class neighborhood playground. Ironically, the commercial sector has stepped in during the late twentieth century to create the perception that "free play" can be purchased by anyone—for a small price. . . .

The Sites under Study

. . . My observations of playgrounds in suburban settings stem from my attendance of playgrounds in a racially mixed but mostly middle-class section of Oakland, California; while I also draw upon observations of playgrounds in Oakland's Lake Merritt Park and Rockridge, I focus most heavily on the small playground in my immediate neighborhood, where I went at least once a week for a period of two years with my young child. This playground is actually in Piedmont, a small city surrounded by Oakland that has higher property values and taxes than Oakland, and thus is known for excellent schools. Rental properties are rare in Piedmont; I had one of the few. It is thus a very settled community. The playground was frequented by mothers with young children, infants to seven years old.

The playground had baby swings, a wood structure with opportunities for climbing and sliding (slide and pole), a steering wheel, a small tunnel, and rocking spring structures that look like vehicles. The entire playground was a large sandpit, encouraging the most child play. . . . Next to the sand area was a wood chip area with picnic tables. Benches surrounded the gated playground, which bordered on tennis courts and a large, open field. . . . Because the playground was nestled in a hill, it had cement walls, upon which mothers would also sit. The cement wall around the hollowed-out area rose dramatically, inviting children to walk along it until they were perilously high. . . .

. . . While the playground's water fountain was supposed to be an adult-defined device for refreshment and respite from play, children wanted to play with the water and bring water into the sand area. Mothers were never sure that playing with the water was acceptable. I noticed that mothers more often allowed children to climb and play at the fountain when only a few of us were there. When the playground was busier, mothers vocally told the children that the fountain was only for drinking or filling buckets—not for sensory play, which was probably viewed as unsanitary. In the two years that I visited this playground, I never saw anyone actually drink from the fountain.

The indoor place of study was McDonald's PlayPlace in Richmond, California, an area more socioeconomically diverse but equally racially diverse. The PlayPlace was located near a popular (Hilltop) mall in the Bay

Area, which radiated discount strip malls and provided the context for the McDonald's PlayPlace, freestanding but proximate to a strip mall with discount and other "big box" stores. The location of the McDonald's PlayPlace in the center of commercialism could not more fully symbolize its difference from the public playground of Piedmont, which bordered school and adult recreation (tennis courts) and thus served to signify the status of the playground in residential, suburban culture. The McDonald's PlayPlace was a place where mothers took their children for a (quick) break from running errands and shopping expeditions, a convenient way for children who had been cooped up in the car to blow off steam and eat at the same time. The public playground, by contrast, signified the leisure of play and restful recreation time among mothers with children; there was very little hurrying and a mood of lingering, time revolving around the routines of the children (mothers went home at naptime, lunch, dinner, etc.). The suburban playground lay at the heart of community organization, organized around the upbringing of children and the opportunity for adults to participate in this upbringing. The McDonald's PlayPlace lay at the heart of busy shopping days; mothers checked their to-do lists and receipts while conversing with one another, wolfing down French fries, and occasionally imploring their children, when briefly surfacing from the play structure, to do the same. . . .

Panoptic Play in the Park

. . . Like Stephen Smith (1998) in his book *Risk and Our Pedagogical Relation to Children: On the Playground and Beyond*, I feel that the ubiquitous park benches signify "a certain relation of the adult to the child" (Smith 1998, 46), and that playgrounds are not spaces removed from the traffic of adult life as they were intended to be, but metaphors for cultural meanings and spaces that ritualize, reflect, and shape ideologies of adulthood and childhood. To Smith, the playground is a matter of risk-taking, and this risk "thematize[s] our interactions with children" (Smith 1998, 5) because adults want children to practice risk-taking in a controlled setting, ultimately to prepare them for the riskiness of the larger world. He argues that we adults see the children's activities on the playground based upon our recollections of the activities we performed as children; thus from our vantage point of knowing the risky world better than children, we are in a position to encourage them in risk-taking. The park bench, in his argument, encourages passive sitting on the sidelines rather than productive, active encouragement of risk-taking; children *need* to feel the posted presence of adults, he says. I agree with Smith's contention that the ring of park benches is a space set apart from the child's playing field; children do not play on the benches—the benches are "something which [the children] approach only when wishing to break away from the activity at hand to seek consolation, reassurance, or some other contact with the adult sitting there" (Smith 1998, 48). However, the social dynamics within the ring of mothers on the park benches changed the meaning of the function of the playground, from a space for children to a space for mothers, from a space for encouraging risks to a space perpetuating the objectification of mothers as they engage in self-discipline through surveillance of one another.

The social discourse among the mothers in the ring revolves around the children, but by sharing their experiential knowledge, the mothers reveal that they self-monitor their own abilities at mothering. The first question asked of a newcomer is, "how old is your son/daughter?"—code for "how long have you been in our circle?" As a friend put it after she brought her first child to the playground, "I feel among the initiated. Mothers ask me questions about him and share their experiences and reflections upon their own children at his age." The moment the mothers discover that you are new to their circle (that your child is your first child), they distribute both advice and admonitions: "That's an awfully little baby to put on that swing," "She's eating sand—can that be good for her?" "The sun's in her eyes—did you bring a hat?" etc. My husband never receives such comments, even when he swung our daughter too high and she fell out. He recalls that the mothers shook their heads but said nothing. I, on the other hand, have learned that if I give my child girl scout cookies and offer them to other interested children, other mothers are quick to produce healthier snacks and, by doing so, dramatize their nutrition values. Without soliciting stories, I have been told of countless childrearing experiences from mothers I've never met, from messy divorces to selection of childcare to the discovery of food allergies. Stories narrate the direct observation of the children. One day I watched my three-year-old try to imitate two vivacious eight-year-old twins on the monkey bars. I soon heard the story of their premature births and the special services they required, a story that spoke of the mother's perceptive early intervention and success, proven by the clear abilities of her healthy, skilled daughters. In their research on health-seeking among mothers, Tardy and Hale (1998) recently "discovered" that the informal networks of mothers at the playground provide mothers with the opportunity to seek and share information about children's health and well-being. This could easily be discovered by merely taking a child to such a park on a sunny mid-morning, and *just sitting* on the bench.

Maternal self-monitoring through narrative practice thinly veils a heated competition between mothers vis-à-vis their children's abilities and achievements. The discourse progresses to what a child can and cannot do, always measured against direct observation of the child. "Does he/she do this yet? Is she/he potty trained? Does she take ballet? Is she going to summer camp?" Stories that prove the abilities of one child or another are shared and one-upped by the next mother. My own child wears glasses, which often sparks the concerned question among mothers of "how did you know?" accompanied by frantic looks toward their own children, revealing the fact that this question is really a question about their own knowledge and perception of children. Their efforts to validate their mothering and knowledge by story-telling and questioning reveal a real need among the mothers for cultural valuation. They lack cultural recognition for their difficult, everyday decisions and interventions, and they and the community must create their own job-performance review. The idea that parents become possessive of their children's behavior on the playground, viewing that behavior as a reflection of self, is the recent subject of a humorous *New York Times* article, "My Kid's Never Been Bad and Other Sandbox Tales" (Lee 2000). The idea that children's "sandbox" performances reflect upon parents to such an extent that parents rewrite the scripts and redirect their children's social roles suggests that the playground provides a space in which "our internalization of idealized and mythic parenting requirements is at work to preserve gender distinctions" (Aitken 2000, 124). Stuart Aitken believes that child development theory assumes and refuses to problematize the assumption that "parents, for the most part, love their children and will do the best they can to provide for a set of universally understood needs in the face of oppressive societal structures" (Aitken 2000, 123). The playground becomes a space in which those parenting requirements are performed, contested, and reified by community. It is a public stage of a screenplay written by nineteenth-century domestic ideology.

When there is conflict on the playground, the ring watches the mother's performance in discipline, and very elaborate rules apply to the performances of helping negotiate toy-sharing and turn-taking. When a child violates another child, the mother apologizes to the other mother. When a child seizes another's toy, the mothers are quick to intervene, one giving the perfunctory speech on "that doesn't belong to you; I brought your sand bucket," and the other praising the value of sharing. The kids completely ignore them, and it's clear that the mothers are really discussing and performing their values. Elaborate systems of turn-taking are verbalized by mothers regarding swings, slides and other equipment. Should a child be hurt, he or she is descended upon by a flurry of band-aids and first aid equipment. My child has been offered hand sanitizer, Kleenex, and lots of food as the women embrace their hostessing role by carrying their domestic preparations to the park. As an article by Sheldon Himelfarb (1994) suggests, and my own experience seconds, mothers spread paraphernalia across the park bench. Snacks, toys, jackets, strollers, and even back supports pepper the seats of the ring on any sunny day. They forge a kind of domestic apparatus on the playground, bringing their domestic authority to organize their children's bodies and space. The ring becomes an extension of domesticity, bringing the nuclear family's privatization of mothering into public view, where it is reviewed and approved.

Maternal performances reveal a sense of competition in mothering, signifying the fact that mothers struggle to authenticate the performance of their role for the suburban community. In particular, issues of discipline bear carefully orchestrated performances; the question of what's fair between children seems more relevant to the involved mothers than the children in question, who already have a clear sense of what they think is fair. As I watched a negotiation over the sharing of a Barbie and Ken doll (two girls wanted Barbie, and nobody wanted Ken), I was struck by the way in which both mothers ritualized the rhetoric of valuing choice. One mother told her daughter to either share the doll or put the doll away, while the other mother told her crying daughter that she should realize the owner's right to not share or they would have to go home. When the owner decided to share Barbie, her mother beamed and gazed directly at the other mother, saying "good choice" to her child, a rhetoric that seemed to have little to do with the child's actual ability to choose, but which had earned her recognition in the playground for enforcing a democratic style of rule. The ways in which mothers use language practices to create boundaries of inclusion and exclusion (they speak neither to fathers nor to babysitters) mirror the ways in which girls on the playground do, as researched by Goodwin (2002). Many researchers of peer groups note that while overt bullying is typically a male practice, girls have more subtle ways of expressing aggression toward one another, including gossip, exclusion, and rule-negotiation (Goodwin 2002; Hawkins, Pepler, and Craig 2001; Opie and Opie 1960). In *Gender Play*, Barrie Thorne (1993) observes a girl tell a boy that he cannot play with the girls because he is a boy. The mothers of this playground do not need to make this explicit.

I believe that the ways in which my experience of various playgrounds differs from Smith's has to do with the fact that I am a mother and he is a father. This is the subject of an article in *Parents' Magazine*, written by a father. In "Laws of the Jungle Gym: Mothers' and Fathers' Playground Behavior," Himelfarb (1994) humorously writes of his observations of gender differences:

> Every day I would arrive at the playground with Danielle and a ball. Most of
> the other dads also traveled light, usually with some form of sports gear. In
> contrast, each mom showed up toting a bottomless carryall much like Mary
> Poppins had. Instead of five-foot coatracks, however, these bags disgorged
> diapers, juice, milk, rash cream, powder, a change of clothes, bandages for
> imaginary "owwies," and usually enough snacks for everyone in sight. What
> is it, I wondered, that makes mothers come to the playground equipped to
> spend the night if necessary, while dads aren't good for much more than the
> time it takes to play a game of hopscotch? (Himelfarb 1994, 245)

He continues by noticing that the mothers actually talk to one another,
"sharing intelligence on everything from schools to stretch marks. They even
swapped phone numbers! We dads, on the other hand, hardly exchanged a
word. We were either on the playground totally immersed in games of kick
ball or tag, or else on the sidelines equally immersed in newspapers" (Himelfarb 1994, 245). His conclusion: that dads regress and become kids again on
the playground, a conclusion not unlike Smith's paternal sense that the playground is an organized space to get kids to take the risks that "adults" recall
finding valuable in their own childhoods.

The ring of mothers that surround me reflects a ritualized reification of
the role of women in the ideology of middle-class, suburban life, organized
around the upbringing of children. As maternal eyes are focused inward on
the behavior, play, and abilities of the children, the community imagines that
it is seeing itself—its future, invested by each mother—reflected back, and is
measuring its standards and practices from the panoptic ring. The center of
the structure, inhabited by the child, is play, the child's job. As Viviana Zelizer
(1985) argues, industrialization and subsequent child labor laws, ushered by
middle-class reformers, saw the transition from children as economic values
to liabilities—but emotionally and spiritually "priceless." Rural and urban
ideas of children as workers, contributing to family subsistence and daily
life, shifted to the dominant ideology of "the child's work is to play." Play is
imagined as the antithesis of work because play focuses on means rather
than ends, although some, such as Roger Hart and Selim Iltus (Project for
Public Spaces), feel that this opposition between play and meaningful work
has hurt children, disabling their sense of agency and meaningful purpose in
the world. Most play theorists actually feel a greater continuity between play
and work (Frost 1992). The ring around this ideal of "non-working" children
is the community of "non-working" women, idealized as unpaid mothers
devoting "priceless" labor to the upbringing of a child.

The public playground of open space, reserved for leisured use of equipment, symbolizes the degree to which there reigns a belief that adults' and

children's worlds are and should be separate. Further, women are the ones responsible for maintaining the boundaries. The ring of mothers believes itself responsible for mediating the child's exposure to the outside world. The suburban community is implicitly organized to protect the children by surveillance, its eyes focused inward in the circle rather than outward into the world beyond children. The word that kept floating into my mind, as I watched these mothers, was "hover." Their hovering, perhaps, registers the degree to which public space has been equated with danger to children, and the extent to which they feel that they alone protect children, unsupported by the public sphere. In the children's perspective, however, the ring of mothers is the embodiment of social authority. Ultimately, the mothers serve as a social gaze that perhaps models the way in which children learn to control their own play and interactions with one another.

The Commercial Playplace:
Children Sprawled in Tunnels and Tubes

The suburban residential structure can be contrasted with the commercial structure of McDonald's PlayPlaces, where the elaborate tunnels and passageways, as well as the burial of balls, hide the children from the parents' gaze and prevent the competitive social discourse and surveillance of maternal performance that I have found in the outdoor public playground. Although located in the suburbs, the commercial playplace serves to symbolize not suburban residential structure devoted to the discipline of children but a structure devoted to pleasure and consumption. Having served as a market researcher for McDonald's for several years, I have heard countless mothers reflect on PlayPlaces as a place to provide them a break from maternal performance. The structures remove the children from their sight as the mothers happily eat their food. The tables for the parents are not set up to survey the children, but to attend to the adult(s) across from them. Unlike the play*ground*, McDonald's PlayPlaces symbolize commercialism, urbanism, and modern (enclosed) rather than rural (open space) life. The tunnels look like the pipes or ducts to be found under the streets, where children once played and faced real dangers. Many children can move through the structure simultaneously, so rules of turn-taking or waiting in line are less relevant. Except for when the mother decides it's time to leave, very little interaction between children and mothers takes place.

Although I observed a mix of middle- and working-class families, the structure suggested a real separation of adult and child social worlds, reminiscent of Nasaw's reports of lower-class urban children playing on the streets: "As long as the children did not disgrace themselves or their families, get into trouble with the police, abandon younger brothers or sisters, or get hurt, their parents left them alone" (Nasaw 1985, 24). This was partly due to the perception that adults were everywhere and would come running if a child got into trouble. Likewise, parents of today feel that commercial spaces share their adult responsibility. Because of this, supervision of the children is very tenuous. Many mothers actually wish that McDonald's would hire a play supervisor, alleviating their responsibilities. Both children and parents often overlook the rules. For example, older children notoriously ignore the height limit and jump into the ball pit, hurting younger children. I witnessed such an event, and it is impossible to either find or reach a child when they are in the structure. Adults are specifically excluded from the small entry-ways to the equipment, and oftentimes parents pay absolutely no attention. In fact, the mother whose child got hurt was not even in the same room as the play structure.

It really is amazing how the structure of McDonald's PlayPlaces imitates the structure of early twentieth-century street play. When I observed a child climb to the top and then get scared, I also observed a sibling rather than parent go to help her, replicating the "little mothers" of working-class street children. Parents simply cannot comfortably fit through the tubes. The sibling in question took the smaller child to the restroom to wash her bloody nose. The mother followed, less actively involved. Small lookout points exist at the ends of many tunnels, such that children who climb there can look out at their parents, unknown to their parents, who are often busy organizing the rest of their shopping expedition, talking, or eating. In contrast to the outdoor public playground, the noisy McDonald's PlayPlace seemed the center of democracy; mothers, fathers, grandparents, babysitters, and older siblings all took their one-to-eight-year-old children to the PlayPlace. The appeal of McDonald's also seemed to cut across social class. Conversations of adults range from planning birthday parties to grocery shopping to a new film, rarely coalescing on issues of childcare or development. Many mothers came to meet a girlfriend with children; more than a few pairs of mothers seemed to be discussing husbands or partners. Collecting children for departure was an enormous production, not because people had brought their domestic apparatus (this is a place of food purchase, after all), but because children did not want to go. The children would say, "in a minute," and disappear again, or negotiate "just one more time!" They might even claim to still be hungry, which put their caregivers in a particular position (they could not deny basic needs like a plea for hunger). The children would ask for a milkshake or an ice-cream, which would inevitably lead to more play time.

McDonald's was a place of unbridled consumption. Although the children actually seemed to eat very little, any interactions between parents and children were negotiations about how many more bites of food the child should have before disappearing again. The children seemed to have a type of consumer power, dictating what food they wanted, how many bites they would eat, and what kind of sauce for their nuggets. This felt uncannily like Nasaw's description of how the candy store functioned for older children in early twentieth-century New York. Consumer power was "the best substitute for freedom" (Nasaw 1985, 118) that the children could find. Candy store owners allowed children with a nickel to take as much time in the store as they wished, just as one could buy a sixty-nine cent ice cream and play in the PlayPlace all day long (but with a parent nearby). This raises broader questions about the role of stores in today's children's play. Does the fact that the commercial sector is creating playplaces mean that children feel a unique cultural recognition in public space? Do they, or will they, regard places of consumption and exchange as their American playgrounds? Are public playgrounds destined to go the way of the apples at Halloween, viewed as potential carriers of razor blades?

At the very same moment that education is questioning the function of recess in public school (Frost 1992; Pellegrini 1995), places of consumption claim to recognize "the child's right to play" and they see this as attracting a family market, mothers and other caregivers being important consumers. The response of a family-targeted chain like McDonald's implies an implicit knowledge that children play everywhere in adult spaces, so why not meet child and adult needs simultaneously? That is, if the children are going to play with the napkin dispensers and salt shakers anyway, why not give them a place to play while their parents eat? I sympathize with this attitude, impressed as I have been by my own children's abilities to colonize adult market space (Payless shoe store is a particular favorite). The colorful, massive displays of material goods seem to unleash an almost uncontainable juvenile energy, beyond all degrees of rationality or decorum. My findings corroborate McKendrick, Bradford, and Fieldler's (2000) study of birthday parties in commercial playplaces. They find that parents cite convenience as the primary motive for the birthday party in the commercial sector, identifying the curious fact that commercial playplaces rather than parents now lead celebrations of rites of passage and instruct parents in the proper ritualizing of the birthday. They conclude that commercial playplaces are more for parents and only secondarily for children. The growth of commercial playplaces in urban and semi-urban areas seems to signify the historical culmination of middle-class efforts to contain free play: "As Jane Jacobs predicted so forcefully two decades ago, streets cleared for the respectable have become free fields for predators. . . . In the destruction of the street life of the laboring poor, a critical means of creating urban communities and organizing urban space has disappeared" (Stansell 1982, 332). With the middle-class perception that women must be ever-vigilant with their children in the semi-urban Bay Area comes an opportunity for corporations to stand for the safety that playfulness requires. And so they symbolize the middle-class maternal function with taglines such as "Chuck E. Cheese's, where a kid can be a kid."

Conclusion

Just as gender is known to be something people perform (Butler 1993, 1999), and just as femininity and the female body are known to be subject to particular scrutiny and gazes (Bordo 1993), mothering is a product of social negotiation between adults as well as between adults and children. Mothers are even conscious of this; Holden and Ritchie (1991) show how battered women report that they parent differently, depending on whether or not their partners are present. The study reported here is neither longitudinal nor experimental (the researcher did not manipulate environments), but merely observations of social performances in community spaces devoted to play. I believe the topic of investigation challenges researchers with factoring the complex social life of mothers into analysis of the lives of children. Magazines for mothers, such as *Parenting*, *Natural Mother*, etc., recognize the value of female social networks in mothers' day-to-day lives, which probably defines their appeal as well. Maternal performances in the public park encode systems by which middle-class mothers govern themselves and one another; through this governance, they also enact and perpetuate governance of children, a governance that the indoor commercial playground disrupts or disables, because consumer-based playplaces are interested in stimulating unbridled passions and desires (the id, if you will), not in subjects disciplining themselves.

The performance of gender and class values is crucial in the theater of the playground, among the mothers who tend the young children, but also among children themselves. What will happen as commercial sectors take a larger role in perpetuating the concept of childhood? Already, corporations are forming relationships with schools and both funding and helping design spaces such as gymnasiums. It is crucial for childhood studies scholars to consider the relationship between children's and women's issues. The success of commercial playplaces should teach us to ask a valuable question: in a culture that equates the child's right to play with someone's—usually a mother's—need to watch, who is disciplining whom?

Bibliography

Aitken, Stuart C. 2000. Play, Rights and Borders: Gender-Bound Parents and the Social Construction of Children. In *Children's Geographies: Playing, Living, Learning*, edited by Sarah Holloway and Gill Valentine, 119–38. New York: Routledge.

. . .

Bordo, Susan R. 1993. *Unbearable Weight: Feminism, Western Culture, and the Body.* Berkeley: University of California Press.

. . .

Butler, Judith. 1993. *Bodies That Matter: On the Discursive Limits of "Sex."* New York: Routledge.

———. 1999. *Gender Trouble.* New York: Routledge.

. . .

Foucault, Michel. 1995. *Discipline and Punish: The Birth of the Prison*, translated by Alan Sheridan. New York: Vintage Books.

Frost, Joe L. 1992. *Play and Playscapes.* New York: Delmar Publishing.

. . .

Goodwin, Marjorie H. 2002. Exclusion in Girls' Peer Groups: Ethnographic Analysis of Language Practices on the Playground. *Human Development* 45 (6): 392–415.

. . .

Hawkins, D. Lynn, Debra J. Pepler, and Wendy M. Craig. 2001. Naturalistic Observations of Peer Interventions in Bullying. *Social Development* 10 (4): 512–27.

Himelfarb, S. 1994. Laws of the Jungle Gym: Mothers' and Fathers' Playground Behavior—About Fathers. *Parents' Magazine.* 69 (11): 245.

Holden, George W., and Kathy L. Ritchie. 1991. Linking Extreme Marital Discord, Child Rearing, and Child Behavior Problems: Evidence from Battered Women. *Child Development* 62: 311–27.

. . .

Lee, Felicia R. 2000. My Kid's Never Bad and Other Sandbox Tales. *New York Times*, September 10. New York and Region Section.

. . .

McKendrick, John H., Michael G. Bradford, and Anna V. Fieldler. 2000. Time for a Party! Making Sense of the Commercialisation of Leisure Space for Children. In *Children's Geographies: Playing, Living, Learning*, edited by Sarah L. Holloway and Gill Valentine, 100–117. New York: Routledge.

. . .

Nasaw, David. 1985. *Children of the City: At Work and at Play.* Garden City, NY: Anchor-Doubleday Press.

. . .

Opie, Iona, and Peter Opie. 1960. *The Language and Lore of Schoolchildren.* Oxford: Clarendon Press.

. . .

Pellegrini, Anthony D. 1995. *School Recess and Playground Behavior: Educational and Developmental Roles.* Albany: State University of New York Press.

. . .

Postman, Neil. 1994. *The Disappearance of Childhood.* New York: Vintage Press.

Project for Public Spaces. Their Work Is Child's Play (Interview with Roger Hart and Selim Iltus). Project for Public Spaces. *www.pps.org/topics/design/hart_iltus_play.*

. . .

Smith, Stephen J. 1998. *Risk and Our Pedagogical Relation to Children: On the Playground and Beyond.* Albany: State University of New York Press.

Stansell, Christine. 1982. Women, Children, and the Uses of the Streets: Class and Gender Conflicts in New York City, 1850–1860. *Feminist Studies* 8 (2): 309–35.

. . .

Tardy, Rebecca W., and Claudia L. Hale. 1998. Getting "Plugged In": A Network Analysis of Health-Information Seeking Among "Stay-at-Home Moms." *Communication Monographs* 65 (4): 336–57.

Thorne, Barrie. 1993. *Gender Play: Girls and Boys in School.* New Brunswick, NJ: Rutgers University Press.

Wellhousen, Karyn. 2002. *Outdoor Play Every Day: Innovative Play Concepts for Early Childhood.* Albany, NY: Delmar.

. . .

Zelizer, Viviana A. 1985. *Pricing the Priceless Child: The Changing Social Value of Children.* New York: Basic Books.

6

"I Saw Your Nanny"

Gossip and Shame in the Surveillance of Child Care

Margaret K. Nelson

For all the recent publicity concerning nannies in the popular press (Kantor 2006b), in fiction (Weldon 2007) and nonfiction best-sellers (Davis and Hyams 2006; Hansen 2005; McLaughlin and Kraus 2007), and in academic scholarship (Ehrenreich and Hochschild 2004; Macdonald 1998; Tronto 2002; Parrenas 2001; Wrigley 1995), one might believe that the bulk of working parents rely on this form of care. Nothing could be further from the truth: the vast majority of preschool children are either in a relative's care (40.2 percent) or in an organized care facility (22.7 percent). Only 3.7 percent of preschoolers are being cared for by a nonrelative in the child's home, and only 15 percent of employed parents who rely on paid care for children under five hire nannies for that care (Johnson 2005). Even so, nanny care excites special interest and curiosity, in part because it highlights the challenging question of whether we can purchase love. It makes us confront head-on the issue of racial and class inequalities, and it provokes childhood fantasies about real and fictional caregivers. Nanny care also provides a focus—the nanny herself—for society's acute anxieties about the care and well-being of vulnerable children while leaving unexamined the broader social processes that produce these vulnerabilities.

In *Other People's Children*, Julia Wrigley (1995) made visible the structural and ideological contradictions of nanny care that result in, among other processes, parental use of surveillance (via nanny cams) as a way to handle their anxieties about what happens when they aren't there to watch interactions between the nanny and their child. When Wrigley wrote in 1995, nanny cams were relatively new. More than a decade later, this surveillance technique has become more widely available and been sufficiently publicized to the point that it is now part of everyday speech and awareness. Meanwhile, information about additional monitoring innovations has shown up in newspaper articles and advertisements: a device that enables video conferencing with a nanny from a parent's workplace (Womack 2006); an online service, *Whereismybaby.com*, that uses a GPS device to monitor the movement of a baby's stroller (Nanos 2006); and surveillance companies that highlight their ability to track information about a nanny's background when "checking references isn't enough."[1]

In August 2006, a website appeared that sought to involve the public in this essentially private solution of close monitoring. Without changing the nature of the relationship between caregivers and care recipients, or between employers and their employees, and without doing anything to make child care a truly public issue, I Saw Your Nanny (*Isawyournanny.blogspot. com*, hereafter referred to as ISYN) invites the public to extend the gaze of the nanny cam by reporting on nannies as they go about their everyday business in public places. Jane Doe, the website's founder, explains her goals for this site: "So often mothers and other nannies have commented that they wished they had an avenue to contact the parent of a child they saw being mistreated by the nanny. We want to be that resource."[2] Nannies and mothers, she suggests, need no longer sit passively on the park bench gossiping among themselves (Blackford, Chapter 5); they can now *do something* if they see a situation they find troublesome. Indeed, they are not limited to just monitoring the performance of women they assume to be nannies and informing parents of any troublesome practices they observe. They can also shame the nanny herself by bringing her into a public spotlight—and, implicitly, they can shame the mother as well.[3]

ISYN is not unique in taking surveillance and shaming to this new level. Rather, it is in line with other surveillance sites that seek to monitor and control behavior of others by subjecting them to public shame (Scott 2007; Montgomery and Beck 2007; Proudfoot 2007; Swartz 2007). Browse the Web and you can find sites that publicize the license plates of bad drivers (*aboveaveragedriver.com*; *platewire.com*) or of individuals parked illegally in handicap spaces (*caughtya.org*), sites that post pictures of men who leer or whistle at women (*HollaBackNYC.com*), and sites that post pictures of people talking loudly on cell phones (*RudePeople.com*), among others. In a *Wall Street Journal* article, Henry Jenkins, director of the media studies program at MIT, argues that "the embrace of the Web to expose trivial transgressions in part represents a return to shame as a check on social behavior" (Saranow 2007).

The public shaming that occurs on Internet sites raises significant questions about just whose values are reflected in the definition of certain behaviors as offensive, and about just how fair or evenhanded the "judges" are in identifying individuals as being guilty of specific "offenses." Just as individuals who stop a mother on the street and ask about her relationship to a daughter who appears to be of a different race or ethnicity make this gesture on the basis of a biological notion about how "real" families are created (Jacobson, Chapter 4), individuals who report on the "offensive" behavior of others are equally likely to be working from their own biases and misconceptions, including, perhaps, a misconception about who is a nanny and who is not. Thus we have to ask whether those who seek to shame nannies (and by extension, to shame the mothers who hire them) on ISYN start from very particular and very class-bound norms concerning what constitutes appropriate care, and whether they are selective in their perception of who is at fault for deviating from those norms. These are the questions at stake in this chapter.

ISYN

The ISYN website itself initially had a "down-home" appearance with relatively unsophisticated graphics; it has since become somewhat more sophisticated. The first two links provided are for reporting child abuse and the sex offender registry, thus framing the site as a whole as being concerned with risks facing young children. Moreover, like the old milk carton campaigns about missing children, it assumes that those risks come from outside the family.

The "action" on the site has two major components. One of these is the observations of nanny behaviors, contributed by individuals moved to participate in this surveillance site and edited and posted by Jane Doe. Most of these postings are "negative" sightings in the sense that the observer has a concern about a particular interaction between a presumed nanny and a child in her care.[4] The second major component consists of the comments that appear on each of the individual posted sightings. This commentary appears to contain a high degree of flaming, defined as "a hostile expression of strong emotions such as swearing, insults, and name-calling" (Lee 2005, 285). This flaming is directed at a variety of targets: at the employers ("How about not hiring the bargain basement nanny. Move to a better neighborhood and spend some real money on a nanny that doesn't have to be on welfare at the same time taking care of your neighborhood's kids."); at the original poster ("Mind your own business! This is supposed to be about children in physical and mental danger! Not about nannies having affairs with their bosses!"); at the other commentators ("You are such a racist. . . . And before you call someone a coward, you might want to think about signing your disgusting posts with your name!"); and at the nannies who occasionally write in ("You sound like a low-rent hoochie nanny").[5] Because of the flaming, the practice of reading conversations without entering into them—what is known as "lurking"—often turned into an unpleasant experience.

Although the ISYN site did not immediately take off, in the seventh week it received twenty-six postings. The frequency of postings remained at a fairly high level for another month before dropping off somewhat toward the end of the research period to a fairly steady rate of between ten and twenty-four postings a week. On average, during the five months of study (from mid-August 2006 to mid-January 2007), these postings received sixteen comments apiece. In an interview in March 2007, Jane Doe said that the site was getting ten thousand "hits" a day (Scott 2007).

By signing onto advertising arrangements with Google and CrispAds, ISYN also became the heir to considerable advertising support and gave the appearance of having the endorsement of those advertisers. And the media played its role: less than six months after its inauguration, the site had been mentioned in a number of different publications, including the *New York Times* (Kantor 2006a), *New York* (Nanos 2006), *Newsday* (Terrazzano 2007), the *National Post* (Patrick 2006), and the *Miami Herald* (Goodman 2007).

Methods

In what follows I analyze the postings of nanny behavior for a twenty-two-week period and the commentary these postings elicited for every third week of that period (a total of seven weeks). In all I report on 201 sightings and 1,043 comments. The sightings originated in twenty-one different states, with a predominance of New York (48 percent), followed by California (18 percent). The most frequent location for a sighting was a park (42 percent), followed by a store or mall (23 percent), and then the street (10 percent); other sightings took place in libraries, recreational centers, restaurants, schools, or amusement places (e.g., theater, zoo, or aquarium).

I coded the sightings according to whether they were positive or negative (that is, "good" or "bad" nanny sightings); I then additionally coded the negative reports by the nature of the "offense." I coded the comments with categories indicating relevance, the degree to which commentators agreed that an offense had taken place, and the location of blame for that offense. In addition, I explored (in a more qualitative way) the kind of solutions various groups of commentators offered for the "problem" of bad nanny care.

Unfortunately, although there is considerable information offered about the location of the sighting and the characteristics of the individuals involved (namely, the nanny and the children), those reporting offer relatively little information about themselves. We thus have no way of knowing just who is doing the observing or whether that individual's characteristics make a significant difference in the content of their observations. The same lack of identifying information characterizes the majority of participants in the blog commentary: most commentators simply sign their responses as "Anonymous." Occasionally, however, commentators indicate such things as whether they themselves are nannies or mothers and, if the latter, whether they work outside the home. There is thus sufficient information of this type to make assessments about how various individuals respond to the postings.

Race/Ethnicity and Class
in the Awareness of Problems

For the most part, the identification of an individual with a child as a nanny rather than as a mother depends on the observer's perception that the nanny is of a different race/ethnicity than the child and often, apparently, on the perception that she is also of a different social class from the children for whom she is providing care.[6] As observers report on nanny behavior, they make the nanny herself into a caricature of either bad or, occasionally, good behavior; the children are transformed into more complex beings whose behavior is explained and who can evoke the observer's empathetic response.

Race and Ethnicity

Slightly under half (48 percent) of the nannies are identified according to race or ethnicity in the postings. Almost one-third (29 percent) of those who are not given an identification of race/ethnicity outright are identified by some marker (e.g., "speaks Spanish," "European looking," "attractive dark skinned, black hair Nanny") that suggests a racial or ethnic designation. When these "ambiguous" cases are included, two-thirds of the nannies are identified by race/ethnicity: of these one-third are black,[7] one-quarter are Hispanic, one-third are white (including European), and a small percentage are "Other" (e.g., biracial, Filipino, and Indian). Presumably the New York dominance in the sightings has much to do with this particular racial/ethnic configuration.

Children are less often identified by race/ethnicity than are the nannies:

only 11 percent of the children are outright accorded a racial designation, and among these the vast majority (78 percent) are said to be white. When we also include implicit indicators of race/ethnicity (blond hair or blue eyes), 41 percent of the children are accorded a race/ethnicity; among these, 90 percent are presumably white. When race/ethnicity is available for both the nanny and the child, difference prevails: in only 7 percent of the cases are the nanny and child explicitly identified as having the same race/ethnicity (6 percent both white; 1 percent both Other). The most common configuration (beyond that of neither nanny nor child being identified by race/ethnicity) is a black nanny caring for a white child.

Social Class

In addition to racial/ethnic identification, the class location of the nanny is indicated implicitly by her occupation (she is employed in a job that generally carries low wages; Wrigley 1995) and also by her deportment, build, makeup (or its absence), and style of dress:

> [Your nanny] wears no make up, [has] green eyes, and carried around a large "bunchy" brown leatherish bag. . . . She also wears a grew [sic] windbreaker that has sweatshirt style sleeves but [is] nylon looking, shiny gray fabric on the bodice.

> Your nanny: Possibly Polish, plain looking, mousy hair, no make up, wears matching sweatsuits (not the fashionable kind).

The comments about dress are connected in some instances to indications about appropriate behavior. A nanny is not supposed to be dressed as if she is going "to work" in the same way that, presumably, the child's mother might be. As the postings below suggest, commentators also believe nannies should avoid making themselves too attractive:

> She has a perpetually annoyed look on her face and is a very dark complected AA who obviously takes great pride in her figure (tight jeans, etc.). If she smiled, she would probably be attractive.

> Seen last on Monday afternoon. Nanny takes care of boy named "Joshua."[8] The nanny has an accent, possibly Swedish or German. Blonde. Dresses in very tight clothing. . . . She obviously has a nice figure but wears her jeans so tight and her shirts so low.

The nanny's class is also indicated by references to a nanny's activities. If she is shopping in Daffy's (where the slogan is "high fashion, low prices"), the assumption is made that she is making purchases of her own: "Daffy's is a hoochie store. No employer buys anything at Daffy's. Except a gift certificate for the nanny for Christmas!" By contrast, if she is shopping at D'Agostino ("Supermarkets of Distinction"), the assumption is made that she is buying something for her employer's family rather than for herself:

> I was in line behind your Jamaican nanny yesterday as she paid for
> your groceries. She paid with cash and used your D'ag member savings
> card. . . . The interesting part of this occurred when the cashier informed
> the nanny that she had earned enough points for a free turkey and asked
> if she wanted to get it now. The nanny paused with a weird look on her
> face. Then she said she would like to get it but wouldn't be able to carry it
> at present with what she already had, so she asked if they could hold the
> turkey for her and she would come back for it after 6 PM. I'm guessing that
> nanny is snatching that turkey up and [will] take it on the cross town bus
> home to the Bronx.

Race is highly fraught in the United States, and its mere mention on ISYN frequently evokes a response. Occasionally respondents, drawing on a stance of "political correctness," suggest that it is unnecessary (or even inappropriate) to point out race: "Wow—why all the creepy racialized descriptions? 'young Jamaican nanny with braids pulled into a side ponytail' and the innocent 'toe [*sic*] headed child.'" It may be in order to ward off these attacks that so many of the sightings code the race/ethnicity of the nanny with the other indicators (hair color, language, and skin color) discussed earlier.

By way of contrast, class identifiers are seldom contested as being inappropriate ways of describing people, although they are on occasion. For example, in response to the sighting concerning the nanny and the turkey, one respondent said, "What nanny shops at DAG?" and received a response challenging the explicit classism: "What a bigoted remark! Because she is a nanny she can't shop at DAG? Maybe it is the closest market to where she is." Children's social class location is indicated by their accoutrements (e.g., the name brand stroller or their hand-held electronic toys); by the brand name of the clothing they are wearing (e.g., "dressed in GAP clothes"); by the activities in which they are participating (e.g., tennis lessons or ballet class); and by the location of the sighting itself (e.g., the Pierre). These identifiers do not arouse the ire of respondents.

Gender

Although class and race/ethnicity are signified (and contested), the gender of the nanny is not explicitly offered unless a male caregiver is being described; female nannies are the unmarked category, and although observers do not say that they are talking about a woman, they use female pronouns. Unlike nannies, children's gender is usually assigned and noted (presumably for the purposes of helping parents identify their own children): 28 percent female, 44 percent male, and the remainder unclear (often because the child is too young to determine gender easily).

What Behavior Is Being Observed?

Although Jane Doe might originally have desired only "bad" nanny sightings, over time the site has morphed into a more varied form of commentary. During the twenty-two-week period of observations, I coded the postings first as to whether they identified a sighting at all (rather than some other commentary), and then whether the sighting was of a "good" or a "bad" nanny. The majority of the sightings are, indeed, of nannies who are considered to have committed some offense: 88 percent of the nannies have engaged in behavior that the observer finds offensive. Moreover, posters frequently suggest that the bad behavior seen in public represents just the tip of the iceberg: "If this is how she treats him publicly, how does she treat him privately?" In so doing, the posters potentially condemn the vast majority of nannies and generalize the problem of bad nanny behavior to include most of what happens out of the public eye. And of course, the sightings also put all nannies on notice: nannies in public should know that they are under surveillance and vulnerable to shaming.

Table 6.1 shows the full array of "offenses" for which nannies are outed on the site. Coding these problems was complex; creating general categories involved assessments about whether specific actions represented child endangerment or merely questionable behavior, such as being inconsiderate or swearing. From the responses these sightings received, it is clear that many would not agree with my classifications. For example, smoking (outside and away from the baby) is seen by some respondents as an endangerment issue rather than a behavior issue ("smoking around a child is abusive"). Similarly, some respondents view "feeding inappropriately" as outright physical abuse ("I don't think a Ho Ho is an appropriate snack for a child under the age of two"; "Dr. Pepper is full of caffeine. This cannot be a good thing for a two year old. Bad Nanny."). The difficulty of coding these—and the disagreement

Table 6.1
Nanny "offenses" reported on ISYN (grouped by nanny's race/ethnicity)

Offense	All Number of reports	All Percentage of total reports	Black Number of reports	Black Percentage of total reports	Hispanic Number of reports	Hispanic Percentage of total reports	White Number of reports	White Percentage of total reports
Ignoring child	55	32	11	34	12	50	5	29
Leaving child unattended or wandering alone	30	17	6	19	6	25	2	12
Keeping child in stroller	4	2	1	3	1	4	0	0
Not interacting with child	11	6	2	6	2	8	2	12
Talking on phone	10	6	2	6	3	13	1	6
Being gruff, impatient, or mean	60	35	14	44	8	33	4	24
Possible endangerment	21	10	3	9	1	4	2	12
Feeding child inappropriately	6	3	0	0	0	0	0	0
Over- or underdressing child	4	2	0	0	1	4	0	0
Allowing child's bad habits	6	3	1	3	0	0	0	0
Sleeping while on duty	1	1	1	3	0	0	0	0
Possibly drinking	1	1	0	0	0	0	1	6
Handing child off to someone else	3	2	1	3	0	0	1	6
Physical abuse	7	4	1	3	2	8	2	12
Causing problems for employer	10	6	0	0	0	0	0	0
Cheating with husband	1	1	0	0	0	0	0	0
Stealing from employer	6	3	0	0	0	0	0	0
Planning to leave	1	1	0	0	0	0	0	0
Gossiping about family	2	1	0	0	0	0	0	0
Nanny's character or behavior	20	12	3	9	1	4	4	24
Smoking	3	2	1	3	0	0	1	6
Swearing	2	1	1	3	0	0	0	0
Behaving suspiciously	6	3	1	3	1	4	1	6
Being inconsiderate to others	1	1	0	0	0	0	0	0
Seeing a man on the side	5	3	0	0	0	0	0	0
Other character issue	3	2	0	0	0	0	2	12
Total	173	100	32	100	24	100	17	100

Note: Detail may not sum to totals because of rounding.

particular postings engendered—is further evidence that no uniform norms exist concerning child care.

As Table 6.1 shows, the most common single criticism was that the nanny was gruff, impatient, or mean to the child without (necessarily) engaging in direct physical abuse:

> If you have two (beautiful) blondish girls approximately 1 & 3 who were at the Bronx Zoo . . . at around 11 AM, I witnessed your nanny while I was at the zoo with the children I nanny for. The child who looked to be about one dropped her sippy cup and the nanny was very gruff with her. . . . The three year old could not see much from her vantage point and she kept asking to "get down." The nanny told her . . . it was "too much hassle."

The second most frequent subset of comments has to do with ignoring the child, either letting the child wander around the park alone or not interacting with the child:

> Your son is David, 3 years old. Your nanny is approx. 40's dark hair, does not speak English, as far as I can tell. Every time I go to the park, on weekdays and weekends, David is there playing by himself and being COMPLETELY ignored by the nanny. It's a fenced neighborhood park next to a softball field and recreation center. She puts on huge headphones blaring music and stares into space while David wanders around the park alone. He's really hungry for attention and is a sweet, articulate little boy. I wouldn't trust this woman with my dog.

Combined, these two sets of responses (gruffness and not interacting) account for over two-thirds of the postings. Additionally, 21 percent of the postings refer to some kind of "possible endangerment" of the child, including handing the child off to someone else, feeding the child inappropriately, allowing bad habits, sleeping in a car (while the child slept in a car seat), possible drinking, and over- or underdressing a child for the weather. Only 4 percent were complaints about outright physical abuse (e.g., pinching, slamming a child down into a seat). The remaining postings concerned character issues on the part of the nanny that might have no relevance for the child's care (12 percent) or other behaviors that might cause difficulty for the employer but were not directly relevant to care (6 percent).

Two points are worth noting about these postings. First, the postings make a sharp distinction between the rights to personhood on the part of the nanny and the rights to personhood on the part of the child. The posters clearly indicate a belief that the nanny is seen not as an individual perform-ing a job but as someone who *is* the job. She is expected to embrace the job wholeheartedly and to love the job (or at least appear to) (Hochschild 1983):

> The thing here, I think, is that you want someone who shares your parent-ing philosophy to watch your children. You're paying someone to take care of them like you'd want them to be taken care of if you could make them your number one priority, all the time.

> Nannies do not always need to be laughing, but they ALWAYS need to be kind. A calm, direct voice can be appropriate, but a sharp tone is not. If they cannot manage the difference they should not be a nanny.

The nanny is not "allowed" boredom, conversation with other nannies, or cell phone use; she is certainly not allowed impatience, haste, or attention to her own needs. The nanny is never identified as being an authentic person with her own needs and desires. Personhood is denied as well by the absence of an explanation or excuse that would explain the behavior being reported in the postings; that is, rather than contextualizing the behavior in any way that might account for why the nanny is using a "sharp tone" or why she is talking on the phone, the posters hold nannies to a standard of behavior that requires constant interaction with the child, who is always put first. In short, the nanny is supposed to be the "perfect" surrogate for the mother and, like other workers in the service industry, ever ready to put the needs of the clients before her own. Moreover, the postings suggest that she can have no backstage area; her full engagement is required for the entire time that she is on duty: "That nanny is on the clock eating her cone. She damn well better do so in a nice manner."

While the nanny's personhood is effaced, the posters impute particular feelings and selves to the children they describe. Often there is an obvious identification between the poster and the child:

> I could see the fright in his eyes and in the little one's looking up at her from the stroller.

> I wish I knew Matthew's parents so I can tell them how lonely and hurt their child seemed.

> [Your nanny] left your sweet daughter, Melissa, age 5, to play by herself the entire time [she was in the playground] . . . I was there with a number

of other mothers and our children, and we all felt terrible for Melissa, who seemed extremely lonely and desperate for attention.

The empathetic description of the children's reactions to the nanny not only reinforces the negative description of the nanny (if she weren't doing something wrong, why would the child be scared?) but also reinforces the notion that children are fragile and in need of careful handling.

The second point worth noting about the postings is that the exhortations on behalf of the child follow specific class-bound standards for child rearing (Demo and Cox 2000; Hays 1996). Drawing on her own intensive ethnographic research, Lareau (2003) describes the middle-class style of child rearing as "concerted cultivation" and locates its key element in the fact that the parent "actively fosters and assesses [the] child's talents, opinions, and skill" (31). By way of contrast, Lareau characterizes the child-rearing style of the working class and the poor as fashioned around providing basic care for the child and allowing the child to grow. Children reared according to the precepts of what Lareau calls "the accomplishment of natural growth" spend their days differently than do middle-class children. They are more likely to be found "hanging out" and interacting with playmates of different ages (including kin) rather than in supervised activities, and the language they hear from adults often takes the form of "directives" commanding obedience rather than reasoned explanations.

The vast majority of the nanny sightings report on the absence of behavior that might be associated with middle-class "concerted cultivation" (or as Sharon Hays [1996] calls it, "intensive mothering"). Indeed, the behavior for which nannies are faulted—not responding to each gesture with reasoning, giving orders, leaving children alone to wander around the park, and keeping children confined to a stroller rather than encouraging their exploration—might fit well within the classification of "accomplishment of natural growth." The reports thus might well tell us as much about the class location of the observer as they do about any significant threats facing children from being in the care of a particular nanny; observers find fault on the basis of their own class-based notions of appropriate care.

Not All Perpetrators Are Alike

This class bias toward the notion of what constitutes a problem in child care is accompanied by a racial bias in the observation of problematic behavior; indeed, the postings suggest that the offense is in the eyes of the beholder and that a nanny's race/ethnicity determines which form of problematic behavior the observer perceives. (See Table 6.1.)

Taken as a whole, black nannies are somewhat less likely to receive bad postings as a proportion of all postings about them (79 percent) than are other nannies. Among these postings, almost half of the offenses the black nannies are perceived to have committed involve being gruff, impatient, and mean toward their charges. Of course, it is hard to know what stands behind these observations, but it is possible that behavior is perceived as being gruff or mean when it comes from someone who incites fear and guilt among members of the majority population or from someone who does not show the expected deference or subservience (Rollins 1985). It is also possible that a stereotype—the "mammy" (Hale 1998; Smith 1949)—shapes these responses so that observers are particularly attentive to differences from what a cultural icon would lead them to expect.

In contrast to black nannies, Hispanic nannies are more likely to receive bad postings as a proportion of all postings about them (97 percent). Among these bad postings, Hispanic nannies are most often faulted for ignoring the child and for talking on the cell phone: "These twins are walked to the park most nice days. The nanny then sits on a bench and eats her bagel and gabs on her cell phone." Indeed, Hispanic nannies are regarded as being involved in behavior that accords with a stereotype of Latin people as outgoing and talkative:

> The upscale neighborhoods of LA are filled with nannies who go to the park nearly all day with very young babies and toddlers and chat with each other or on their cell phones in Spanish the entire time, with their backs to the children. It is obvious to me that they spend their time being paid to socialize. I don't speak Spanish, and the people I talk to at the park are the children. I am the one scooping up the baby who is about to be hit by the swing, or about to fall off the side of the slide. I am the one comforting the child who has gotten hurt, and asking them where is your mommy or nanny?

(Interestingly, the fact that the poster cannot speak Spanish herself in the example above may make her feel a sense of exclusion from the group and the conversation.)

White nannies are cited for bad behavior (as a proportion of all sightings concerning them) more frequently than are black nannies (83 percent versus 79 percent), but considerably less frequently than Hispanic nannies (83 percent versus 97 percent). Among all three groups of nannies, however, white nannies are least likely to be seen as gruff or impatient. Among our cultural icons stands the Mary Poppins character, who is simultaneously stern and loving; the low level of gruffness reported might indicate that similar behavior is interpreted as being strict rather than mean. However, white nannies are not off the hook: they are most often identified as displaying a poor "character" (such as smoking or being engaged in some form of "suspicious" behavior). Hence it appears that a different standard is at work with white nannies than with black or Hispanic nannies; assumed social class seems to play a greater part in this standard than is the case with black or Hispanic nannies.

Not All Victims Are the Same

Interestingly, some slight evidence exists that children are perceived as being subject to different offenses depending on their gender. Although by and large the problems are the same, girls are perceived as being more vulnerable than boys to being "snatched"; they are more often observed being handed off to someone (5 percent versus 0 percent) and more often observed wandering alone (26 percent versus 15 percent). It may be that boys' wandering is not observed because it is more culturally appropriate as gendered behavior.

In short, class, race/ethnicity, and gender enter into the observations that are posted on ISYN, with nannies being identified by race/ethnicity and class but not by gender, and children being identified by class and gender and less often by race/ethnicity. Each of these variables frame the observations in other ways as well: nanny behavior is seen as problematic when it does not conform to a style of child care that prevails among the middle and upper classes; nannies are presumed to commit different offenses depending on which racial/ethnic group they are identified as being part; and the identification of certain problems may well depend on the gender of the child.

Having said as much, however, I do not mean to dispute the characterizations or to suggest that problematic behavior has not occurred. Many of the reported interactions between the nannies and their charges sound unpleasant, if not downright mean. But the patterns of these observations challenge the premise of an impartial judge who can shame according to community-wide norms. The fact that the shaming is contested on the blog also challenges the notion that community-wide standards or norms exist.

Responding to Surveillance

Judging the Offense

On average, each posting receives sixteen responses. It was as hard to code these responses as it was to code the postings themselves. The largest single response category includes comments that are irrelevant to the posting itself but follow some thread topic (38 percent). An additional subset (9 percent) ask questions. Some of these request more information about the incident, and others ask, "How do you know it is a nanny treating the children this way and not their own mother?" This latter response implies that if a family member were engaging in the reported behavior it would be deemed as being less offensive; paid caregivers are held to different standards than parents.[9] For example, commentators readily make excuses when the offender might be a mother having a bad day. They also propose that the offender might be a grandmother with a different style of care ("Either your description is incomplete or you're nuts. It sounds like the kid refused an instruction from his Grandmother, who has a stricter philosophy of child rearing than you do. Children will often not stay where they are supposed to or leave when you ask them to, and grabbing them by the arm is the only way."). These comments suggest that it is not necessarily the caretaker's behavior that is the problem, but the assumed relationship to the child of the person performing the care. They suggest as well that what is being purchased is intended to be "good care," not just care.

Among those responses that *are* directly relevant to the actions in the posting (that is, when irrelevant responses are excluded), almost half (45 percent) of the respondents agree that some offense has, indeed, taken place, and 7 percent of the respondents think that the offense was serious enough that the poster should have intervened. In addition, a small percentage of respondents believe that an offense has taken place but that the fault lies less with the nanny than with the parents, who either employed an inadequate caregiver or were so foolish as to leave their children with a caregiver at all. An occasional respondent blames the children themselves for being difficult to care for.

Very few respondents (8 percent) disagree with the poster's assumption that there was a problem, although a few respondents (10 percent) accuse the poster of making assumptions or intruding into a situation that was possibly benign. One-fifth (20 percent) of those commenting on a posting seek to explain the nanny's behavior or actually defend the nanny against the charge that she has done something wrong.

Differences in Assessments of the "Nanny Problem"

Most of those who comment on a posting do not identify themselves; indeed, the authors of only 13 percent of the comments could be identified in some way. Among those who do identify themselves, there are differences in the kind of responses given to the sightings. Stay-at-home mothers (SAHMs) and nannies are more likely to defend the nanny for her behavior than are mothers who identify themselves as working outside the home (37 percent and 35 percent, respectively, compared to 14 percent), and they are less likely than working mothers to agree that an offense has occurred (35 percent and 41 percent, respectively, versus 64 percent). SAHMs and nannies are also more likely to shift blame onto parents (18 percent and 17 percent, respectively, versus 7 percent), but they have different reasons for doing so: nannies are more likely to blame parents for making unreasonable demands on nannies, and SAHMs are more likely to blame parents for leaving their children in the care of someone other than the mother. There is also an undercurrent in the comments from both SAHMs and nannies (more frequently made explicit in the comments authored by the latter) that some of the problems are brought on by the children themselves (children can be annoying and difficult), that taking care of children is hard work, and that it is not necessary (and may even be inappropriate) to respond to every single need expressed by a child.

In short, all types of respondents on ISYN agree that nanny care frequently constitutes a problem, but they differ in their willingness to defend the nanny and offer different explanations for the problems that are identified. These differences emerge along lines relevant to one's position in the world of nanny care. SAHMs and nannies themselves—individuals who are involved in the direct care of children day in and day out (what Fisher and Tronto [1990] call "taking care")—are more willing to defend nannies: they understand that child care is hard work and that occasionally individuals act in ways that outsiders might view as constituting a problem. These two groups, however, part company on the question of whether anyone can ever substitute for a mother. Those who hire others to perform that care (what Fisher and Tronto call "caring about") are more critical of nannies and more insistent that nannies always be ready to respond to a child's needs and desires; however, like nannies themselves, they want to believe in parental substitutes. Interestingly, the alternative of a day care center is almost never raised by any of these respondents, even though that setting has been shown to have fewer "accidents" than other settings (Wrigley and Dreby 2005). Thus, although some commentators do contest the use of nannies, taken as a whole the comments reinforce the notion that a nanny is the only viable alternative to a mother's care.

Differences in Solutions to the "Nanny Problem"

Three groups of commentators—parents employing nannies (PENs), parents not employing nannies, and the nannies themselves—have sharply different ideas about how to solve the "nanny problem." PENs offer a number of different solutions. One solution focuses on an attempt to create class sympathy by turning the nanny into a member of the family:

> My experience has been the better I treat the nanny and include her as part of the family, the better for me and my children. My oldest child is 16 and I have had only two nannies in my life, (the current one has been with us nine years) so I know of what I speak.

> When we decide to bring a nanny into the care-giving process for our children, we are not hiring an employee. We are adding a member to the family, a member with the emotional authority and responsibility of a parent—and I think we have a moral obligation to accord that member of the family the same care and understanding (and, yes, tough love, too) we accord to any other family member.

Whatever other functions it fulfills, it is clear that the interest in making a nanny a member of the family involves the possibility for heightened surveillance: "I want to know everything I can about the person in my home, and that is why I chose carefully and made her a part of my family."

A long tradition of scholarship has examined the "member of the family" perspective (Macdonald 1998; Romero 1992, 2001; Colen 1986; Rollins 1985; Parrenas 2001). As Colen (1986, 60) notes, "The ideology of the family is used to manipulate the worker. . . . It is used to encourage people who are not family members to perform tasks or to tolerate treatment that may be exploitative." Similarly Romero (2001, 1657), citing Rollins (1985), notes that the occupation of domestic worker is "characterized by everyday rituals of verbal and spacial deference." This incorporation may also isolate the nanny from her own family and allow employers to ignore the other constraints in her life.[10] Not surprisingly, then, by and large nannies reject the notion of incorporation into the family. They want a job with good working conditions, but they do not want to be treated as a member of someone else's family: "A nanny is not a member of the family. I love the children I care for, and have a friendly relationship with the parents, but it is a JOB! If you want a great nanny who will be responsible, and do a professional job, you need to understand that."

As an extension of the incorporation strategy, PENs believe that by encouraging middle-class behavior (Wrigley 1995) they can transform the nanny into both a better worker and someone more like themselves:

> I am a WOHM [work-outside-the-home mother]. On my lunch hour, I take a jog in the park any chance I get. I would LOVE it if my nanny was so much into exercising that she wanted to do this! . . . I think to encourage your nanny to be physically active at work (even if it is indoors while the child sleeps) is only going to make the nanny happier and improve her job performance.

> My nanny takes my child to the gym with her. She drops her at the daycare program. I got my nanny the gym membership. It is the same gym that I go to. I have an awesome nanny who works long days and is a live in. I would do anything to keep her.

Some parents seek to hire nannies who already resemble them in terms of class (and race/ethnicity) and thus to overcome the possibility of different child care approaches. What parents refer to as a "real nanny" is identifiable by her professional credentials: "I required an education in early childhood development and many years of experience. I hired a real nanny, not a babysitter."[11] Parents who employ this strategy also boast about what they pay for their nannies and challenge the notion that "real nannies" exist outside of metropolitan centers. Real nannies become the ultimate luxury item and are carefully selected and carefully guarded from those who might want to nab them: "As a professional woman who has had a professional nanny in my employ for the past 6 years, I totally agree. Professional Nannies are in short supply. Anytime someone meets my nanny for the first time, they want to know where they could find someone like her. [Real nannies] are truly the gems of the childcare industry!" Some nannies also assert a class status, aligning with the parents who employ them in the notion of real nannies. But where the parents are likely to talk about credentials and references, nannies are more likely to talk about character and good working conditions: you get a good nanny by hiring a good person and then treating her well.

Finally, PENs believe in greater surveillance. Parents report on their own tactics of surveillance (e.g., going through private belongings and using nanny cams), and they encourage everyone to engage in very careful checking of references. Parents speak with pride and enthusiasm about all of these practices:

I caught my nanny red handed in my top dresser drawer and I didn't sue
her. I acted outraged but forgave her because when she left her boyfriend's
backpack here, I went through every compartment on the thing.

One time she was feeding [my son] homemade (by me) alphabet pasta
soup and she picked up, with her fingers, and scooped up with her hands
(the same way you would clear a table of crumbs) the pasta that spilled
out of his mouth and onto the table top and placed it back in his bowl and
fed it to him. This I got to see on our nanny cam. Seeing that was pretty
disturbing.

Indeed, by reporting on the effectiveness of surveillance and the problems with the absence of surveillance, the site itself encourages greater
surveillance.

By way of contrast, nannies generally reject the notion of surveillance as
a solution to the problem of "bad" nannies: "If my employers don't trust me,
I'd rather they just let me go than that they spy on me. If you feel the need to
spy on your nanny, you shouldn't be taking the chance of leaving your children with them. The safety of your children should come first." Of course,
nannies cannot simply oppose surveillance; they do, however, suggest that
the sneaky component be eliminated: "As a nanny I feel it is completely okay
to have a nanny cam as long as you are upfront about it."

Unlike PENs and nannies, parents who do *not* employ nannies (and especially SAHMs) worry about any care other than parental care:

Maybe the baby is colicky and if [the mother] were at home, someone
would complain that her baby was crying all day. Maybe, just maybe the
nanny feels stressed and knows this way she will not hurt the baby physically or emotionally. Some babies cry. Just giving her the benefit of the
doubt, though only the mom of the baby would really know. There's a
reason I stay home with my kids. This is it.

I agree—stay at home with your babies—they need you. Don't let greedy
corporate America tell you a woman can have it all—career, kids, money,
3 cars, vacations, $400 shoes, etc, because it's the kids who suffer. You
can't do it all—you're too tired when you get home from work, aren't you,
and then the kids go off to bed. Besides, if you can afford a nanny you can
afford to stay home. You may have to cut back here and there, but it's so
worth it in the long run. I worked in graphic design for years, I gave it all
up to be a SAHM, and I love it. There is always time to make money. Your
kids are only little for so long—don't miss it.

Just as positions in the world of nanny care shape perceptions of and explanations for perceived problems, these positions also shape potential solutions: whereas parents employing nannies believe in both surveillance and the possibility that one can hire a "good" nanny, nannies themselves place the least trust in surveillance, while stay-at-home mothers place the least trust in nannies.

Conclusion

In *Everyday Surveillance*, Staples (2000, 153) says of the new surveillance practices, "Taken together, these 'small acts of cunning' constitute the building blocks of what I would argue is a rapidly emerging disciplinary society; a society increasingly lacking in personal privacy, individual trust, or viable public life that supports and maintains democratic values and practices." But as Blackford (Chapter 5) and others show, there is nothing new about gossip and busybodies, surveillance, disciplining, and even attempts to shame others. One can assume that much of what is made visible on ISYN went on without the Internet and other new technologies. Indeed, as Gumpert and Drucker (2001, 116) note, "Public life has traditionally offered opportunities to watch and be watched. . . . Surveillance of a human rather than technological nature is as old as community itself."

Yet, Gumpert and Drucker (1998, 417) acknowledge as well that there *is* something new when new technologies are involved: "Just as computer-mediated communication provides new ways to socialize, it includes new threats to individual privacy. The new ways of being public may also threaten publicness itself, though, creating a web of connectivity that is empty of the real connectedness that sustains community." This general concern applies well to ISYN. Sharing information that leads to shaming on the Internet differs from sharing information and shaming in the context of community in several ways. Not least of these is that Internet "gossip" allows for anonymity; it thus ceases to be a transactional process in which the gossiper is also held accountable, even as the spread of the information may serve the same general purpose of social control as does "ordinary" gossip. The new gossipers, while lauding or touting their benign intentions (and while occasionally alerting parents to real abuses), can operate outside the realm of true civic responsibility. Rather than act in any kind of constructive way to make the world a better place for children—or to take genuine responsibility for another's child—the posters simply report behavior to the world at large and then go on their merry way. Doing so anonymously means that they claim no responsibility for whatever follows; they cannot be held accountable to the children, to the nanny, or to the employer. Moreover, the information is spread out to a broad audience. However, that information may reflect not a general set of standards that prevail within a given community but rather individual (class-bound) standards writ large as if they were universal.

As a second difference, whereas face-to-face gossip might be self-correcting over time (the content of communications that begin with "I heard" or "Did you know that" can be contested by those with greater knowledge), Internet gossip may be contested (some respondents challenge the notion that an offense has occurred), but it cannot be corrected unless the nanny herself speaks. In addition, whereas the "official" punishment of shaming takes place as a result of a "fair hearing" (or as fair a hearing as our current judicial system can create) in front of a jury of one's peers or an impartial judge, Internet shaming occurs without any kind of hearing at all. Indeed, the postings are sent out as if they are objective descriptions of the facts of the matter.

Yet, as this discussion has shown, the notion of an offense is in the eye of the beholder. Children are viewed as being at risk (and the nanny viewed as having committed some "crime") if they are not treated with a middle-class style of concerted cultivation, or if they are offered food (Ho Hos, Dr. Pepper) that does not meet some observer's standard of appropriateness. Moreover, the race/ethnicity of the nanny seems to determine what kinds of problems are noticed: nannies are more often perceived as being gruff if they are black, engaging in too much sociability if they are Hispanic, and having character flaws if they are white. In addition, the sex of the child makes a small difference: girls are more often seen as being at risk of being handed off to a stranger or being left to wander alone.

Finally, the publicizing of offenses on the Web also raises the question of what the goal of this shaming is. Do those who post sightings on ISYN mean to educate the offender (as "shaming" punishments are designed to do; Garvey 2007) or alert the parents to concerns about the care they have selected? Even if the goal is to have an effect on the individuals involved (that is, educating the offender and alerting the parents), the ultimate effects might be quite different, including heightening suspicion about an entire class of workers and about a broad range of practices that might otherwise go unnoticed.

To be sure, an observer's position in the world of nanny care shapes her or his perceptions and ideas about possible solutions: those who do employ nannies believe that increased surveillance offers the key to improving nanny behavior, nannies themselves believe the solution to potential problems lies within the good character of the nanny herself, and stay-at-home mothers believe that only parental care will ensure that a child is being well cared for.

Of course, each of these "solutions" is individualistic in its own way; none provides a resolution to the broader problem of how we care for the children of parents who work outside the home (Wrigley 1995). These solutions, however, are where the "retreat of the state" (Katz 2001) has left us. Simply put, we can snoop, we can rely on assessments of character, or we can stay home and care for our own children. Whichever we choose, the gender relationships of care remain uncontested—all the major players are still women. And whichever we choose, we leave intact privatized responsibility for care, and substitute gossip and shaming for any meaningful significant collective responsibility for the care of children.

Notes

I thank Adam Fazio for his careful coding of the ISYN data. I also thank Cameron Macdonald and Anita Garey for their helpful comments on early drafts.

1. This quote comes from a 2007 advertisement for one such service, Intelius. The ad also shows a picture of a nanny putting a child in a car; the nanny's T-shirt reads, "Nanny for hire; 3 drunk driving convictions." These surveillance and conference technologies are also used by day care centers.

2. According to one article (Scott 2007), "Jane Doe" is a thirty-seven-year-old personal assistant in New York, a former nanny with no children of her own.

3. An attempt to develop interest in an alternative site that shamed mothers directly has been relatively unsuccessful. As of June 2007, I Saw Nanny's Employer (isawnannysemployer.blogspot.com/), which seeks to post "reports of mommies treating nannies unfairly," had received only four "sightings," and another imitation site, I Saw Your Mommy (isawyourmommy.com), had zero postings.

4. There are also positive sightings, indicating behavior of which the observer approves. Responses to an occasional poll (for example, at Christmas nannies were asked to write in about what gifts they had received from their employers), general commentary about missing or abused children, and other related topics round out the postings.

5. As is often the case for e-mail and blogs, writing on ISYN sometimes contains misspellings and erratic capitalization. In what follows, rather than using "sic" when the error is trivial and the meaning is clear, I correct errors. Hence "MIind your own business! This is supposed to be about children in physical and mental danger! NOt about nannies having affairs with their bosses!" becomes "Mind your own business . . . Not about nannies . . . " However, when the meaning is ambiguous, I retain the original spelling. I do not correct grammatical mistakes.

6. Occasionally in the comments, this "difference" is contested by women who point out that they themselves have children of different races, or that because they are young they are occasionally mistaken for their own children's nannies. On the whole, however, the assumptions of race/ethnicity difference prevail.

7. I combined those who were cited as being African American and those who

were cited as being black or as coming from a Caribbean Island into a single race/ethnicity.

8. I changed the names of all children in these sightings; I did not want the chapter itself to serve as a source of further shaming.

9. The privacy and autonomy of the family is preserved implicitly even as the site itself invades the privacy and autonomy of families. Ironically, those families whose private affairs are usually most protected from outside surveillance because of the location of their home (e.g., private yards and gated communities), and because they are less likely to come into contact with judicial system or public welfare, become visible by hiring someone who is *not* in the family.

10. Although nannies occasionally refer to their own lives—their children, their significant others—other posters almost exclusively see the nanny as if she is totally free from other constraints. For example, when a nanny seemed to be "handing off" the child to another nanny, most of the respondents believed this was entirely inappropriate, although one respondent grudgingly acknowledged that nannies might have their own responsibilities: "Everybody needs an occasional window on a workday to take care of something." Similarly, when a nanny asked a woman sitting in the park to watch her child while she went to the bathroom, some respondents suggested that maybe she had a legitimate reason for not wanting to take the child in the bathroom (feeling sick, extremely bad period), while others suggested that nannies had to care for the child always and could not use their own judgment.

11. Interestingly, discussion about this question of just who was a "real nanny" engendered the most racist/classist comments as respondents blamed others for hiring "bargain basement" nannies.

References

Colen, Shellee. 1986. "With Respect and Feelings": Voices of West Indian Child Care and Domestic Workers in New York City. In *All American Women: Lines That Divide, Ties That Bind*, edited by Johnnetta B. Cole, 46–70. New York: Free Press.

Davis, Susan, and Gina Hyams. 2006. *Searching for Mary Poppins: Women Write about the Intense Relationship between Mothers and Nannies.* New York: Hudson Street Press.

Demo, David H., and Martha J. Cox. 2000. Families with Young Children: A Review of Research in the 1990s. *Journal of Marriage and the Family* 62: 876–95.

Ehrenreich, Barbara, and Arlie Russell Hochschild. 2004. *Global Woman: Nannies, Maids, and Sex Workers in the New Economy.* New York: Owl Books.

Fisher, Berenice, and Joan Tronto. 1990. Toward a Feminist Theory of Caring. In *Circles of Care: Work and Identity in Women's Lives*, edited by Emily K. Abel and Margaret K. Nelson, 35–62. Albany: State University of New York Press.

Garvey, Stephen P. 2007. Can Shaming Punishments Educate? *University of Chicago Law Review* 65 (3): 733–94.

Goodman, Cindy Krischer. 2007. Resources to Aid and Support the Working Mom. *MiamiHerald.com*, May 9.

Gumpert, Gary, and Susan J. Drucker. 1998. The Demise of Privacy in a Private World: From Front Porches to Chat Rooms. *Communications Theory* 8 (4): 408–25.

———. 2001. Public Boundaries: Privacy and Surveillance in a Technological World. *Communications Quarterly* 49 (2): 115–29.

Hale, Grace Elizabeth. 1998. *Making Whiteness: The Culture of Segregation in the South, 1890–1940*. New York: Pantheon Books.

Hansen, Suzanne. 2005. *You'll Never Nanny in This Town Again*. New York: Crown.

Hays, Sharon. 1996. *The Cultural Contradictions of Motherhood*. New Haven, CT: Yale University Press.

Hochschild, Arlie Russell. 1983. *The Managed Heart: The Commercialization of Human Feeling*. Berkeley: University of California Press.

Johnson, Julia Overturf. 2005. *Who's Minding the Kids? Child Care Arrangements: Winter 2002*. Current Population Reports No. P70–101. Washington, DC: Department of Commerce, U.S. Census Bureau, October.

Kantor, Jodi. 2006a. Memo to Nanny: No Juice Boxes. *New York Times*, September 28.

———. 2006b. Nanny Hunt Can Be a 'Slap in the Face' for Blacks. *New York Times*, December 26, U.S. section.

Katz, Cindi. 2001. The State Goes Home: Local Hyper-vigilance of Children and the Global Retreat from Social Reproduction. *Social Justice* 28 (3): 47–56.

Lareau, Annette. 2003. *Unequal Childhoods: Class, Race, and Family Life*. Berkeley: University of California Press.

Lee, Hangwoo. 2005. Behavioral Strategies for Dealing with Flaming in an Online Forum. *Sociological Quarterly* 46: 385–403.

Macdonald, Cameron L. 1998. Manufacturing Motherhood: The Shadow Work of Nannies and Au Pairs. *Qualitative Sociology* 21 (1): 25–53.

McLaughlin, Emma, and Nicola Kraus. 2007. *The Nanny Diaries*. New York: St. Martin's Griffin.

Montgomery, Linda, and Christine Beck. 2007. Guerilla Snooping. *Seattle Times*, January 30.

Nanos, Janelle. 2006. Busting Mary Poppins: Spying on the Babysitter Has Never Been Easier. *New York*, October 21.

Parrenas, Rhacel Salzar. 2001. *Servants of Globalization*. Stanford, CA: Stanford University Press.

Patrick, Kelly. 2006. Web Site Posts Nannies' Misdeeds: Anonymous Criticism. *National Post*, September 30, Toronto edition.

Proudfoot, Shannon. 2007. Tattlers Using the Internet as a Weapon: Websites Expose All: From Leering Men to Sub-par Service. *Calgary Herald* (Alberta), January 22.

Rollins, Judith. 1985. *Between Women: Domestics and Their Employers*. Philadelphia: Temple University Press.

Romero, Mary. 1992. *Maid in the U.S.A.* New York: Routledge.

———. 2001. Unraveling Privilege: Workers' Children and the Hidden Costs of Paid Childcare. *Chicago-Kent Law Review* 76: 1651–72.

Saranow, Jennifer. 2007. Online Vigilantes Are Watching You. *Wall Street Journal*, January 15.

Scott, Marian. 2007. All Eyes on You: Cellphone Cameras and the World Wide Web Have Created a New Kind of Public Shaming for Wrongdoers, from Litterbugs to Bad Drivers to Negligent Nannies. *Gazette* (Montreal), March 3.

Smith, Lillian. 1949. *Killers of the Dream*. New York: Norton.

Staples, William G. 2000. *Everyday Surveillance: Vigilance and Visibility in Postmodern Life*. Lanham, MD: Rowman and Littlefield.

Swartz, Tracy. 2007. The Wide World of Cyber Snitching. *Chicago Tribune*, May 31, RedEye edition.

Terrazzano, Lauren. 2007. Ways to Watch Your Nanny. *Newsday*, February 15, Nassau and Suffolk edition.

Tronto, Joan C. 2002. The "Nanny" Question in Feminism. *Hypatia* 17 (2): 34–51.

Weldon, Fay. 2007. *She May Not Leave*. New York: Grove/Atlantic.

Womack, Sarah. 2006. Nannycam Keeps Working Mother in Touch with Children. *Daily Telegraph* (London), October 4.

Wrigley, Julia. 1995. *Other People's Children*. New York: Basic Books.

Wrigley, Julia, and Joanna Dreby. 2005. Fatalities and the Organization of Child Care in the United States, 1985–2003. *American Sociological Review* 70: 729–57.

Part III

Who's In, Who's Out: Monitoring Family Boundaries

The chapters in this section explore the process of constructing family boundaries at different moments in a family's history. The monitoring of family boundaries is used to include or exclude not only particular individuals (*in*—famous fifth cousin Albert Einstein; *out*—untrustworthy Uncle Joe) but also particular kinds of people or potential people (*in*—child from a sperm donor with a high IQ; *out*—cousins from "the wrong side of the track"), particular characteristics (*in*—Irish genealogical line; *out*—fetuses with two X chromosomes), or particular relationships (*in*—half-siblings from a shared gamete donor; *out*—a sibling's same-sex partner). In constructing and patrolling family boundaries, issues of care and control become relevant as current family members assess both the past actions and the potential future actions of given (or imagined) individuals in order to decide where they will be placed relative to a constructed family boundary line.

7

The Social Impact of Amniocentesis

Rayna Rapp

Editors' Note: We have selected three excerpts from Rayna Rapp's Testing
Women, Testing the Fetus: The Social Impact of Amniocentesis in America
*(2000). In the first of the three excerpts, Rapp talks about women who decide
not to have an abortion following the diagnosis of a certain, or occasionally
ambiguous, anomaly in fetal development.[1] In earlier sections of this discussion, Rapp explored "structural reasons that influence women to forgo prenatal testing, and more individuated, personal concerns contributing to a decision not to use amniocentesis . . . [and] noted the strong class influences on
the structural positions pregnant women occupy in relation to the provision
of medical services, and their comfort and confidence in understanding the
risks and benefits of them." She also "plotted the points along the trajectory
of technological use—before a genetic counseling appointment, during, and
after one at which the decision to opt off the conveyor belt may occur" (183).
She continues:*

. . . But there is another, much rarer refusal of this technology, as well:
Women who accept an amniocentesis and, learning of "bad" or "positive"
results, decide to continue their pregnancies. It is to the decision-making
processes of such women that we now turn.

But first, three things should be said in contextualizing these decision-
making stories. The first is that responses to the receipt of a "positive diagnosis" are the subject of [another discussion (Rapp 2000, chapter 9)]. Here,
I only preview the topic, focusing on those who choose to continue their
pregnancies, in effect rejecting the next step in the use of a reproductive

technology. The second caveat is that there is no way to evaluate the representative status of the stories I tell here: No records are kept either federally or by state on the outcomes of amniocentesis; New York and California probably have the best approximations of statistics concerning both the use of amniocentesis and the birth of babies with chronic conditions (Meaney, Riggle, and Cunningham 1993; Cunningham 1998). In principle, those two sets of statistics could be studied in tandem, but the task is arduous and therefore expensive. In a world of health cost accounting and severe cutbacks, there is no incentive to undertake this particular, rather arcane task. Thus, my best approximation of numbers comes from speaking with epidemiologists and biostatisticians in those states, and genetic counselors, the front-line workers on these issues. According to all, the decision to keep a pregnancy after receiving the diagnosis of a serious condition is relatively rare. But it is not possible to evaluate precisely how rare . . . (cf. Palmer et al. 1993). A third and related point is this: The decision rests in large measure on the diagnosed condition. Most people hold firm opinions about Down syndrome long before they encounter amniocentesis; they thus feel entirely competent to make a decision to continue or end a pregnancy in which this condition has been diagnosed. When Down syndrome is diagnosed, abortion rates run high, 90 to 95 percent in local clinical studies (Palmer et al. 1993). But most of the other conditions for which the test can provide diagnoses—chromosomal problems ranging from the severe and deadly, like trisomy 13, to the ambiguous, like the sex chromosome anomaly, Turner's syndrome—are usually unknown to a pregnant woman and her supporters before they receive the news that their fetus "has something seriously wrong." Response to disability news, couched at first in entirely biomedical discourse, is thus a complicated affair, engaging a lot of hard work toward understanding and evaluation on the part of both genetic counselors and their pregnant patients.

Pat Carlson, who enlisted help from her Mormon roots when she wanted to keep a pregnancy in which Down syndrome had been diagnosed, was thus quite unusual in deciding to keep her pregnancy after a positive diagnosis.[2] But she was *not* exceptional in the way in which both prior reproductive history and religious resources entered into her decision-making process. Before coming to her decision, Pat did a lot of work. Her obstetrician suggested an abortion as he delivered the bad news, but Pat stalled for time. She left his office in a daze, and while walking around her neighborhood, she noticed a home for retarded adults. She immediately made an appointment to visit the place. She said, "You know, it was kind of nice. They looked pretty happy, they had jobs, they went bowling. It really made me think about it." Unmarried, a divorcee with a grown child who had survived two miscarriages and the death of a premature baby who lived only three days, Pat's reproductive history made her value this pregnancy as a "miracle." She used the Mormon church to sustain her decision to keep the pregnancy in the face of her obstetrician's objections. . . . Migdalia Ramirez's story also contains unusual elements. Sent for genetic counseling and amniocentesis at the tender age of 15, Migdalia, a Puerto Rican, was a devout Catholic who considered abortion to be "killing." But she was also the older sister of a girl with severe spina bifida whose disabilities had made a profound impression on Migdalia and her mother. As Migdalia described it:

> My sister, she can't walk, she can't see, they left her blind at City Hospital, my mother is still in a lawsuit. When I got pregnant the first time, I was very young, 15, 16 when I had my baby. I talked with my mother, she really wanted me to have the tests, I wanted it too, she had such a cross to bear. God gave it to her, but it's a lot of work. It was hard for my mother to carry that cross, to take care of a child like that, especially when my father walked out on her. Oh, we love my sister, it's just that God made her special, it's a cross to bear. I was only concerned if my own baby couldn't walk or talk. I just talked it over with my mother, no one else, and together we decided about that test. The test wasn't hard, they explained it good, they took a bit of the liquid, I wasn't worried, I just didn't want my baby to be like my sister. I don't know what I would have done if it had been like my sister, I think I would have had an abortion. My mother and me, we're against abortion, so maybe I would have carried that cross, like my mother did. But then again, it's a case where I think I would have had an abortion.

Migdalia's fetus didn't have spina bifida, for which she had requested prenatal diagnosis. It did, however, have Klinefelter's syndrome, one of the sex chromosome anomalies involving growth problems, sterility, and, possibly, learning disabilities and mild mental retardation. Migdalia's reaction to the news is instructive:

> I wasn't too concerned when they said he'd be normal. Just that he might be slow-minded, but he'd look normal in appearance. I have faith in God, I'll be there for my son. And I have my mother helping me all the way. He's gonna be normal, he'll see and walk. That's all I care about. As long as he looked normal, acted normal, I'll be there for him. And I didn't mind if he maybe was a bit slow. And as it turns out, he isn't, he's quick to pick up everything. Back then, I talked it over with my mother, she thought so too: What's the use of killing it if he'll be normal, he'll walk?

Like many other women for whom religion provided orienting meta-phors and beacons, Migdalia's narrative is richly embroidered with her Catholicism; it also highlights her close relationship with her mother. In deciding to keep her pregnancy after Klinefelter's syndrome had been di-agnosed in her fetus, Migdalia wasn't unusual; counselors estimate that less than half the women receiving this diagnosis choose abortions (cf. Robinson, Bender, and Linden 1989). Her decision has a very strong context: Intimate knowledge of one disabling and worrisome physical condition in her sister could be contrasted with a disability that "didn't show." It was the relative invisibility of the consequences of her son's atypical chromosomes that made them normal in her estimation. Indeed, "normal" was a concept she person-ally and actively produced under the shadow of her sister's condition. For Migdalia, both spina bifida and Klinefelter's syndrome have concrete, spe-cific meanings.

Donna Moran's positive diagnosis was delivered by sonogram, not by amniocentesis. A 45-year-old mother of four and the emotional center of a breakaway Catholic commune in rural upstate New York, she saw a local midwife only episodically in her fifth pregnancy and intended to give birth at home. Both she and the midwife felt that the baby was not moving properly; in her seventh month of pregnancy, she agreed to travel to a nearby town for a visit with an obstetrician who owned a sonogram machine. He quickly lo-cated the problem and delivered very bad news: The fetus was anencephalic, lacking a portion of its brain and skull. This condition, inevitably fatal, is one of the few bases on which an abortion can be obtained after the legal cutoff date (in New York State, twenty-four weeks). Most legal and ethical scholars are in accord: The suffering entailed by this condition for both mother and child merits abortion. But Donna was clear in her decision: She would carry the fetus to term and accept God's mercy in taking the baby quickly to Him. Her labors began in the eighth month and, since the fetus had no upper skull with which to push, ended after much stress in an emergency cesarian. The baby lived for several days; the mother's recovery was arduous and pro-longed. Here, the meaning attributed to a reproductive tragedy was highly religious. Donna saw her own suffering and the suffering of the baby as a test of God's mysteries. Additionally, she was surrounded by a group of commu-nards with whom she had constructed an alternative, rural, spiritual life for most of two decades. Donna's story and its interpretation came to me from one of those communards, who expressed awe at the spiritual strength and physical endurance of someone she saw as a true "earth mother." She also felt strongly that Donna had been exploited by an unself-conscious male bias present in her own commune: The role of mothering and maternal suffering was taken as central to a higher order. While I do not know enough about this case to venture an alternative or lengthier commentary, it strikes me that some of the same themes obtain—strong religious orientation, strong social support, prior (confident) reproductive history—that were present in other cases of women deciding to continue pregnancies marked by positive diagnoses.

In one case, I was present as a positive diagnosis was produced. Working in the lab one February afternoon, I observed a technician as he found something ambiguous on the #9 chromosomes of the sample he was scoping. After using the laboratory protocol to check twice and then three times the number of cells usually examined for a normal diagnosis, the case went to the head geneticist, who agreed: There was additional chromosomal material on the top, short arm of the #9s. She initially called it "9P+," "9" for the pair of chromosomes on which it was located, "P" to designate the short arm, and "+" to indicate additional chromosomal material. First, she scanned the literature for an interpretation. Then she phoned the head obstetrician at City's prenatal clinic, in charge of the case, and made an appointment for the woman to be called in. Over the course of a week's research, the geneticist located some clinical reports on trisomy 9, the closest known condition to which this case might be assimilated (her reasoning was not frivolous . . .). In all those cases, babies born with trisomy 9 had physical anomalies and were mentally retarded. Armed with a provisional diagnosis, the geneticist met with the genetic counselor, who then counseled the mother. When the mother decided to keep the pregnancy, the genetic counselor asked the geneticist to meet with the mother. After a second consultative counseling session, the mother remained quite firm in her decision to continue the pregnancy.

The baby was born in early June, and in late July the geneticist contacted the new mother through her obstetrician, asking if she would be willing to bring her child to the genetics laboratory for a consultation. The mother agreed. On a Wednesday afternoon, the "trisomy 9" came visiting: He was a six-week-old Haitian boy named Etienne St-Croix. His mother, Véronique, spoke reasonable English and good French. His grandmother, Marie-Lucie, who carried the child, spoke Creole and some French. The two geneticists spoke English, Polish, Hebrew, and Chinese between them. I translated into French, ostensibly for the grandmother and mother. Here is what happened: The geneticist was gracious with Véronique, but after a moment's chitchat asked to examine the baby. She never spoke directly to the mother again during the examination. Instead, she and a second geneticist, both trained in pediatrics, handled the newborn with confidence and interest. The counselor took notes as the geneticists measured and discussed the baby. "Note the oblique palpebral fissure and micrognathia," one called out. "Yes," answered

Véronique in perfect time to the conversation, "he has the nose of my Uncle Hervé and the ears of Aunt Mathilde." As the geneticists pathologized, the mother genealogized, the genetic counselor remained silent, furiously taking notes, and the anthropologist tried to keep score. When the examination was over, the geneticists apologized to the baby for any discomfort they had caused him, and one asked the mother a direct question: "I notice you haven't circumcised your baby. Are you planning to?" "Yes," Véronique replied, "we'll do it in about another week." "May we have the foreskin?" the geneticist queried. "With the foreskin, we can keep growing trisomy 9 cells for research, and study the tissue as your baby develops." Véronique gave her a firm and determined "yes," and the consultation was over.

Walking Véronique and Marie-Lucie to the subway to direct them home to Brooklyn, I asked what she had thought about the experience: from the amnio to the diagnosis to the genetic consultation. She replied:

> At first, I was very frightened. I am 37, I wanted a baby. It is my husband's second marriage, my mother-in-law is for me, not the first wife. She wanted me to have a baby, too. If it had been Down's, maybe, just maybe I would have had an abortion. Once I had an abortion, but now I am a Seventh-day Adventist, and I don't believe in abortion anymore. Maybe for Down's, just maybe. But when they told me this, who knows? I was so scared, but the more they talked, the less they said. They do not know what this is. And I do not know either. So now, it's my baby. We'll just have to wait and see what happens. And so will they.

Here, marital and kinship relations clearly influence the decision to continue a pregnancy after positive diagnosis; so does religious conversion. But at the center of this narrative lies another important theme: diagnostic ambiguity. Biomedical scientists work from precedent, matching new findings with old. When presented with an atypical case, they build a diagnosis in the same fashion, comparing the present case to the closest available prior knowledge in clinical archives. While the geneticists are confident that this child will share the developmental pattern reported in the literature for other children with very similar chromosomal patterns, the mother was quite aware of the idiosyncratic nature of the case, its lack of clear-cut label and known syndrome. She therefore decided that the contest for interpretation was still an open one. This is a dramatic instance of interpretive standoff between biomedical discourse and family life.

But in some sense, all positive diagnoses appear ambiguous to pregnant women.[3] An extra chromosome spells out the diagnosis of Down syndrome, but it does not distinguish mildly from severely retarded children, nor does it indicate whether this particular fetus will need open-heart surgery. A missing X chromosome indicates a Turner's syndrome female but cannot speak to the meaning of fertility in the particular family into which she may be born. Homozygous status for the sickle-cell gene cannot predict the severity of anemia a particular child will develop. All such diagnoses are interpreted in light of prior reproductive histories, community values, and aspirations that particular women and their families hold for the pregnancy being examined.

This problem of ambiguity—inside of biomedicine and inside of family life—is one encountered by genetic counselors with a fair degree of frequency. Virtually all counselors I interviewed mentioned mosaic conditions when I asked about difficult cases. In mosaic diagnoses, cells are both normal and atypical in varying proportions. Roughly speaking, the greater the density of atypical cells, the greater the likelihood of disabling conditions which are known to geneticists and can be described to potential parents. But some conditions may exhibit mosaicism in one cell line without profound clinical expression at the level of the whole organism, that is, the child. This is true, for example, of mosaicism on chromosome 20, where the atypical findings may come from the amniotic membranes rather than from the fetus. Yet when experts find a single mosaic cell line they cannot know which organ system of the body will be affected or unaffected. And sometimes a known condition—for example, Down syndrome—may be present in mosaic patterns on the cellular level, producing a child who is "slow" but still coded by the relevant caretakers in her life as "normal." Mosaic diagnoses are thus hard to explain and harder to interpret. Their inherent ambiguity leads some women to continue pregnancies in which they have been diagnosed, especially if the number of atypical cells is relatively small or the genetic counselor can say of a particular condition with some degree of confidence, "It rarely has profound clinical significance." Women receiving mosaic diagnoses are among the most likely to stop the technological conveyor belt, preserving their pregnancy and preparing for the birth of a child whose cellular "fortune" has been read but whose clinical future they understand to be truly unpredictable (Robinson, Bender, and Linden 1989).

Existentially speaking, of course, we *all live* with truly unpredictable clinical futures; the existence of prenatal diagnosis has simply added a new twist to that impasse in the human condition. Now, it is possible, indeed necessary, for those who would have the chromosomes of their fetuses "read" to know something about possible problems and limits a coming child may face *in vitro*, without having encountered those problems and limits as they unfold *in vivo*. The difference between a biologically described organism and a socially integrated child is, of course, enormous. And it is within this gap between laboratory-generated descriptions of disabilities and potential disabilities and their consequences for family life as a child develops that some women receiving positive diagnoses choose to operate. Those who opt to continue a pregnancy after any positive diagnosis must consciously face what the rest of us confront only episodically: The hard work of redescribing and reinscribing a powerful biomedical definition into the more complex and variegated aspects of personhood, childhood dependency, and family life. In this situation, the structure of chromosomes initially looms large as a defining characteristic of what a child's future may bring. Women who continue pregnancies after positive diagnoses thus expend considerable agency reducing the significance of chromosomes in order to welcome a child on grounds other than biomedical normalcy.

As I have tried to show . . . women with strong religious affiliations, strong kinship or other communitarian social support, or strong reasons anchored in their reproductive histories are most likely to decide against the biomedical information amniocentesis brings as a basis for accepting or rejecting a particular pregnancy. These patterns hold true across differences of income, lifestyle, and job description, which provide rough measures of socioeconomic class. But other patterns of amniocentesis use and rejection are highly class-structured: Access to information and respectful health care surely conditions how prenatal testing is perceived and valued. Moreover, those without advanced scientific education are most likely to reject testing altogether, although many women from working-class and working-poor backgrounds also choose to be tested. And the problem of male privilege or even male dominance in decision-making also intersects these patterns of use. Such socially structured trajectories cannot be reduced to a reflexive response to any particular diagnosis; in other words, they hold no automatic or predictable intersection with the biomedical diagnoses described in the course of laboratory life (to borrow a felicitous title from Latour and Woolgar 1979).

Editors' Note: In this next section, Rayna Rapp examines the reasons why some women decide to terminate a pregnancy following the diagnosis of a certain, or occasionally ambiguous, anomaly in fetal development.[4] Rapp refers to these decisions as "forced choices," and she discusses women's attitudes toward what she calls "the chosen loss."

Forced Choices

The delivery of a positive diagnosis inevitably forces the pregnant woman and her supporters to make a decision to continue or end the pregnancy. The full impact of that decision-making process is, of course, multifaceted and complex; it provides the subject of this chapter. But one of the first things that struck me when I began interviewing women who had been through this painful process was that my sample divided dramatically into two groups: those who more or less knew that they would choose abortion if a serious condition were diagnosed in their fetuses, and who therefore "decided" instantaneously upon hearing bad news; and those who needed to work their way through the problem step by step, arriving at the abortion decision as the conclusion of a more protracted process. The two strategies condense multiple differences, including the very significant difference between understanding common and arcane or ambiguous diagnoses, discussed below. But in addition they reflect sociocultural influences on women's comfort and trust in biomedicine, including diagnostic technology, and the prior knowledge, attitudes, and beliefs that pregnant women and their supporters hold about specific disabling conditions, as well as about childhood disability in general.

The use of abortion after a serious positive diagnosis seems almost automatic, if nonetheless painful for some women, especially under two conditions. One is the diagnosis of Down syndrome, with which they feel familiar. This diagnosis is the single most common one made through amniocentesis, and accounts for almost half the chromosome problems detected. While there are no national figures for abortion rates following positive diagnosis, epidemiological and biostatistical experts estimate that more than 90 percent of women receiving this diagnosis go on to abort (Drugan et al. 1990; Hsu 1989). One Midwestern study found that 93 percent of the women receiving what the physicians characterized as "severe" prognoses, including all autosomal (nonsex chromosome) trisomies, of which Down's is the most common, decided to abort (Drugan et al. 1990). These suggestive studies correlate well with data collected in England, where national statistics on abortion following a positive prenatal diagnosis are kept. There, 92 percent of those receiving this diagnosis chose to end their pregnancies (Alberman et al. 1995). The second factor which seems to influence an "automatic pilot" response to a serious diagnosis is attachment to an upper-middle-class, or middle-class, Jewish background:

Decision, what decision? It comes with the territory. If you're having am-niocentesis, you're having an abortion when they find something wrong. (Leah Rubinstein, 39, white homemaker)

We talked it over before deciding to have amnio. If I was going to have it, we would already know that I was going to have the abortion. People always have their opinion, and people were saying, "If it's Down syndrome, you don't want to have to live with that for the rest of your life." I can tell you a lot of compassionate stories about friends with mentally retarded kids. And I know if we just had a kid with that problem, with no testing, we'd do the right thing, we'd love that child and raise it well. But the bot-tom line is, we agreed that we want to avoid this problem if we can. (Fran Goodman, 34, white nonprofit community service worker)

And, of course, while virtually every Jewish woman in my sample had this response, they were not alone. Many others also told stories in which deci-sion-making was instantaneous, almost always with Down syndrome and, sometimes, with other conditions as well:

And when the doctor told me, that was the first instance when I knew that I was going to have an abortion. I made up my mind instantly, I checked in the hospital right away. . . . It was the only thing I could have done. I mean, it was the only thing I could have done. (Nancy Tucker, 36, white college professor)

An unambiguous decision does not entail less suffering:

Sure, it was the best decision I could have made under the circumstances. It was a perfectly right, clear decision, but an enormously painful one. (Diana Morel, 28, Puerto Rican secretary)

I feel fine about the decision, I'm fine with it. Nothing could have been more obvious. It's just that my heart is permanently broken. (Donna deAngelo, 38, white homemaker)

Most of my respondents had prior knowledge about Down syndrome gleaned from neighbors, friends, and kin who had children with this, or another, form of mental retardation. Seven were teachers or social workers whose professional life had brought them into contact with families with disabled (usually, mentally retarded) members. Sylvia Lin, 43, a Japanese-American special-education teacher, said, "I told my husband, 'Down's, that means practically nothing.' Because I've seen them very retarded, and I've seen them practically normal."

Other women also had more nuanced understandings of this, and other disabilities:

> I knew enough to know not to worry about Down's babies. They're cute, they get by. But you really worry about what happens when they grow up, when you get old, when you die. Who takes care of Down's babies then? (Harriet Genzer, 41, white editor)

> I had an autistic brother. My mother put everything she had into him; it ate up her whole life. Maybe the kid would do well. But what about me? (Megan Johnson, 41, white writer)

And some expressed self-criticism of their own aversion to keeping a child with the diagnosed disability:

> I'm not proud of this, but to be honest, I don't want to cope with a mentally retarded child. My mother did volunteer work in the schools, with MR kids. She's deeply against abortion. But she's not against abortion for this. I guess some of her attitudes must have rubbed off on me. The thing that entrances me is having a smart child. (Sally Hart, 38, white college professor)

The Chosen Loss

Knowing (or thinking one knows) about a condition undoubtedly strengthens the resolve of decision-making. But it doesn't lessen the pain of loss. Ending a wanted pregnancy is a multifaceted, complex process which all the women with whom I spoke consistently identified as a profound loss. The emotional recovery after what is medically labeled a "selective abortion" is lengthy. Women and their supporters experiencing this process share an existential territory with all who survive the death of loved ones; they also have much in common with those recovering from any pregnancy loss or stillbirth. But their experience is also distinct because it is a chosen loss (Black 1994; Kolker and Burke 1994). The idea of "choice" is one to which women returned again and again, especially highly educated, middle-class women. Said Pat Gordon, a 37-year-old white college professor, "I felt like a voice in a Greek chorus, chanting, 'Your choice, your choice, your choice is upon your shoulders.' I felt like a minor figure in a major tragedy."

Yet for some, the very notion of "choice" is unbearable and must be abolished from the vocabulary of grief: When I asked about decision-making, I heard again and again, from women of diverse backgrounds, "I had to have an abortion" or "It was a forced choice." Some were even more explicit:

> I'd prefer the doctor told me the baby was dead. I kept secretly hoping it would die before we got to the hospital. Then I wouldn't be part of causing this loss. (Nivia Hostos, 26, Puerto Rican administrative secretary)

> Don't speak of it as an abortion, that's disgusting. This was a loss. I did what I had to do, I couldn't help myself. It's a loss, not an . . . (Harriet Genzer, 41, white editor)

Others acknowledged their ambivalence about what one woman who identified herself as "a rabid pro-choicer" nonetheless called "being an accomplice to a murder." And some spoke of the pain in having to have a choice at all:

> When I was going to Dr. R's office to have the laminaria put in again and again, I kept thinking: No one is forcing me to do this. I'm making my own choice. This is awful. It's the single most awful thing that's ever happened to me. But it's my choice, and I'm making it. (Michelle Kansky, 38, white public school teacher)

Indeed, the seriousness of "choice" was a theme that occurred repeatedly as women spoke about decision-making:

> Because I had a very serious relationship with that child, and to be carrying it around, wondering whether I was gonna kill it or not was just very serious, I mean, it's feeling like you're going to murder something that you're very close to that's inside of you, when you have the choice not to, and you're choosing to, you know, you're choosing the most difficult thing. (Margaret Thompson, 34, white psychologist)

Many expressed gratitude about having had a choice, despite the deep pain that accompanied its exercise. Knowing about a profound problem in a fetus and being able to choose to avoid bringing it to term was, in their estimate, better than living with the consequences of its birth. "It's better to know than not to know, better to have the choice rather than not to have the choice at all," said Marilyn de Soto, 34, Puerto Rican social worker.

Yet contained within this discourse of choice are the seeds of at least two other themes, which bear mention. One is the subtle, perhaps fetishizing aspects of individualism implied in the concept of choice. Because the fetuses who are diagnosed grow within individual women's bodies, the sociodemographic circumstances of their development—older mothers, accessible, new reproductive technologies, the "background rate" of "birth defects" in all populations—may be harder to spot. This theme was brought home to me in the words of an African-American nonprofit education administrator who was also a single mother. Much of our conversation concerned the benefits and burdens of being on one's own as a professional and a mother. Yet when I used the language of "choice" to her, Doris Paul immediately responded, " 'Choices, choices.' 'Decisions, decisions' would be more like it. Because we're always called to crossroads and tests, they aren't things we seek, they're situations that befall us. And we go on, just the same."

Her reminder of the matrix within which individuals find themselves confronting decisions is apt, for it turns down the volume on individual volition, beckoning us to also attend to the structured situations over which individuals have very little control, but within which they regularly operate and compose their lives. This message was likewise echoed by a medical professional who wrote about her experiences with abortion after early prenatal diagnosis. For Rose Green (a pseudonym), the "choice" masked the non-choice of having produced an unhealthy child (Green 1992).

It is this second theme of "having produced an unhealthy child" against all odds and desires that also bears discussion. When I spoke with her a few weeks after she had terminated a pregnancy upon learning that her fetus had Down syndrome, one white lawyer quoted a recent popular book on pregnancy loss, which includes a chapter on abortions after prenatal diagnosis: "The father was speaking of a double whammy of grief [in Kohn and Moffat 1993]. That's right. First you've produced this defective child, then you've gone on to have a devastating abortion. Who could possibly understand?" And others went on to speculate about the meaning of making a fetus that couldn't live, or couldn't live normally, especially when the diagnosis included mental retardation, a profound dilemma for the many constituencies who value normal intelligence:

> I feel pity for my husband. All he can think about, the thing that torments him is: He's smart. I'm smart. The other kids are smart. How could this have happened to one of our children? (Donna deAngelo, 38, white homemaker)

> After this, I really understood adoption much better. Because it can't be predicted how your child will be from getting your genes. And you don't

need your kids to be genetic copies, they might be unlike you anyway. After all, there we were, two perfectly accomplished, intelligent, competent adults. And we'd made a baby who could never grow into those things we most valued. For some, I know it's guilt. For me, it was astonishment. And overwhelming grief. (Pat Gordon, 37, white college professor)

And there was anguish expressed at having produced the "wrong" child. . . . For example, Fran Goodman, 34, white nonprofit community organizer, said, "I always wonder when people hear [that we aborted a fetus with Down syndrome], there's still this thing like, 'Can't you have a healthy baby?' There's just a little piece of me which thinks they're wondering."

Diana Morel, a young Puerto Rican secretary, suffered a doubly devastating loss: First, she experienced the stillbirth of her first child from spina bifida, closely followed by an abortion when her next pregnancy was revealed on sonogram to be carrying a fetus with Epstein syndrome, a rare and inevitably fatal heart insufficiency. Yet she spoke to almost no one about her disorientation, grief, and depression: "I'm ashamed. I'm ashamed that they'll blame me for the damages I made."

Editors' Note: Finally, in this last section, Rapp explores both boundary issues and how women take into account the needs and concerns of their already living children as they make decisions about testing and decisions about abortion.[5]

Becoming Un-pregnant

Women also described a range of feelings concerning their responsibility for the death of a desired fetus. While some stressed an achieved understanding of responsibility . . . others felt guilt. . . .

The problem of taking responsibility arose starkly for some women who—either voluntarily or without volition—immediately threw themselves back into work. I heard about this issue across the class spectrum, from professional lawyers and social workers, from freelance writers, secretaries, and hospital housekeepers. The return to work usually implied having a story of the pregnancy's end, a problematic issue in boundary maintenance. This problem of drawing a line between those who "deserved the truth" and those who "just needed to know I was hurting" was an issue that arose in all the interviews. It is deeply linked to attitudes about politics (most obviously, abortion politics) and religion. It is also linked to questions of social support and isolation. . . . And it reflects the shift of "women's work" into the social service sector, where many jobs are highly public or visible. Many of the women I interviewed were teachers, social workers, secretaries, or hospital employees. They worked in busy offices and classrooms, where they encountered scores of colleagues and members of "the public" every day. In such circumstances, pregnancies are highly noticeable and frequently discussed. So, then, are their unexpected endings. A story thus had to be constructed in which was condensed a statement about a dense range of issues: Individual attitudes toward disability, abortion, responsibility (or guilt), and the relatively private or public nature of grief and mourning. Some women spoke openly about their diagnoses and abortions; others spoke only of a "loss." And most used a "mixed strategy" of elaborating the story for one circle of friends and relations, while giving less detail to a wider group:

> So I took off two weeks, and they told my kids [in the classroom] that the baby came out too early and died. And that week, they showed a film about the Ethiopian famine, and one of the kids asked if they could buy a starving baby and give it to Mrs. Kansky. They had to be told something, you can see it really affected them. (Michelle Kansky, 38, white public school teacher)

> I told my boss, and he told a few others, and they told the rest. Mostly, we just referred to my loss. I knew who knew, and I wanted them to know. But for months, the others, the others who didn't know, they kept asking me, "What'd you have, what'd you have?" It was hard having to keep saying that I lost the baby. (Marilyn de Soto, 34, Puerto Rican social worker)

One other problem involving boundary-keeping narratives also arose in women's stories of mourning and recovery. Women who had other children took them into account throughout the decision-making process and the termination of their pregnancies. Indeed, one of the strongest differences among those I interviewed occurred between women expecting (and thus losing) their first child, and those with children at home. Childless women tended to fantasize perfect babies; their loss included the loss of an imaginary experience of new motherhood. They thus mourned the loss of a romantic motherhood, along with the specific pregnancy. Women who had children were less romantic in imagining life with the child who would have resulted from the diagnosed pregnancy; they already knew the burdens of caring for perfectly ordinary, healthy offspring. The mothers recovered more rapidly from their grief, in part because they had child-centered responsibilities which kept them moored to the earth; they could rarely find the time to focus on their own pain.

Another Voice?

Their attentiveness to the needs and reactions of other children should be underlined: Too often, the politicization of abortion is inscribed in a discourse of individual "selfishness." . . . But in the interviews I collected, women usually positioned their abortion decisions in relation to the way they imagined their intimate others would be affected. The most salient of these were their other children. Many expressed fear that a sick baby would absorb an unfair share of the family economy of love and time. Others were quite explicit about how having a disabled child would affect their families:

> When the decision came through I told my husband, I just said, 'We cannot take the time. We're working parents, that's what we are. We'll never see Antonia again if we have to take care of this sick baby. We've got to end it, and end it now.' (Iris Lauria, 29, Puerto Rican hospital housekeeper)

> Some people say that abortion is hate. I say my abortion was an act of love. I've got three kids. I was 43 when we accidentally got pregnant again. We decided there was enough love in our family to handle it, even though finances would be tight. But we also decided to have the test. A kid with a serious problem was more than we could handle. And when we got the bad news, I knew immediately what I had to do. At 43, you think about your own death. It would have been tough now, but think what would have happened to my other kids, especially my daughter. Oh, the boys, Stephan and Alex, would have done ok. But Livia would have been the one who got stuck. It's always the girls. It would have been me, and then, after I'm gone, it would have been the big sister who took care of that child. Saving Livia from that burden was an act of love. (Mary Fruticci, 44, white homemaker)

Such comments provide a healthy antidote to the discourse of "selfishness," substituting a more embedded sense of maternal responsibility and relationality in its place. But they also suggest that altruism toward other household members is the reason for the decision to end a diagnosed pregnancy. This important corrective then performs invisible work of its own, muffling cultural attitudes toward disability and the voluntary limits of maternity. But . . . standards for acceptable and unacceptable children, and the meaning of specific disabilities, are always culturally constructed. Though public support is strong for keeping abortion legal when "defective" or "damaged" fetuses are diagnosed, far less consensus exists on which disabilities are grounds for abortion (Drugan et al. 1990; Goldberg and Elder 1998). For some women and their supporters, the mental retardation accompanying chromosome trisomies is reason enough, while for others, physical stigmata are more upsetting. . . . In some times and places, infanticide or fostering is prescribed for babies born with socially inadmissible conditions; in contemporary America, a medical procedure appears to offer a cutting edge in defining the limits of what women and their families are willing to accept. A discourse of "altruism" toward others thus masks an important discussion of whether, and under what conditions, women feel entitled to refuse specific pregnancies as a way to refuse specific disabilities in their children, and to refuse the surplus labors entailed in caring for them. At the same time, the possibility of positive effects—the acceptance of difference, the learning of compassion—which siblings of a disabled child might experience is never imagined. "Maternal altruism" thus papers over a terrain carved out by political demands for both reproductive rights and disability rights, even as it provides a more realistic portrait of the complexity with which many women approach an abortion decision.

In addition to including their other children in the constellation of decision-making factors, women also had to find appropriate ways to discuss the end of a pregnancy with them. Age-appropriate stories were constructed, with young children often being told some version of, "The baby was sick, and it died, and mommy went to the hospital to take it out." Older ones might be told more specifically what happened, such as, "We found out the baby was going to be retarded and might die from a heart problem. So the doctor helped us to end this pregnancy. Daddy and I are very sad, and we miss the baby. But its life would have been very difficult, and that would have made it hard for all of us."

In the small literature on the social impact of abortions after positive prenatal diagnoses, other researchers have commented on the "transient but real signs of distress" which the ending of the pregnancy—whether officially discussed or not—invoked in young children (Goldberg and Elder 1998; cf. from a child's perspective, Scrimshaw and March 1984). Conversations reported back to me included children's comments, such as:

Mommy, what happened to your breasts? They're not so nice now. (3-year-old boy)

My son, now he takes his friends to his room, I hear him saying, "In this house, we are not happy, we are very sad. Because our baby was sick, and it died. And my mother had to get it taken out, and we all really, really wanted that baby. So we're sad." And he's 7. (Donna deAngelo, 38, white homemaker)

My little one only wants to know, "Will I catch that?" and I have to explain that it happens before you're even born, and no, she can't catch that at all. The big one is more concerned with me: She sees me crying, she wants me to stop crying and to have another baby. (Carolyn Williams, 36, African-American postal worker)

Some parents are obviously more comfortable explaining their abortion or their grief than others. But all who had children felt the impact of their situation on them.

Notes

1. Excerpt from pp. 183–90 of Rapp 2000.
2. Pseudonyms were used to protect the confidentiality of the pregnant women, mothers, children, and their supporters.
3. The point is made throughout Rothman 1986. It was also pointed out to me separately by Shirley Lindenbaum and Emily Martin.
4. Excerpt from pp. 222–29 of Rapp 2000.
5. Excerpt from pp. 245–49 of Rapp 2000.

References

Alberman, E., D. Mutton, R. Ide, A. Nicholson, and M. Bobrow. 1995. Down's Syndrome Births and Pregnancy Terminations in 1989 to 1993: Preliminary Findings. *British Journal of Obstetrics and Gynaecology* 102 (6): 445–47.

Black, Rita Beck. 1994. Reproductive Genetic Testing and Pregnancy Loss: The Experience of Women. In *Women and Prenatal Testing: Facing the Challenges of Genetic Technology*, edited by Karen H. Rothenberg and Elizabeth J. Thomson. Columbus: Ohio State University Press.

Cunningham, George. 1998. "An Evaluation of California's Public-Private Material Serum Screening Program." Ninth International Conference on Prenatal Diagnosis and Therapy, Los Angeles, June 11.

Drugan, Arie, Anne Greb, Mark Paul Johnson, Eric L. Krivchenia, Wendy R. Uhlmann, Kamran S. Moghissi, and Mark I. Evans. 1990. Determinants of Parental Decisions to Abort for Chromosome Abnormalities. *Prenatal Diagnosis* 10 (8): 483–90.

Goldberg, Carey, and Janet Elder. 1998. Public Still Backs Abortion, but Wants Limits, Polls Say. *New York Times*, January 16.

Green, Rose (pseudonym). 1992. Letter to a Genetic Counselor. *Journal of Genetics Counseling* 1 (1): 55–70.

Hsu, Lillian. 1989. *Portrait of the Prenatal Diagnosis Laboratory, a Tenth Anniversary Report*. New York University Medical School, June 10.

Kohn, Ingrid, and Perry Moffat. 1993. *Silent Sorrow: Pregnancy Loss, Guidance and Support*. New York: Dell.

Kolker, Aliza, and B. Meredith Burke. 1994. *Prenatal Testing: A Sociological Perspective*. Westport, CT: Bergin and Garvey.

Latour, Bruno, and Steve Woolgar. 1979. *Laboratory Life: The Construction of Scientific Facts*. Beverly Hills, CA: Sage.

Meaney, F. John, Susan M. Riggle, and G. C. Cunningham. 1993. Providers and Consumers of Prenatal Genetic Services: What Do the Data Tell Us? *Fetal Diagnosis and Therapy* 8 (suppl. 1): 18–27.

Palmer, Shane, Joanne Spencer, Theodore Kushnick, John Wiley, and Susan Bowyer. 1993. Follow-up Survey of Pregnancies with Diagnoses of Chromosomal Abnormality. *Journal of Genetic Counseling* 2 (3): 139–52.

Rapp, Rayna. 2000. *Testing Women, Testing the Fetus: The Social Impact of Amniocentesis in America*. New York: Routledge.

Robinson, Arthur, Bruce G. Bender, and Margy G. Linden. 1989. Decisions following the Intrauterine Diagnosis of Sex Chromosome Aneuploidy. *American Journal of Medical Genetics* 34 (4): 552–54.

Rothman, Barbara Katz. 1986. *The Tentative Pregnancy: Prenatal Diagnosis and the Future of Motherhood*. New York: Norton.

Scrimshaw, Susan, and D. M. March. 1984. "I Had a Baby Sister but She Only Lasted One Day." *Journal of the American Medical Association* 251 (6): 732–33.

8

Turning Strangers into Kin

Half Siblings and Anonymous Donors

Rosanna Hertz

The release of my book *Single by Chance, Mothers by Choice* (2006) prompted me to follow through on a commitment I had made to the women I interviewed.[1] I invited them to a party at Wellesley College's bookstore. Sophie was among the women who came that day, and she brought her son, Sam, age ten.[2] She was anxious to share news about the discovery of her son's donor siblings.

Sophie had selected artificial insemination with an unknown donor as her route to motherhood because she believed that this method would minimize any legal entanglements with parental kin. She therefore presumed that she would not be including her son's biological paternal kin within her family's boundaries, because they would not be known to her. Her imagination stretched only to the donor and his legal family, however, and not to other children created from his seminal fluid.

When Sam was about seven years old, Sophie learned about a sibling registry website, and a startling possibility arose for locating a new category of paternal blood kin: *donor siblings*. Knowledge of this sibling registry website presented choices Sophie thought had ended when she selected an anonymous donor. Prior to learning of the website, the borders of Sophie's family lay dormant. Now, however, she could decide whether to search for donor siblings who traced themselves to the same seminal fluid she had purchased. And if these new kin should turn up, Sophie would have to more actively patrol the border of family life and decide whether to include these people within it. Moreover, if she chose affirmatively, she would also have to monitor the interactions between her family and these new additions. The quality and content of the interior of family life would also need watching.

The story of Sophie's response to this new possibility, supplemented by blog commentary, provides an in-depth case study of the discovery of donor siblings and boundary maintenance from the mother's standpoint.[3] I argue that as much as mothers and children may want to embrace "new paternal family," women heighten the security around their watertight mother-child family before deciding to open up the boundaries to the child's discovered donor siblings. Because donor siblings have no precedent in constructing families, mothers and their children are cautious, and there is a lot of back-and-forth surveillance of the half siblings and their mothers. I use the information Sophie shared with me in a follow-up interview to illustrate the process that is set into motion as families discover half siblings and their parents. Margaret Nelson (2006) refers to this dynamic of creating social ties while maintaining boundaries as one aspect of "doing family."[4] The case under investigation here demonstrates that ties and boundaries emerge through strategic interactions. Mothers and their children, separately and together, try to figure out, first, whether to extend family membership to donor siblings and their relatives and, second, what direction these new relationships will take.

People-Finding Websites

"Shared identity" sites provide a connection for strangers who share something in common. In recent years, an incredible number of such sites have sprung up on the Internet, including identity sites for people who are contemplating single motherhood. In addition to providing information on such hot topics as sperm banks, these sites also encourage chats about common concerns, such as how to tell the prospective grandparents about the process of becoming pregnant, experiences with a particular sperm bank, and the use of known versus unknown donors. "People-finding" websites allow an exchange beyond simple information and foster a sense of intimacy between members. Such sites have developed to help people locate others in virtual space whom they hope to meet in the physical world.[5] While bulletin boards in the supermarket or in organization offices (such as the Red Cross) still exist as physical places to post want ads, missing ads, or sales ads, these websites—existing across time, place, and space—allow individuals to search worldwide. The Internet has also expanded the ability of people to search for their genealogical roots and existing family connections—a new technology serving a time-honored activity. Recently, however, the Internet has been used not only to search for family connections that may have been lost but also to find and possibly forge connections with people who share the same anonymous sperm donor, and even to find the donor himself.

The search for a child's donor siblings is an interesting twist on the general idea of locating people. To support the goal of finding donor siblings, Wendy Kramer and her son Ryan, age twelve, founded *www.donorsiblingregistry.com* in 2000. Wendy, like the other individuals who register on her site, gave birth using an anonymous donor after purchasing sperm from a major sperm bank listed on another website. She had no idea that she had the right to search for her son's half siblings or donor.[6] Wendy learned from the sperm bank that other children were born from the same donor as Ryan. Although Ryan knew that his anonymous donor was not likely to be found, he wanted to meet his half siblings. Wendy, with whom I talked as I wrote this chapter, told me that she wanted to honor her son's wish:

> I told my son, "I can't guarantee that we will find your donor, but maybe we can find half siblings." We hatched the idea to try to meet some part of the paternal side of the family. If he could connect to other siblings, he said to me, "at least I could see the invisible side of myself in someone else and that would help answer some of my questions."

In this new world, a sperm-bank-assigned donor number becomes the means of locating others who share the same donor.[7] Just as new surveillance technologies decrease privacy (e.g., when a workplace monitors behavior such as using e-mail for personal matters [Fox, Anderson, and Rainie 2005]), this use of technology breaks down yet another barrier of privacy: personhood. Assigning people numbers has historically made them less than human, even if the numbers serve as a way to keep track of donors. In an ironic twist, the numbers that disassociate men from their gametes are used to connect the children who were sired from those gametes, and sometimes even to connect those children to the donors themselves. As these new websites break down the system of genetic anonymity, they can forge the most intimate of ties to newly discovered family members.

These new family members are without precedent and constitute an entirely new category of kin. Although half siblings are not new—they exist through extramarital affairs, through remarriage, and through relinquishing a birth child for adoption—another parent is part of the equation in these more conventional situations. These normative models are disrupted, however, when the donor's personal relationship with various mothers is not the basis for the creation of half siblings. Nor are donor siblings equivalent to long-lost kin. We hold the belief that there is always room in our hearts should someone claiming family membership show up on our doorstep. Such people are welcomed as family because they can trace their own genealogy back to common ancestors with those who are already family members. This is particularly true in the case of family members lost to circumstances beyond the family's control (e.g., slavery, the Holocaust, or immigration). This long-lost person has a place in the family, and he or she claims that place by showing up as the grandson of my grandmother's first cousin, the daughter of my uncle's third wife, or any other relation imaginable.

By contrast, the claim to family membership by donor children as offspring or siblings has no social basis and is purely biological. "Long-lost kin" has always been linked to the actions of individuals; donor siblings are "just" biological, and the idea is harder to grasp than the concept of families that include friends who become "aunties and uncles." While the idea of social kin (i.e., families we choose) is generally accepted, we have not accepted the idea of purely biological kin. In short, no cultural paradigm has existed for understanding the relationship between donor siblings, in which a donor number serves as a stand-in for a shared relative, a genetic father.

However, the public was soon to learn about this new possibility for kinship, and it was about to become a reality for many people. A *60 Minutes* segment that aired on television in March 2005 heightened the visibility of Wendy and Ryan's website.[8] As of December 2006, Wendy reported that her website had 7,002 members and estimated that one-third were single moms, one-third were lesbian couples, and one-third were heterosexual couples. Also as of December 2006, there were 2,764 matches, mainly between donor siblings. In addition, four hundred donors had registered, and some of these donors had located their genetic children. The largest match so far, Wendy told me, was one donor and fifteen offspring.[9]

Registering on a website is voluntary and does not obligate anyone to reveal his or her identity. However, whether or not registrants follow through on contacting their donor siblings, registering signals the wish for further information about children conceived through a particular anonymous donor. Despite the thrill of using the Internet as a source to locate potential paternal kin, it also can be a risky venture with the possibility for a less than "happily ever after" ending.

In this chapter, I discuss how locating a shared donor entails a form of familial border patrol: Will genetic kin be turned into "real" kin and kept? Or will they be relegated to a "shadowland," solely a curiosity satisfied? I explore these questions using the story of Sophie and Sam.

Earlier Stages: The Watertight Family Always Included the Donor

Long before the issue of donor siblings arose, Sophie, like other middle-class women who choose to conceive using artificial insemination from an anonymous donor, had engaged in two stages of making choices and intense monitoring. She had selected a donor by carefully studying her options, and she had observed her child closely to craft an image of the donor she had selected. The possibility of meeting her son's donor siblings threatened to disrupt some of these accomplishments.

Selecting a Donor

Having tossed out the rulebook in order to become mothers, women who select an anonymous-donor-assisted route to motherhood do not rely solely on the sperm bank's selection to decide on a specific donor.[10] Instead, they develop sorting rules to pick among available donors. As part of their selection process they read paper profiles and turn the abstract stranger into a likable character.

Why a woman selects one donor over others is hard to puzzle out. The way a woman evaluates the many aspects of the donor profiles, calculating how the donor addresses her personal taste as well as her needs, means that there's much more to the choice than just pure, hard facts such as medical history. Almost all women look first to race as a primary determining factor, particularly since the sperm bank has already ruled out men with poor medical histories.[11] Most women choose someone whose appearance is similar to theirs, because they prefer that their child look like them. One woman, Corina Joseph, said, "If my child's only going to have one parent, he might as well look like that parent."

Women also look to the answers on the donor questionnaire to try to create a persona to go along with the physical descriptions. The personal taste of the woman determines how she perceives the importance of the various answers. Sophie laughed when she read that one donor was "proficient at playing the tape deck" (his musical talent), and so she decided right then and there that he was the donor for her. Ultimately, then, the women use these bare-bones profiles to turn a stranger into a likable, real person. The social questions anchor the man in the otherwise abstract world of donor profile descriptions.

Women realize that their child will invariably question the absence of a physical father in her or his life, and thus they make their decisions with an eye to positive and enticing information they can pass along to their child. Through the persona gleaned from the paper profile and other information, a woman can offer her child an identity that includes an imagined father figure (Hertz 2002, 2006). The mothers simply want to be able to, as Nadine Margolis said, "tell [their] kids about him, that he was a nice person, which was better than 'he had blonde hair' or 'green eyes.'"

A woman's selection process thus includes monitoring information to pass onto her children and finding socially acceptable bits of the donor's identity that can be comfortably inserted into the future family. However vague, the donor will thereby "live," to varying degrees, in the mother and child's life together.

Crafting the Donor in a Child's Image

A second stage of monitoring emerges once the child is born. Close observations of the child's gestures, expressions, behaviors, and likes and dislikes help women reconstruct the father. As the child grows, his or her unexplainable traits—from physical attributes to character, behavior, and interests—become attributed to the anonymous donor. That is, "he" may be the source of the child's traits that do not seem to emerge from the maternal line. In this way, the anonymous donor takes on a persona of his own. Although this creation may be more fiction than fact, the mother and child take comfort in giving this father role some meaning in their lives. Once the donor is acknowledged as being unlike other children's fathers, the mother and child begin to create an imagined man who is a positive yet invisible presence. The "nice" man who helped them to become a family makes him a worthy human being, if not an idealized one. In short, as the woman examines and monitors her child, she also transforms the donor into a man and crafts him in her child's image. The presence of the genetic father is a physical reality experienced by the mother through the children. She embraces the donor through embracing her children.[12] Yet without a visual image, women can only guess at the characteristics of the donor they observe in their children. As Nadine Margolis told her twin toddlers, "Mommy's never met him. . . . But he must be very smart and very handsome because look at you." Donor siblings, however, introduce the potential to both affirm and disrupt the mother and child's construction of the donor father.

Working Through the Idea of Donor Siblings

Like Ryan, Sophie's son, Sam, was very curious about his donor. As a precocious seven-year-old, he figured out that his donor's number was a clue that could lead to his paternal kin. As Sophie explained:

> He was very curious about the donor, just the sort of abstract idea that there is a donor, that is very important to him—he hasn't made him into a person. . . . He said at age seven, "Well, if you went to a sperm bank and got

sperm you can't be the only woman who got sperm from this donor." And I said, "You are right." And he said, "So I must have siblings," and he continued, "I want to meet them. How can I meet them?"

Sophie wanted to help her son search for more answers to his paternal identity, which could also confirm the talented, successful paternal line they had crafted. Although she shared Wendy's wish to help her child, Sophie was not sure how she felt about what Sam had figured out. She had created a watertight family (mother-child dyad) with a particular explanation that might be challenged rather than confirmed by the discovery of half siblings. She knew that trying to locate the donor siblings would set into motion a series of events that would require inspection, control, and possibly the need to re-think paternal kin. Sophie had thought the borders of her family were tightly sealed when she selected donor insemination as a route to parenthood. Now, without even the help of a kinship terminology, Sophie would have to figure out how to "name" children who share only biological heredity with her son, and whose mothers are not part of a socially recognized kinship structure (such as polygamy). Since they do not fit within a cultural paradigm for understanding the social relationships of kinship, Sophie would have to be even more vigilant in how she filled the void of paternal kin. The paternal line would have to measure up to what she had crafted. That is, the donor children would have to share traits that everyone could agree come from the paternal line. Sophie hoped that the fantasy of paternal kin would live up to the reality. However, compared to the possibility of meeting blood relatives who are real and physically available people, the imagined father became a less satisfactory link.

Still, Sophie was not willing to grant these blood relatives automatic family membership; she needed to see whether they were worthy. Although she was not exactly sure what "test" they would need to pass, she knew she would have to restrain herself and Sam from automatically welcoming them as kin. Was a sibling claim based on seminal fluid from the same unknown source enough to open the borders of her family life? Although she would have embraced the donor, or at least the donor in the form of the man she and Sam had crafted, there were no guarantees how other donor siblings would turn out. Sophie's embrace of the donor was premised upon her reasoning that "family" shares genetics. Even though there was no relationship between Sophie and the anonymous donor to make them kin, the donor was her child's biogenetic father, or "bio-dad," to use another woman's term. The unanticipated consequences of scientific development and technical know-how created for her a new set of questions about who is and who is not kin.

Nevertheless, Sophie was curious about these donor siblings and, with great trepidation, called the sperm bank she had used:

> I thought, "Shoot—this opens up something so unknown, and I don't know how to put it in my brain." I called the local bank. They told me to call the national bank. It was their catalog that had the donor I had chosen. The administrator I spoke to at this bank said, "Yes, this has become a common question—one that we didn't anticipate. We have this sibling registry." And she told me how I could get onto the registry. She was surprised that Sam was only seven at the time he asked this question because kids don't usually ask until they are twelve or thirteen. So I went to the website and signed up and waited. There was nobody else already registered under this particular donor number and Sam would ask periodically if I checked the website—it wasn't actively on my mind.

Sophie registered on the website because of Sam's push to know more about his paternal kin, thickening the stock of information he already had. Donor siblings were more science fiction than reality for her, as they stood outside anything she knew. Were they the "real thing" or a substitute for paternal kin? Sam legally had no paternal kin; even his birth certificate said "father unknown." However, if individuals who shared the same genetic matter from a common donor came forward, would Sam gain a deeper understanding of himself and, somewhat like Pinocchio, feel transformed?

You've Got Mail

As much as Sophie wanted to help her son search for paternal siblings, she worried about protecting her family's borders from the invasion of strange donor children related to her child. As odd as it might seem, they shared a common thread: the donor's number gave them a genetic tie that she could not overlook. Slowly, however, Sophie began to apply bits of conventional relationship norms as a basis for kin ties. Doing so also meant that she had to change her views on motherhood by coming to terms with the fact that she was not the only woman to have children from her particular donor. Women do not think about other children sired from "their" donor; instead, when they purchase seminal fluid, they think about it as theirs alone. A mother's decision to sign up on websites to meet her child's half siblings entails accepting that the donor is not exclusively hers and that his act of kindness, commercialized by a sperm bank, has resulted in producing other children.

In rethinking motherhood, Sophie was already engaged in a form of monitoring the boundaries of her family since the act of registering the donor's number could electrify the borders of kinship prior to an e-mail answer. Sophie explained that it took two years to receive an e-mail response:

> Two years later we got an e-mail, when Sam was nine. [It said] "Dear Sophie: We have two children by donor number 1360 and we would like to make contact." The "we" is a lesbian couple who turned out to have two children by the same donor as Sam. I waited a little while because I had to digest the news, and then I told Sam, "I have big news." He thought it was work-related, and I said, "It is even bigger news: we heard from somebody who has two girls from donor number 1360." He was ecstatic, jumping up and down. I was more stunned, I was more ambivalent. I had hoped for my sake I never heard from anybody. This was unknown and I was uncomfortable—I didn't know how I would process the information—there is not a cognitive slot for this kind of relationship.

Sophie wanted to feel the same joy as her son over finding "family," but she was at a "moment of pinch," or discrepancy between what she wanted to feel and what she actually felt (Hochschild 1979, 562). She reminded herself that her confusion at that moment was okay, as her situation was uncharted territory. She redoubled her efforts to be cautious since there was much at stake—meeting these people could disappoint her and Sam's expectations of close kinship or result in the unraveling of her fabrication of her son's donor family. Indeed, one of the reasons women like Sophie turn to anonymous donors is because it is a way to take control of their lives, after years of feeling that motherhood is dependent on a man and marriage. Women say that an anonymous donor is less "messy" than a known donor because a known donor might change his mind and want more of a relationship with the child than the original contractual agreement specified. Now Sophie, in spite of her previous choice of an unknown donor, had the potential for a messy situation. This possibility made her uncomfortable. She alone was the gatekeeper, patrolling the borders of her small family: "I kept thinking, what if they have one digit off, because then they would mean nothing. This news could mean everything or nothing. It is so abstract. If they have the right number my son has two sisters and if they are one number off my son has nothing. It just seemed so enormous."

Sophie knew that she had to reframe her thinking if she wanted the possibility of paternal kin for her son. The ideology of "two sides of a family" (maternal and paternal) outweighed her other concerns. Although she never said so directly, the family narrative that "male and female gametes make a baby" was the catalyst for responding to the e-mail.[13]

Sophie was relieved that the e-mail sender was not part of a hetero-sexual couple. This way none of the three children had a social dad, an important parallel between the siblings. A social dad might trump a genetic donor and make the half siblings less important to some of them. Sophie explained the social importance of a paternal tie with no legal "dad" who can offer up his family as a paternal substitute: "Since neither of our kids had dads, that seemed to be an important issue. It was important to me in terms of Sam's comfort or the feeling of Sam feeling comfortable with his sisters. Sam's not having a dad is a significant part of his identity and not necessarily bad, but he is fully aware of it. The sisters shared the same position as he did by not having a dad, but also having the same donor."

This news allowed Sophie to feel more comfortable because both families shared one of the same circumstances. Rapidly more of Sophie's fears dissolved: "I sent them a picture of Sam. And then they sent me pictures in the follow-up e-mail. And then it was absolutely unquestionable because the older daughter looked just like Sam. We were all amazed by the resemblance."

Siblings as Windows

Sophie immediately realized that Sam's half siblings were indeed his, and that there was no chance of being "one digit off." She was in awe of the donor's genetic imprint clearly stamped and immediately recognizable in the children's photos. When I asked specifically what traits they shared, she told me, "They both really like math, they both are really kind—being nice is really important to them. [The other mother and I] would have phone conversations, and I would go, 'Oh my God, Sam, too.'" Sophie could see even more similarities in the photos: "The way they hold their bodies, the way they move their bodies, the gesture and facial expressions are the same. It is remarkable." The unanswered gesture that caught a mother's attention now appears in the half sibling, confirming its belonging to the paternal side.

Sophie could now see the donor through the siblings. Meanwhile, Sam had a revelation of his own: he could see himself in his half sisters. He no longer had to rely only on his mother for assurance and help in imagining how his donor might see him. Now he had sisters who would reinforce the self-identity he wanted. He saw traits in his half siblings that he recognized.

Photos were not enough, however; he wanted to meet the girls to find out firsthand what else they might have in common.

As Wendy, the founder of the donor-sibling website, told me (and as various Internet blogs confirm), some families only exchange photographs, and that is enough. Others decide to extend the relationship to another level of intimacy. Sophie and Sam's decision to meet the other family would disclose even more common ground between the children.

The Frontier of New Families: Opening the Borders

Sophie was initially ambivalent about Sam's having paternal kin, but her son was eager to meet the other family. She didn't want to let him down, but she also wanted to make sure this family passed "the test" before meeting them. Talking on the phone was a way that she could keep a distance while gathering information. Sophie wanted to like the family because these were the people raising the only paternal kin Sam knew. When Sophie picked up the phone to call them, she was nervous about how to proceed, even though she hoped for a genuine connection. The phone conversation was a search for finding commonality so that she could share her son's enthusiasm and reduce her vigilance. Sophie was listening for something that would lead her to incorporate these strangers into her family or at least give her a reason to want to get to know them more. Sophie relayed the conversation to me this way:

> She [one of the donor siblings' mothers] seemed to be right on the mark in what was important and interesting, and she spoke about Sam's siblings in ways that I talk about him, emphasizing the same aspects of what is important about him as a person. She asked questions that I thought were interesting, and there were similar values in terms of describing their personalities. We both selected the same traits to explain our children to each other. We were amazed at the same sorts of things about our children. I especially liked that we both approached the issue of having really smart children in the same way—it seemed important to say they were smart but not braggy.

Sophie was intrigued and comforted by the fact that she and Jess and Amanda, the mothers of the half siblings, shared "similar values in terms of describing their personalities." That similarity is part of what enticed Sophie to pursue the relationship. She needed something familiar and affirming to help her want to open the borders of her family to include this family. And

Sophie found this affirmation in her new knowledge that the donor siblings were also "bright" children. If the donor siblings shared the traits of the imagined father that Sophie and her son had crafted, then she would further her claim that the donor was a "good man." It would help her confirm that she made a good choice when she sorted through the paper profiles to find the right donor.

Sam and the older daughter (age seven) talked by phone once their mothers finished talking, and the children continued to talk by phone weekly. Since both families lived on the East Coast, they decided to meet in a public spot between each family's home. Sophie recalled that day in detail, as it gave her clarity on how she felt about her son's newfound family.

> We decided we all really liked each other. I really liked the way they were with their kids (balance between letting them do what they want and setting limits). I loved Sam and [the] girls together. All three of us [mothers] were very cautious. But we really are in this relationship on behalf of our children. It had to do with our kids, not us. We all had a stake in this relationship between the kids, but as the day went on I realized we (myself and the girls' two moms) shared a lot in common, and I thought, "I like them." At one point I said to Jess, "Oh my God. We are so lucky," and she said, "I know." And she said that she said the same thing to Amanda. They are women I could be friendly with. We all had the same concern: would we get along and like one another? And how would we negotiate this because we were going to have to have a relationship on behalf of the kids, because they are siblings.

These families bond around their social similarity (e.g., shared values, social class, employment status). Of course, the women who turn to sperm banks as a route to motherhood often share the same social class position from the start.[14] Still, it is possible that Sophie might not have liked this family, or that the family might not have liked her and Sam. For instance, if Sophie had been homophobic or if Sam's half sisters had a social dad that made Sam feel jealous, Sophie might have revised her position, deciding after one meeting not to make additional plans. Sam and Sophie also could have disagreed about liking this family.

While finding donor siblings relieves women of the "emotional labor" of imagining the paternal donor, at the same time mothers must monitor these new relationships.[15] Sophie and Sam met Sam's donor sibling family a second time over the summer in Boston at Sophie's home. This time they recognized that they were establishing a level of closeness reserved for kin members. As much as these families were "choosing" one another to be kin

(Weston 1991), they were creating the presence of paternity based on so-cially engineered relationships that have no legal basis or even definitive sci-entific basis. For instance, no one suggested taking a DNA test or viewing the donor profiles to make sure they matched:

> It was really easy and relaxing and the kids were adorable together, really acting like siblings: got into a little fight—they were siblings. The level of comfort and the ongoing relationship is amazing. We all presume the relationships are important, but also intimacy was there immediately. This relationship is very important and the children say they love each other. Sam said, "I don't miss my father any more now that I have sisters." So, this has been profound for him to discover something about his paternal side and have a connection on that side. It ends what in some ways is a mystery: who is this guy? He can see himself through viewing his sisters.

Sam and Sophie stayed at Jess and Amanda's house on the third visit together, and it was during that trip that Sophie realized, as she told me, "I have fallen in love with [Jess and Amanda] and their children." However, So-phie also reminds herself that she needs to be vigilant and delineate between her child's kin and her own kin:

> My family boundaries are very solid and unambiguous. Sam is not their son and they are not my daughters. It does not even feel like they are nieces. They feel like my son's siblings, and this is a new psychological construct. I do not feel like I am in any way their parent, like I might to an extent if I had stepchildren. I am not a stepmother. These children are none of my business as a stepparent role assumes some degree of respon-sibility and authority, and I don't feel like I have either of those. . . . Now, almost a year later, [this situation] feels natural and normal, but for quite a while—I remember the very first time Sam and I spoke with them, and he said, "I am emotionally exhausted," and I said so was I. This is so new that I had to carve a new place in my mind for these relationships to go.

Sophie's story thus suggests that donor siblings change the interior of family life for single mothers who choose artificial insemination from an anonymous donor. Instead of guessing about paternal traits, other donor kin substantiate (or refute) Sam's socially constructed paternal identity. Sophie and Sam have formed a new kind of extended family with Jess and Amanda and their two children. Yet they may not be close kin. Donor siblings and their respective mothers may become important to each other, but they may remain distant kin. Even though Sam and his half sisters are close genetic relatives, and even though Sophie does embrace the girls and their mothers as family, a year after receiving the initial e-mail, she still locates them more as distant cousins. She knows they will stay in touch and visit sporadically, but they will not be family members that routinely tell each other everything, nor will her feelings toward these children be as close or similar to the closeness she has with her best girlfriend's children. These women are not co-mothers to each other's children, yet Sophie is grateful for their presence in her and her son's life. In short, Sophie's monitoring (and Sam's immediate acceptance of the girls) led her to conclude that these are good people. But they are also "Sam's siblings and their parents," not Sophie and Sam's kin.

Not All Happy Stories

Wendy and Ryan have not been so lucky. All matches are not "love-fests." Twice they heard about potential half siblings, but neither case had resulted in a meaningful or exploratory family connection, despite a common donor. One teenager figured out she was Ryan's half sister, but her mother forbade her from further contact with Ryan. For now that teenager has obeyed her mother, who does not want their nuclear family disrupted. The mother, single when she had her daughter, had married, and her husband had adopted Ryan's half sister, accepting her as his own child. Male infertility caused another couple to become pregnant using a donor, which produced two half siblings who were toddlers at the time of my research. The wife saw Ryan on television and wanted him to know she had birthed two children related to him. She and her husband were not sure when or if they would tell their young children about the use of a donor to create their family. The mothers in these donor-sibling families are vigilant keepers of a certain kind of blood-kin nuclear family, even if that family was created by seminal fluid from a donor. These are examples of tightly woven secrets and legal ties that the adults do not want to alter. Ryan remains hopeful that other siblings will someday appear.[16]

Conclusion: Reimaging Kinship through "Extraordinary Extended Families"

Sophie's decision to become a single mother may have initially been a choice about a route to motherhood that appeared to give her control over family life and to reduce the amount of monitoring she would have to do. However, even though she engaged in monitoring when she selected a donor and then again when she noticed behaviors in her child that might be linked to biological paternal traits, it was the surprising possibility of searching for donor siblings that presented Sophie with a new issue of monitoring. Donor siblings might mean that she and her child would open up the borders of their watertight family to a potentially messy situation. Borders are monitored in order to watch the coming and going of people who fall into different categories (whether temporary or permanent occupants). Activity on the border (such as contact through the Internet) presupposes that some people might want in, and allowing outsiders in can be risky. Donor siblings might reinforce the mother's or child's vision of paternal kin; however, real individuals might also provide revisions or alternatives to imagined donors. Donor siblings might also provide additional ways for a child to figure out pieces of his or her self-identity, which previously rested only on the mothers' assessments; this new information might not be welcome.

Donor siblings share biogenetic matter and nothing else. This is a "pure" case in which blood roots family. This basis of family emerges at a time when other sociological directions (such as fictive kin, chosen kin, etc.) have become a test tube for family inclusion. That is, "social kin" challenge the traditional idea of family relatives as related only by blood or marriage (and adoption). The claim (and obligation) of donor siblings as relatives is without any shared family history or initial consensus as part of a socially chosen group, making this new blood family difficult to grasp. The women, who cleverly traced paternal blood kin through the Internet, have good reasons for worrying about how and in what ways to embrace these strangers as relatives. Donor siblings ended up as genetic kin arbitrarily, a by-product of the rise of reproductive clinics.

It is the children that join these mothers together in a loosely knit family, not as co-parents but as women who share children from the same purchased product. A biological connection might allow donor siblings temporary family membership while they go through a trial period before possible acceptance. However, genetics alone does not make people kin. For example, donor siblings who only exchange photos over the Internet establish shared genes that satisfy curiosity and nothing more. They may say they have found half siblings, but "sibling" is a social relationship as well as a biological one. We have no language for Internet lookers, those individuals who leave after seeing their physical resemblance in another person. Even if these individual families meet, they are still not automatic family. Donor-sibling families gauge each other (as a group and as individuals) as they try to find consensus about how they will be together. The possibility exists that they will not agree. The process of learning about new kin makes family a complicated interplay of genetics, social interaction, and cultural expectations.

So far Sophie's decisions are in line with the needs and desires of the others involved. However, the possibility of conflict is huge. Sophie and Sam could have disagreed about liking the new kin. Or if both Sophie and Sam did not like this family, they could have kept their names on the website list hoping another family, one they might click with, would answer their request. Sam may want to meet other donor siblings, but his mother may not want the added responsibility of multiple families and relationships to manage with more donor-sibling kin. When do the mother and child take their names off the list and stop searching for more donor siblings? And what if Sophie took her name off the list, but Jess and Amanda did not, and they discovered more donor siblings? Would Sophie and Sam feel obligated to open up the borders of their family to the donor-sibling families discovered by the donor-sibling family they had already embraced?

Donor children who have met their donors or donor siblings have entered a new world in which social obligations and responsibilities are murky. Family citizenship is not automatic. Donor siblings (such as Sam and his sisters) have no legal rights or obligations to one another, nor does their anonymous donor, should he come forward. Further, a sperm donor might have a legal birth daughter and donor children. What is their relationship? Are they half siblings? Genetically they are, but socially how will these families determine the boundaries of who qualifies as kin and in what ways? If the donor meets his donor child, is he just a genetic father, or will he become something more: a dad? And, if so, will the partner of the donor and the donor child's mom weigh in—and what will their relationship be? These have become sociological issues that are at the nexus of how blood kin becomes accepted. Are donor children equal family members, or are they second-class citizens only marginally included at the dinner table? The ways in which families develop guidelines for embracing their genetic kin who fall outside conventional reproductive narratives will be fascinating to observe over the coming years.

Notes

I thank Alyssa Thomas for her research assistance. Peggy Nelson and Anita Garey's excellent comments strengthened this chapter. However, I take full responsibility for the contents.
1. Between 1995 and 2004, I interviewed sixty-five women about their families (Hertz 2006). I interviewed each woman, on average, two to three times.
2. Aside from Wendy Kramer, founder of *www.donorsiblingregistry.com*, all names in this chapter are the pseudonyms I used in my book. Fifteen women became pregnant using anonymous sperm donors, and thirteen women became

pregnant using known donors. I only discuss the known donors as a contrast in limited ways in this chapter.

3. For blog commentary, see, for example, *www.mothering.com.*

4. See also Naples (2001) on death in her family, a lifecycle event that sets in motion a rethinking of inclusion and exclusion of family members as boundaries are redefined and alliances are reworked.

5. For instance, single strangers who desire to attract a romantic partner or date can register on sites such as eHarmony or JDate. The dating sites offer seekers a fast and easy way to find a "match" using their desired qualities and from the comfort of their own home. Slowly, these sites are beginning to replace the local "looking for" magazine ads for single individuals.

6. Wendy and her husband, who divorced when Ryan was one year old, had fertility problems. They turned to donor sperm to have a child.

7. Fertility banks code donors using a number tracking system. Buyers purchase the gametes of a specific donor using this number. Most women buy enough vials to last through three to six months of fertility treatment; no one, however, knew if they bought out a donor's entire "stock." Since the banks are self-regulated, they can decide how long a donor can contribute his gametes. Even if a buyer purchases all the available vials from a specific donor, she has no way of knowing whether the donor will continue to donate. Women do not know whether (or how many) other children were born from that same donor.

8. Sometime after 2000 the major sperm banks also added donor registries, and their website policy statements changed to allow for the *possibility* that, if both donor and offspring expressed interest in contact, sperm bank personnel would try to facilitate this. This is not a guarantee that donors will reveal their identity. See Spar (2006), who argues that human reproduction has become a $3 billion annual industry. An estimated 30,000 children are born in this country each year to mothers who have been artificially inseminated with sperm from an anonymous donor. This multimillion sperm bank industry, built on anonymity, is beginning to talk about proposing a national registry.

9. These websites point to the need for U.S. social policies surrounding donor anonymity. Presently, other countries have established donor registries (such as Britain, Canada, the Netherlands, New Zealand, Sweden, and Switzerland) banning anonymous sperm donors. At age eighteen, a child born using donated gametes can go to the registry, look up his or her donor, and contact the donor. These registries give children the right to know who their genetic father is, placing the rights of the children as the priority. The United States needs to establish a national registry.

10. Sperm banks offer both the men who donate sperm and the women or couples who purchase the gametes legal protection via "a system of bilateral ignorance of paternity among donors and recipients" (Sullivan 2004, 53). The donors leave behind a paper profile and a promise to never lay claim to the children that result from insemination. The women I interviewed settled for this arrangement. Sullivan (2004), who studied lesbian couples, observes that the erasure of paternity easily allows for second-parent adoption among the lesbian couples she interviewed. The second mother can become the second parent

without another person relinquishing parental rights, as I note about known donors (Hertz 2002, 2006). However, only a few states allow for adoption by a second parent. Interestingly, all but one of Sullivan's couples were able to secure "yes" donors, which meant that these children could someday meet their genetic father. The women I interviewed discovered that these donors were in such high demand that they were unavailable. Unwilling to wait for "yes" donor gametes, they ultimately selected donors who would forever remain anonymous.

11. While sperm banks have a large number of white donor profiles, donors of color are few. At the time of my study, the major bank listed Hispanic, Asian and black donor categories, but within each of these broad racial groups there were only two or three donors. Women of color in my study reported few options, something they found frustrating because they wanted donors to share their race.

12. See Hertz (2002) for a conceptualization of Cooley's (1902) "looking glass self" and its importance to these mother-child relationships.

13. I asked Sophie if she asked the girls' moms why they decided to contact her. Sophie told me they were curious because they had friends who had had a positive experience meeting other donor siblings.

14. While we have only anecdotal information, the individuals who purchase gametes are most likely middle- and upper-middle class. They most likely have medical insurance and are able to afford the cost of the gametes and the medical procedures (e.g., new reproductive technologies) that may be necessary to become pregnant.

15. Hochschild (1979) discusses an interactive account of emotional management beyond the scope of this chapter.

16. On prime time television in 2007, after this chapter was written, Ryan did meet a half sibling.

References

Cooley, Charles Horton. 1902. *Human Nature and the Social Order*. Repr., New Brunswick, NJ: Transaction Publishers, 1983.

Fox, Susannah, Janna Quitney Anderson, and Rainie Lee. 2005. *The Future of the Internet*. Washington, DC: Pew Internet and American Life Project.

Hertz, Rosanna. 2002. The Father as an Idea: A Challenge to Kinship Boundaries by Single Mothers. *Symbolic Interaction* 25 (1): 1–31.

———. 2006. *Single by Chance, Mothers by Choice: How Women Are Choosing Parenthood without Marriage and Creating the New American Family*. New York: Oxford University Press.

Hochschild, Arlie. 1979. Emotion Work, Feeling Rules and Social Structure. *American Journal of Sociology* 85 (3): 551–75.

Naples, Nancy A. 2001. A Member of the Funeral: An Introspective Ethnography. In *Queer Families, Queer Politics: Challenging Culture and the State*, edited by Mary Bernstein and Renate Reinmann, 21–43. New York: Columbia University Press.

Nelson, Margaret K. 2006. Single Mothers "Do" Family. *Journal of Marriage and Family* 68 (4): 781–95.

Plotz, David. 2005. *Genius Factory: The Curious History of the Nobel Prize Sperm Bank*. New York: Random House.

Schmidt, Matthew, and Lisa Jean Moore. 1998. Constructing a "Good Catch," Picking a Winner: The Development of Techno-Semen and the Deconstruction of the Monolithic Male. In *Syborg Babies: From Techno-sex to Techno-tots*, edited by Robbie Davis-Floyd and Joseph Dumit, 21–39. New York: Routledge.

Spar, Debora L. 2006. *The Baby Business: How Money, Science, and Politics Drive the Commerce of Conception*. Cambridge, MA: Harvard Business School Press.

Strauss, Anselm L. 1959. *Mirrors and Masks*. Glencoe, IL: Free Press.

Sullivan, Maureen. 2004. *The Family of Woman: Lesbian Mothers, Their Children, and the Undoing of Gender*. Berkeley: University of California Press.

Weston, Kath. 1991. *Families We Choose*. New York: Columbia University Press.

9

The Powers
of Parental Observation

Constructing Networks of Care

Karen V. Hansen

Parents are expected to vigilantly observe their children and those who interact with them; they accept the task of careful monitoring as part of responsible parenting. In turn, others observe parents as they rear their children. Once children are in school, parents have less control over their children's environments and less ability to see interactions firsthand. Nonetheless, parents continue to monitor and screen people as they construct networks of care.

This chapter explores the ins and outs of this process of monitoring as parents exercise their prerogative to include and exclude other adults from their children's lives. Simply being related, being a good friend, or living nearby is not sufficient to qualify a person to become a member of a network of care. However, a shared philosophy of child rearing is indispensable. Parents seek to establish a firm basis for trusting the care of their children to adults they know only superficially, if at all. Screening potential members—kin and non-kin—for networks of care is a long, ongoing, and subtle process.

In this chapter, I investigate a specific kind of network: one focused on helping parents care for their school-age children. As a society in which 79 percent of mothers with children ages six to seventeen are in the labor force and there is an inadequate supply of before- and after-school programs, we face a "care gap" for elementary school children. The Annie E. Casey Foundation (1998) estimates the difference between school hours and parents' working hours to be as high as twenty to twenty-five hours per week. My research explores how working parents in several economic locations construct networks of people (rather than institutions alone) to cover that gap.

I define a network of care as that group of people identified by an anchor—the person at the absolute center of the child-rearing project (in this research, a parent)—that helps rear a child. Some segments of the networks of care operate regularly and predictably; others are on standby, ready to be activated when necessary. Some networks are more robust and pliable; others are thin and brittle. In the end, these networks of care may not furnish the greatest absolute number of hours a child spends with a nonparent (although they may). Nonetheless, the networks are significant because they help to create a larger margin of safety than would otherwise exist for the children and to cultivate a greater sense of possibility in the world for the anchors.

Methods

My objective was to understand the internal processes of networks, something that could be accomplished only through qualitative, in-depth interviews or fieldwork. These networks are not intended to be representative of the anchors' class positions, their particular child-care arrangements, or the division of labor within the network. They are intended to provide insight into the *internal dynamics* of these specialized networks of care, situated in particular social and economic locations.

At the end of my first interview with each anchor, I asked her or him to enumerate those who were involved in caring directly for the children and those who provided emotional or practical support or advice to the anchor. The lists generated by anchors include those involved in the geographic orbit of daily life (Holloway and Valentine 2000): neighbors, grandmothers, friends, uncles, aunts, babysitters, and nannies. The networks include primary caregivers (those who spend a significant amount of time with the child and are high on the list of who to contact in an emergency) and secondary caregivers (those who spend less time with the child and are more peripheral). I then interviewed each person identified about his or her role in the network.

This chapter is based on interviews in northern California with forty people who constitute four separate networks of care. Three networks are anchored by a woman, and the fourth by co-anchors, a man and a woman, who jointly coordinate the care of their children. Of the network interviews, six are with children—three boys and three girls—and thirty-four are with adults, approximately one-third with men and two-thirds with women. All of the network anchors and most of the network members are white; each of the four networks occupies a different class location.

Profiles of Networks

The Cranes: A Culture of Family Resilience

The Crane network extends its long reach across four generations, with Patricia Crane at its heart.[1] The network cares for Patricia's six-year-old son, Robbie, as well as Patricia's mother, Fran, and grandmother, Louise. Patricia now lives with Fran and Robbie in a one-bedroom apartment in a poor section of the city, about two hours from the lettuce fields where she grew up and previously worked. The single-story, mission-style apartment building in which they live functions as a small community, one that has had its share of battles with drug trafficking, addiction, and economic hardship. Patricia's nineteen-year-old son, who has a different father than Robbie, is in federal prison. Patricia's brother, Ben, a foreman at a tree cutting service, lives a couple of doors down from Patricia in the same apartment complex. Patricia's network for Robbie's care consists of her mother; her brother; her next-door neighbor, Tracy Johnson; and the father of her son, Robert Sr. As Patricia tells it, Fran has taken care of Robbie since his birth, and Tracy is the only non-family member who has ever cared for him.

When I first interviewed Patricia, she was working two part-time jobs, one in sanitary maintenance at a truck stop and one as a driver at a car auction. Most mornings, Patricia takes her son to the bus stop across the street from their apartment in the mid-morning. After school, when Patricia is at work, either Patricia's mother, Fran, or her brother, Ben, picks Robbie up at the bus stop and takes him to Fran's house so she can watch him without leaving Patricia's grandmother, Louise, alone. On the mornings that Patricia has to leave early, Tracy takes over Robbie's care. Tracy has become a close friend of Patricia's, and she reported that her four children have embraced Robbie as one of their family. Several evenings a week, Ben cares for Robbie while Patricia works the swing shift. Ben, tall and robust with a winning bright smile, identifies himself as the on-site male role model, although he characterizes his relationship with Robbie as more that of a brother than of an uncle or father.

Patricia's method of constructing a network for Robbie involved moving in order to be near her mother. The move pulled Robbie out of the daily orbit of his father, but not out of his influence or participation. Far from being an absent father, Robert is an active participant in Robbie's life and an important parenting partner to Patricia. He sees Robbie at least one weekend a month and for longer stretches of time in the summer. Patricia says that Robert, who was a close friend of her eldest brother growing up, has been her best friend since high school. And although they have never been married, they have lived together and unequivocally share the project of raising Robbie. He is psychologically involved and emotionally available, and he has his own network ready to provide transportation or whatever is needed at a moment's notice. Both parents agree that when Robbie needs more structure and discipline, Robert's home is the place to be. Robert is Patricia's hedge against having Robbie repeat the mistakes of his older brother.

This network of caregivers struggles with the limitations of its financial resources and its vulnerability to health crises. Paid employment must be molded to the contingencies of life, while government support systems (such as Social Security, disability benefits, and Temporary Assistance for Needy Families), however inadequate, function as a genuine safety net. In this context, family comes first and provides the central stays of support, although it does not operate in isolation (Nelson 2005). As Tracy puts it, she and Patricia have a "buddy-buddy system" that makes each woman's parenting more effective and alleviates some of her respective stress.

The Beckers: A Culture of Helping

The second network, the Beckers, is anchored in a solidly middle-class family in a diverse and large urban center. The Becker network is wealthy in its people resources and moderate in its income. At the center is Dina Becker, a freelance photographer. Her husband, Mark Walde, is a school teacher, and they have two children, Donalyn, age eight, and Aaron, age six. Their system for rearing children is built around a shift strategy (Garey 1999; Hertz 1986; Hertz and Charlton 1989; Presser 1988) and buttressed by considerable kin help. Dina works at home during the day and hands over the children to Mark when he walks in the door between four and five o'clock. Mark then feeds the children, bathes them, and puts them to bed while Dina meets with clients and deals with the complicated details of her work. Because a big part of her business involves shooting weddings, she works most weekends as well as evenings.

It is no wonder that when I asked Dina what word best describes her network, she said "family." A majority of Dina's sizable family of origin lives within a five-mile radius and participates in her network of care. In fact, her network is composed entirely of kin: her mother, her father, her two brothers, and three of her sisters. The critical mass of family members ready and willing to help her out means she does not hire babysitters of any type.

And although she had previously drawn a close friend with same-aged children into her child-rearing project, the friend moved to a different town, thus ending the ease of collaboration and exchange in everyday life. Dina lives in the same city where she grew up. Her childhood home, where her mother and father still live, is less than five minutes away and serves as the geographic center of the Becker network. At a moment's notice, Dina can call her father or brother to pick up her son from school and confidently expect them to cover for her. The Beckers have cultivated a strong sense of familism. Everyone is expected to help each other because it is part of their family culture.

Although I describe the Beckers as middle class, people within the network have a range of resources and, compared to her parents, Dina is downwardly mobile. So rather than experiencing middle-class comfort, she and Mark experience middle-class anxiety—a sense of just barely hanging onto their place on the economic ladder (Newman 1999). In this context her motivation for combining a family network with a shift child-care arrangement with her husband makes sense: "If you have to pay for child care, that would just push us right over the—we would not be able to try for this new house." The network makes more possible and makes life richer for her, Mark, and their children. But the dark circles around Dina's eyes belie her sense of calm. Even with a robust network of sixteen hands, Dina and Mark have traded time with each other for time with the children and for the savings that parental and kin care allows. Marrying Dina meant marrying her family, which in Mark's estimation was a huge bonus. But the shift arrangement means the couple sees little of each other, and it means no down time.

The Duvall-Brennans: A Culture Torn between Careers and Intensive Parenting

The third network, the Duvall-Brennans, is well off financially but stretched extremely thin in terms of people. When I asked Maggie Duvall what word she would use to characterize her network, she said "inadequate." It is anchored by Maggie and her husband, Jack Brennan, both of whom are full-time attorneys. They have two children: Danielle, who is six and in kindergarten, and Scott, who is three and in a day care center full-time. Maggie and Jack are active co-parents and co-anchors of the network, sharing the psychological as well as organizational work of rearing the children and running the household.

Maggie and Jack's caregiving network consists of Jack's brother and his domestic partner, three former neighbors, two friends from Maggie's women's group, and Jack's sister, who lives on the East Coast. The network list is substantial (it includes eight people in addition to Jack and Maggie), but it has limited resilience. As in other studies of middle-class dual earners (Hertz 1986), an air of resignation to the overwhelming demands of career and parenthood hangs over them both. They try to schedule time for exercise and friendship, but neither fits easily into an already full schedule. Their child-care strategy has changed as their children have grown and developed. In light of their needs as full-time attorneys with little workplace flexibility, and in the absence of help from their own families, institutional care was the only dependable solution that would ensure their ability to work and the safety and well-being of Scott and Danielle. Although the children have full-time institutional care, the Duvall-Brennans still need an informal network. Both Maggie and Jack can make the commute to work in about an hour each way if there are no accidents or traffic jams, but there are no such guarantees. After six months in their new upscale neighborhood, they know virtually no neighbors. The slightest disruption to their carefully crafted schedule can and does precipitate an emergency.

The children are in child care or school approximately ten hours a day. At the same time, both Maggie and Jack feel they are "skating" (Jack's term) on their jobs in order to accommodate family life. Because they prioritize family, they do not work the sixty-to-eighty hours per week that is standard for attorneys. They feel they are barely holding their work and family lives together. From their perspectives, they are challenging the office culture and the expected workload by shaving time off both ends of each day and by not taking work home on nights and weekends. As a result, they feel inadequate as workers and as parents.

The Aldriches: A Culture of Philanthropy and Service

The Aldrich network reveals a glimpse into profoundly different circumstances. The anchor, Sarah Aldrich, describes herself as a "woman of means, involved in the community." She grew up in a family whose wealth dates back well into the nineteenth century, and that has wielded influence in education, environmentalism, and politics in the state of California. She is the mother of two children, Kimberly, age fourteen, and Jacob, age eleven. After seventeen years of marriage, Sarah separated from her husband, Alex Brolin, about a year and a half before I first interviewed her. They have a joint-custody arrangement in which the children spend half of their time at each parent's home. The separation made the logistics of child rearing much more complicated, even though Alex lives only two miles away. Like many women with inherited wealth (Daniels 1988; Ostrander 1984), Sarah has numerous philanthropic commitments and responsibilities that amount to more than a full-time job. She works as a trustee on boards of four educational and cultural institutions around the greater Bay Area, and she chairs two of them. She spends at least twenty hours a week as chair of the board of her son's school. Most of Sarah's professional work is unpaid; the exception is her position as the chair of the board of the "family office," a corporate entity that pools investment money from members of the extended family and also organizes collective extended-family vacations and gatherings. Sarah says she has cut back dramatically on her board work since the separation from her husband in order to be home more with the children. Alex, a developer, also has major board commitments, primarily related to environmental issues.

Sarah's network of care includes her full-time nanny (who does not live with the family), her mother, her best friend, the mother of her son's best friend, her husband, and a babysitter who has worked for her approximately once a week for ten years. In mooring her network, Sarah has hired an absolutely top-notch nanny—who also serves as Sarah's right hand—and Sarah goes to great lengths to keep the nanny satisfied with her job by providing good pay and positive working conditions. Sarah's mother, Jane Aldrich, covers cracks in the caregiving system rather than playing center stage. Members of the Aldrich network take the children to and from school, run them to lessons and games, and occasionally babysit. In addition, Kate, Sarah's best friend, makes herself available to discuss the challenges and joys of child rearing. Hired help also assists in running the household—a housekeeper two days a week, gardeners, and the like—but Sarah does not include them as part of her network of care. She describes herself as being at the high end of the delegating-work continuum.

For all this help, the glue of the system is April, the nanny. April is a vivacious thirty-year-old woman who picks the children up from school and shepherds them to their various extracurricular activities—primarily dance for Kimberly and sports for Jacob. Importantly, in the midst of the separation between Alex and Sarah, April is the "stuff pony." That term is her way of describing her responsibility in transporting the children and their belongings back and forth between Sarah's and Alex's houses. In part because of her enormous planning responsibilities, and in larger part because of her solid, loving relationship with each of the children, April is indispensable in making this complex shared-custody arrangement work. She anticipates needs in both households and acts as an advocate for the children.

Like all families with working parents, the Aldriches feel the pinch of inadequate coverage at times, the pull between work and the needs of the children. Sarah Aldrich has effectively set up a network, using her considerable monetary resources and her skills as a loyal and dependable friend, to rear her children and to ease the tensions of a failing marriage.

The Social Construction of Network Candidacy

Who is eligible to be part of a network of care? Parents have a long list of questions and various litmus tests to screen candidates and determine who is worthy of joining their intimate circle and possessing key caregiving responsibilities. Parents observe others closely and make judgments based on how they act and what they say.

Kinship

Across the economic spectrum, the involvement of extended kin is shaped by beliefs about families and about the roles that family members and other adults should play in the life of a child. The simple fact of kinship doesn't elevate someone to be a network member. Even if kinship is privileged in parents' conceptions of potential caregivers, kin have to be screened just like everyone else. The networks vary in how they view asking for child-care help from non-kin as opposed to extended kin. The middle-class Beckers and the working-class Cranes adopt a "family first" approach. They expect family members to provide that help. As Kent Becker, Dina's brother, puts it, "You always got to be able to just call the family." The professional, middle-class Duvall-Brennans, however, are geographically distant from other family members, who do not in any case take a great deal of interest in the Duvall-Brennan children; they operate on a principle of "family in the last instance." The upper-class Aldriches value family history and family ties, but they do not rely on family members for child care, and they expect to pay for the help they need rearing their children. Their reliance on paid caregivers reflects an emphasis on the managerial dimension of child rearing and expresses a confidence in the anchor's ability to influence the children via the babysitter, regardless of how much time she spends with them herself.

Giving family members and family matters priority is not something that happens naturally or inevitably. The Beckers clearly honor family, but this is an ethic the senior Beckers, Peter and Susan, purposely developed with their children. The Becker siblings, in turn, have taught their own children to recognize and act upon the importance of family. Dina Becker's sister Michaela explains the approach: "People will say, like, at certain times, 'After family, there's nothing.' Or, you know, like, 'Family is gonna be with you when you're at your deathbed.'. . . or, like, Lila [my other sister] will say to her kids, you know, 'That's your sister. You need to look after your sister. You are her ally. You guys need to be good to each other.' " The Beckers' strong family culture extends beyond helping in a crisis to encompass routine aspects of daily life. In addition to providing the sort of overt instruction Lila gives her daughter, the Becker clan reinforces the family ethic in frequent, fun-filled family gatherings.

Kinship, however, does not guarantee membership in a network. In all four networks, some biological kin are included as network members, some are not; some kin are trusted, some are not; some kin are considered reliable—sure to be there when times get tough—some are not. Even in networks that embrace the "family first" ethic, genealogical kinship status does not automatically grant kinship privileges and responsibilities. This constructed quality of kin relationships (Schneider 1978; Weston 1991) became apparent periodically in the lack of mention of certain relatives during the interviews I conducted with network members. When I noticed these glaring absences in the list of network members, I asked additional questions. Patricia Crane, for instance, talked freely about her brother Ben, but offered no information about her other three brothers until I inquired directly. She told me that one brother calls her occasionally; she has no contact with the other two. And among her still-living maternal aunts and uncles, Patricia remains in touch with two aunts. One uncle, who lives nearby, she described as "bad news." She has no interest in hearing from him. None of these relatives is part of the landscape of Patricia's everyday life, nor do any participate in her network of care.

Tracy, Patricia's neighbor, who has eight biological brothers and eight biological sisters, is similarly selective in calling on kin for help. She counts only two sisters and one brother as part of her network. Musing over what makes these three siblings special, Tracy said, "Maybe because we have the same mom, probably. I don't know. I don't think so." She went on to say that the two sisters in her network are her best friends. One of her brothers, in contrast, she dismisses as too self-centered to be trusted with her children's care.

> I have another brother here; I'm not close to him. Actually, I can't even stand him. Neither can my other brothers, but he's my dad's son. I can't say that's the reason, because my little sister is my dad's daughter. But that doesn't mean a thing to me. I just can't stand him. . . . He's greedy. . . . He can eat two steaks, two pork chops, a skillet of potatoes, four eggs, and bread. [*laughs*] And my children could stand there and watch him, and he would never offer them anything. Really, he's greedy.

By contrast, Tracy explains how Patricia's approach to the world and to her children has won Tracy's trust. Each views the other as prepared to "do anything" to help. "I like to share things," Tracy explains, "and if I have it, hey, it's yours—just like Patricia. Go right ahead." She claims she developed this generosity with selected people as a defense against her family of origin, which was decidedly *not* generous. She characterizes her father as "a stingy person, and he's out to get whatever he can get. And with my mom, she always took away from me." Even her grandmother, who raised Tracy and her brother for a while, seemed to withhold affection, favoring her brother over her. As a result, Tracy has set her sights on creating a different kind of environment for her own children by selectively choosing the people with whom she rears her children—some kin, some friends.

This process of observing potential network members over time is a fundamental aspect of parental gatekeeping. Which kin end up participating in networks can be shaped as much by the haphazard exigencies of life as by deliberate acts of inclusion or exclusion. Well-liked kin may live at a distance or have too many other responsibilities to participate in networks of care for children. Well-liked kin may also have physical or emotional limitations that would make caring for children burdensome. For example, Sarah Aldrich was mindful of her father's heart condition. He wanted to be more involved with his grandchildren, but he had to be careful about overexcitement.

Friendship

As with kin, not all friends are tapped to participate in networks of interdependence that focus on children, in part because of class-based differences in the expectations of friends. Karen Walker's (1995) research on friendship reveals that middle-class men and women tend to expect friends to be emotionally supportive and share leisure activities, whereas working-class men and women expect material interdependence as part of their friendship. As with kin, a sifting process and different levels of active engagement sort out which friends or neighbors might be both acceptable and willing to help with children.

In U.S. culture as a whole, friendship is seen as voluntary, whereas kinship is viewed as obligatory (Walker 1995; Rubin 1985). And yet the actions and comments of the network members I interviewed reveal the contingent nature of kinship and the steadfastness of some friendships. In three of the networks, the anchors recruited friends because they provide support, advice, emotional stability, and, when possible, hands-on care. Many of the women in the networks spoke passionately about their commitment to, reliance on, and admiration for their friends.

The Dynamics of Inclusion and Exclusion

In building networks, parents and guardians act as gatekeepers, strategically selecting some people and consciously excluding others. Michaela Becker made the point that having a strong, select group necessarily means excluding some people: "The other side of the strong family . . . is that it's not completely open to . . . people from the outside. Which seems contradictory to me. Like, there's such a strong sense of . . . family comes first and all of that. And that we all have that so strongly etched into our skin that, you know, it would be fine to . . . be more inclusive or whatever. But that's not always the case." Currently, marriage and birth are the only ways into the Becker network. Other networks, however, are more open to friends and non-family members. Anchors include and exclude potential members along three dimensions: their sense of affinity and shared values; competence; and proximity and convenience.

Affinity and Values

Anchors exclude and include people on the basis of their feelings of affinity for the network candidates. That affinity grows out of the anchor's reaction to personality and the sense of personal connection the anchor feels and observes between the network candidate and the child. Anchors want to feel confident that the person they allow to care for their child will act as a surrogate, making the same kinds of decisions the anchors themselves would make if they were present. Dina Becker, for example, does not include her husband Mark's family in her network of care because she is uncomfortable with her in-laws' interactive style. Describing the Walde family, Dina said,

> They don't hug each other hello or goodbye much. They never say they love each other. Some of them aren't speaking to each other. Like Mark's brother did not speak to his father before he died, and he rarely spoke to Mark's mother, his mother, as well. Now that his father has died, he's speaking to his mother a lot . . . it's not that they're not nice people. They're just—they're not the same kind of people.

Dina thus excludes Mark's family members from her network of care.

In order to become a member of a network of care for children, a candidate must share the anchor's philosophy of child rearing, especially in the context of a church or synagogue, a school, a workplace, or a neighborhood, where parents must establish a firm basis for trusting the care of their children to adults they know only superficially, if at all (Macdonald 1998; Uttal

2002). Byron Russell, a former neighbor of the Duvall-Brennans' and a member of their network, talked about his efforts to establish consistency across the caregivers of his own children: "We don't want people taking care of our kids who would do it very differently from the way we do it."

Anchors' efforts to determine the trustworthiness of potential network members entail a conscious, deliberate process. When I asked Patricia Crane if she felt comfortable with the way Tracy treats Robbie, she responded, "Oh, yes," and then continued, "That's why only my family and her watches him. Because I've seen how she takes care of her children . . . and that's right in the line of mine. She comes home, they do their homework first, they do their chores, and that's exactly what I have Robbie on—doing his homework, doing his chores, like sweeping." Knowing that she and Tracy shared similar beliefs and values, such as personal responsibility and the importance of children helping out at home, convinced Patricia that Robbie would be in good hands while in Tracy's care.

Sometimes the lack of affinity between an anchor and a potential network member is tied to differences in the way people approach and interact with children. In an extreme case that goes well beyond disagreements over child-rearing style, Patricia excludes another neighbor, Luella, because she has seen how this woman treats her own children and hears the children's cries at night through the thin bedroom walls. "I don't trust her with my son," Patricia stated firmly. "No, no, no, no. Just the ways she talks to her children, I don't like it." She attributed her neighbor's behavior to mental illness, something beyond Luella's control except when moderated by the effects of medication. In addition to observing the way her various neighbors speak to and treat their children, Patricia notices the value they place on discipline, on education, on responsibility—those qualities she believes to be of utmost importance in her son's life.

Sarah Aldrich approaches the matter of affinity differently. She sets high standards for her close friends and for those she hires to help run her household. She expects network members to establish a personal connection with both the children and the other adults in the network, and to exhibit expert managerial skills. In emphasizing the importance of screening for "quality people," Sarah expressed the same concerns as Patricia Crane. Sarah, however, must conduct her screening without the benefit of the kind of intimate information that can be acquired from living on the other side of a thin apartment wall from a potential candidate. Upper-class parents like Sarah effectively control who their children have contact with by virtue of decisions they are able to make because of their class location. These include living in exclusive neighborhoods, sending the children to private schools, carefully selecting children's after-school activities, and meticulously screening the hired household help. Sarah looks for caregivers who are capable, responsible, dependable, organized, high energy, and, importantly, fun. She applies considerable resources to her quest to retain someone with abundant energy and cultural capital.

Commonality of perspective on other topics, such as junk food, also may create a basis for trust. Among the middle-class network members, attitudes toward food registered as a sorting device. With her siblings, Dina Becker's sister Caitlin took for granted shared values about the inappropriateness of giving children junk food: "I don't have to worry when Kent has them—I don't have to tell him what to give them for lunch. He just gives them a reasonable lunch. It doesn't occur to him not to, and we don't have to talk about it." Which values are shared and emphasized varies by network. Nonetheless, whatever the stated passions, pet peeves, and values, they constitute a basis for sorting people under consideration for membership. Shared values about children's nature and child rearing are essential for being included.

Consistent with the social science research on child rearing, those values appear to vary by class. In her study of the lives of working-class and middle-class children, for example, Lareau (2003) observes that working-class families often watch television together in a multigenerational environment, but middle-class families do not. There are, however, several highly contested issues that occur *within* class—and watching television is one of them. In the middle-class networks, television, more than anything else, acted as a lightning rod, drawing out differences between people and serving as the basis for including or excluding potential network members. Unsolicited, members of both the Becker and Duvall-Brennan networks identified attitudes about television as a defining child-rearing issue. In contrast, television did not surface as a top-of-mind issue among the Cranes or the Aldriches.

As proponents of anticommercialism, each of the Becker sisters who have children felt herself to be part of a cultural minority in her neighborhood and in her children's schools. Lila Becker reflected on the support her kin bestow:

> Dina and Caitlin do raise their children, in many ways, the same way [as I do]. And I feel in some ways we're not like many of the people we know here. Just—our children watch less television, eat less junk food. They're just much less media oriented. We don't do quite as many sports. I mean, they do play some. . . . I think my children are a lot more like their cousins than [they are like] many of their classmates.

Here, the extended family provides important psychological reinforcement for the mothers and children in deflecting the influences of mass culture.

The Duvall-Brennans also feel strongly that children are at risk for health and behavioral problems as a result of their saturation in materialist popular culture. The Brennan extended family, however, sees Maggie's opposition to television as a form of provocative extremism. Even Jack's brother, Tom, the family member closest to them and a participant in their network, expressed disdain for the no-television policy:

> The very glaring, obvious thing is they don't believe in television. And I said, "Jack, okay, that's fine. There's a lot of crap on TV. But what's wrong with *Sesame Street*?" And he believes in *Sesame Street*, but Maggie doesn't. [The kids have] never seen *Sesame Street*. [*Sesame Street* characters] taught my kids to read! [*laughs*]

Thus, in the Duvall-Brennan network, values similar to the Beckers' lead not to harmony with extended kin but rather to acrimony and conflict. Whether individuals condone or condemn a particular child-rearing value or belief, the conflict usually is about parenting in general. Tom Brennan comments on what he sees as the flaw in Maggie and Jack's parenting philosophy: "I guess part of my theory is that you can't hide children from something forever. Eventually, they're gonna see television. . . . You can't shelter your children from the big bad world forever. Someday it's gonna be there." Many of the feelings Tom expressed about Maggie and Jack included similarly prickly edges. As a result, while he remains at the top of the back-up list, Maggie and Jack do not call on him routinely. Their clash of child-rearing values creates too much conflict.

Competence

Occasionally, anchors judge potential network members as incompetent to meet the responsibilities that inevitably accompany caregiving. They avoid people who they see as negative role models for their children, such as drug abusers or thoroughly self-absorbed individuals. During my first interview with Patricia, Tracy's mother knocked at the door. Patricia shooed her away, saying she had company. Then, in a hushed voice, she told me that Tracy's mother was a heroin addict. She and Tracy tried to keep her away from their children. "We don't use her," Patricia said.

Patricia's mother, Fran, in talking about her own half-sister's inability to care for their mother, Louise, asserted, "Sherry don't know *how* to take care of her." Fran viewed Sherry's incapacity as arising from her position as the youngest and therefore least responsible sibling in the family. According to Fran, Sherry is "spoiled"—that is, she has never had to pull her own weight in the family: "She's just been spoiled. . . . I was sixteen when she was born. So she had us older kids, you know? And she was just spoiled. . . . She didn't do nothing, no. She didn't have to. Mother didn't make her do nothing, you know? . . . Whatever Sherry wanted, she got [*laughs*]." In Fran's mind, this form of upbringing left her half-sister ill-prepared to meet the challenge currently at hand, and not a good candidate for pitching in with Robbie.

Sometimes kin are excluded because they have conveyed to parents a low level of interest in their children or in the performance of a culturally assigned kin role. Maggie Duvall was not alone when she said, "I love [my mother] dearly, but she's not a grandmother." Maggie has a conception of what grandmothers should do, and her own mother falls painfully short. At another point, she observed, "Both my parents are rather distant grandparents, unfortunately for my children. They are not into children, and they are not into really being a part of their lives, which is too bad." Her former neighbor and network member Byron talked in a similar way about his brother, who lives a thirty-minute drive away: "He's not really inclined. I'd like him to spend more time with the kids, but we don't want to push it." Parents tend to avoid thrusting children on a reluctant family member.

Proximity and Convenience

Beyond affinity and competence lies the issue of proximity and convenience. Research consistently confirms the importance of proximity in constructing networks and activating extended kinship systems. Potential network members' physical distance or lack of time can create social and emotional remoteness and establish a general lack of availability (Fischer 1982; Roschelle 1997; Wellman 1999). In identifying individuals who are eligible and desirable as child-rearing helpers, anchors consider two dimensions of availability. The first involves geographic closeness. Physical proximity affects the convenience of a potential member's participation and his or her accessibility to the anchor's home and to the locations of the children's activities. The second dimension addresses the person's availability in terms of time (Daly 1996). Free time is shaped both by employment and by the individual's interpretation of his or her nonwork time as available for network participation.

While network members emphasize the importance of being nearby, they also make clear that more than geography is involved. Proximity in a network of interdependence includes an element of purposefulness, something I call "*intentional* proximity." Unquestionably, some network association results from convenience, but studies underestimate the intention behind proximity. While some friends and kin live conveniently close, their location alone is insufficient to recruit them into a network. In other cases, living farther away does not preclude people from participating in the network. But such proximity reflects a choice on the part of the anchor as well. For Patricia Crane, economic circumstances prompted her to move geographically close to family members—they need to rely on and help each other. The Beckers consciously choose to live near kin in order to maintain a certain kind of family and enable reciprocity in everyday life. The Duvall-Brennans, by buying into a certain economic stratum, opt out of being geographically close to family and social networks. The Aldriches can import their networks into proximity—by paying others to bridge the gap (such as with the "stuff pony").

Conclusion

In a culture of perceived heightened danger, fears about potential adult untrustworthiness and abuse linger in parents' minds. Parents have to navigate what is real and what is only feared or imagined. Parents intentionally and carefully observe kin, friends, and neighbors as they interact with children—their own and others. They monitor adults' behavior in terms of shared values, trustworthiness, and interest in their children.

Furthermore, parents need help and support for themselves and prefer relying on people who they like and who share their values and approach to child rearing. They consider a variety of potential network candidates, assessing their appropriateness for involvement with children, their interest and availability, and the convenience of folding them into their networks of care. They winnow out reluctant or inappropriate participants. Because relationships are ongoing, they re-evaluate them over time. Thus part of the work of parenting is constantly observing and monitoring their networks of care.

Note

1.   All of the names used in this chapter are pseudonyms.

References

Annie E. Casey Foundation. 1998. "Care for School-Age Children" ("Kids Count" brochure). Baltimore: Annie E. Casey Foundation.

Cochran, Moncrieff, Mary Larner, David Riley, Lars Gunnarsson, and Charles R. Henderson Jr. 1990. *Extending Families: The Social Networks of Parents and Their Children*. New York: Cambridge University Press.

Daly, Kerry J. 1996. *Families and Time: Keeping Pace in a Hurried Culture*. Thousand Oaks, CA: Sage.

Daniels, Arlene Kaplan. 1988. *Invisible Careers: Women Civic Leaders from the Volunteer World*. Chicago: University of Chicago Press.

Faludi, Susan. 2000. *Stiffed: The Betrayal of the American Man*. New York: Harper Perennial.

Fischer, Claude. 1982. *To Dwell among Friends*. Chicago: University of Chicago Press.

Garey, Anita Ilta. 1999. *Weaving Work and Motherhood*. Philadelphia: Temple University Press.

Hertz, Rosanna. 1986. *More Equal than Others: Women and Men in Dual-Career Marriages*. Berkeley: University of California Press.

Hertz, Rosanna, and Joy Charlton. 1989. Making Family under a Shiftwork Schedule: Air Force Security Guards and Their Wives. *Social Problems* 36 (5): 491–507.

Hochschild, Arlie Russell, with Anne Machung. 1989. *The Second Shift: Working Parents and the Revolution at Home*. New York: Viking.

Holloway, Sarah L., and Gill Valentine, eds. 2000. *Children's Geographies: Playing, Living, Learning*. New York: Routledge.

Lareau, Annette. 2003. *Unequal Childhoods: The Importance of Social Class in Family Life*. Berkeley: University of California Press.

Macdonald, Cameron. 1998. Working Mothers and Mother-Workers: Nannies, Au Pairs, and the Social Construction of Motherhood. PhD diss., Brandeis University.

Nelson, Margaret K. 2005. *The Social Economy of Single Motherhood: Raising Children in Rural America*. New York: Routledge.

Newman, Katherine S. 1999. *Falling from Grace: Downward Mobility in the Age of Affluence*. Berkeley: University of California Press.

Ostrander, Susan. *Women of the Upper Class*. 1984. Philadelphia: Temple University Press.

Presser, Harriet B. 1988. Shift Work and Child Care among Young Dual-Earner American Parents. *Journal of Marriage and Family* 50 (1): 133–48.

Roschelle, Anne R. 1997. *No More Kin: Exploring Race, Class, and Gender in Family Networks*. Thousand Oaks, CA: Sage.

Rubin, Lillian. 1985. *Just Friends: The Role of Friendship in Our Lives*. New York: Harper and Row.

Schneider, David, and Raymond T. Smith. 1978. *Class Differences in American Kinship*. Detroit: University of Michigan Press.

Uttal, Lynet. 2002. *Making Care Work: Employed Mothers in the New Childcare Market*. New Brunswick, NJ: Rutgers University Press.

Walker, Karen. 1995. Always There for Me: Friendship Patterns and Expectations among Middle-Class and Working-Class Men and Women. *Sociological Forum* 10 (2): 273–96.

Wellman, Barry, ed. 1999. *Networks in the Global Village: Life in Contemporary Communities*. Boulder, CO: Westview Press.

Weston, Kath. 1991. *Families We Choose: Lesbians, Gays, Kinship*. New York: Columbia University Press.

10

"Show Me You Can Be a Father"

Maternal Monitoring and Recruitment of Fathers for Involvement in Low-Income Families

Kevin Roy and Linda M. Burton

How low-income single mothers and nonresidential fathers sort out responsibilities for taking care of their children remains a keen policy interest in American society. Unfortunately, we have limited insight into how low-income single mothers acquire resources for their families (Dominguez and Watkins 2003). We also have limited insight into how nonresidential fathers maintain involvement with unmarried mothers and their children (Carlson, McLanahan, and England 2004; Waller and McLanahan 2005).

Maternal gatekeeping has been used by researchers as a blanket concept to identify most efforts by mothers to shape men's involvement with their children. Gatekeeping has emerged from studies with a primary focus on coresidential, married couples, most of whom are middle class and European American (Allen and Hawkins 1999; DeLuccie 1995; see Fagan and Barnett 2003 for exception). The term is primarily used to indicate mothers' exclusion of fathers' involvement, including motivations to discourage or deflect men's interactions with children. However, Pleck and Masciadrelli (2004) note that most gatekeeping studies link discouragement of paternal involvement only to mothers' attitudes, and rarely to actual family processes and behaviors.

In previous research (Roy and Burton 2007), we identified a specific family process: "kinwork," or the work that mothers do to maintain family members' commitments that promote children's well-being. Mothers create a set of family scripts that guide social expectations and lead to efficiency and consistency in taking care of family responsibilities (Byng-Hall 1985). This kinscripts framework (Stack and Burton 1993) situates women's work within complex family relationships over time and serves as an alternative approach to the gatekeeping concept. The framework also shifts the focus of study from mother-father relationships to extrafamilial relationships that "regenerate families, maintain lifetime continuities, sustain intergenerational responsibilities, and reinforce shared values" (Stack and Burton 1993, 160; see also Crosbie-Burnett and Lewis 1999; DiLeonardo 1987).

Kinscripts become critical when mothers make decisions to create or dissolve supportive networks for the daily survival and social mobility of their families (Hansen 2005; Nelson 2000, 2005; Stack 1974). They are crafted as accepted standards of behavior that family members must favorably meet as dedicated kinworkers. Mothers may recruit a range of men (e.g., biological fathers, boyfriends, non-intimate friends, and paternal and maternal kin) for involvement if those men fulfill basic kinwork expectations. For most fathers, for example, an established standard is that they accept responsibility for their biological children by contributing resources or time to improve children's life chances in economically disadvantaged communities.

Family members often hold time-proven mental representations of low-income fathers as "renegade relatives" whose transitions in residences, relationships, and employment put low-income families at risk for loss of resources, conflict, and abuse (Edin and Kefalas 2005; Sano 2004; Stack 1974; Waller and Swisher 2006). However, focused recruitment of men into kinwork roles potentially enhances families as well. Men provide financial resources for their children (Gibson, Edin, and McLanahan 2005; Kotchick, Dorsey, and Heller 2005; Mincy, Garfinkel, and Nepomnyaschy 2005; Roy 1999) even through the simple act of paternity establishment and through the subsequent contributions of fathers' own kin (Stack 1974). Low-income single mothers seek from fathers not only guidance for their children but also emotional support or trustworthy caregiving (Jarrett, Roy, and Burton 2002; Roy, Tubbs, and Burton 2004).

What is underexplored in research on recruitment, however, is how mothers gather information to make decisions about recruiting fathers, and how they monitor those fathers once they are recruited. In this chapter, we consider how the work of surveillance is particularly relevant as mothers create or dissolve family membership. This type of monitoring differs from formal surveillance by public organizations, as it is rooted in surveillance of the "borders" of role relationships (Marx 2007). Personal data about fathers may be at the core of mothers' "thin" surveillance methods, especially if unemployment histories, physical mobility, and past experiences (e.g., incarceration, gang activity, and drug use) determine whether men are appropriate parents (Torpey 2007; Zuriek 2007). Moreover, both the ongoing process of monitoring and the act of recruitment bring power into play in family relationships, especially when information on men's behavior leads mothers to let go of them as family members.

In this chapter, we return to our previous analyses (Roy and Burton 2007) to expand on how monitoring shapes "kinscription" (i.e., the recruiting of kin for specific work within a family). We explore low-income single mothers' monitoring and subsequent recruitment of men as open-ended and contested processes, inclusive of these multiple family needs and multiple actors. We examine monitoring as an ongoing process that forms the basis for initial recruitment and continuing validation of men's positive involvement with children. We define recruitment as the negotiation of connections with a range of men (biological fathers, boyfriends, non-intimate friends, and paternal and maternal kin) in order to improve children's life chances in economically disadvantaged communities. In short, paternal monitoring and recruitment are critical dimensions of mothers' efforts at kinscription and efforts to be "good mothers."

Methods

Overview and Participant Recruitment

The data for this study is derived from the ethnographic component of the Welfare, Children, and Families Three-City Study. This multisite study integrates survey, developmental, and ethnographic components to monitor the consequences of welfare reform for the well-being of children and families over a four-year period. (A detailed description of the Three-City Study and a series of reports are available through the John Hopkins University website, at *www.jhu.edu/~welfare.*) Using data from the Three-City Study, we explore strategies that women employ to recruit men's support for children in low-income families.

Families who participated in the ethnographic components of the Three-City Study were recruited between June 1999 and December 2000. We selected 149 families (70 percent of the 249 families in the total ethnographic sample) with nonresidential fathers or father figures during the first year of study (Table 10.1). Families were recruited in Boston, Chicago, and San Antonio, and recruitment sites included formal child-care settings (e.g., Head Start); the Women, Infants, and Children (WIC) program; neighborhood community and youth centers; churches; local welfare offices; and other social service agencies. Multiple neighborhoods in each city were targeted for recruitment, based on compatibility with probability sampling areas used to recruit participants for the Three-City Study survey component.

All families who participated in the ethnography had household in-

Table 10.1

Demographic characteristics of focal mothers (N = 149 families)

Demographic characteristics	Number of mothers	Percentage of total
City		
Boston	48	32
Chicago	42	28
San Antonio	59	40
Ethnicity/race		
African American	62	42
Hispanic	58	39
Non-Hispanic white	29	19
Age of primary caregivers		
15–24	61	41
25–34	56	38
35+	32	21
Education		
Did not complete high school	58	39
Completed high school or GED	33	22
Completed some college or trade school	58	39
TANF status		
Receives TANF	76	51
Does not receive TANF	73	49
Work status		
Working	76	51
Not working	73	49
Total number of people in household		
1–2	20	13
3	29	19
4	35	24
5 or more	65	44
Marital status / living arrangements		
Not married, not cohabiting	100	67
Married, spouse in home	8	5
Married but separated	11	8
Cohabiting, not married	30	20

comes at or below 200 percent of the federal poverty line (U.S. Department of Health and Human Services 2002). Most mothers received Temporary Assistance for Needy Families (TANF), although some mothers whose income was slightly above poverty level represented working-poor families who experienced many of the contextual impacts of poverty in low-income neighborhoods. In the sample examined here, 39 percent of the families were of Hispanic ethnicity (this category includes Puerto Ricans, Mexican Americans, and Central Americans), 42 percent were African American, and 19 percent were non-Hispanic white. Mothers ranged in age (41 percent were fifteen to twenty-four years old, 38 percent were twenty-five to thirty-four, and 21 percent were thirty-five or older) and educational attainment (39 percent did not complete high school, 22 percent completed high school or GED testing, and 39 percent completed some college or trade school courses).

For this analysis, we used ethnographic data collected during 1999, the first year of the Three-City Study. At the time of the study, most mother-father unions included young children. The unions were in tenuous early stages and involved high expectations, bitter disappointments, conflict, and union dissolution. The early phases of data collection were conducted at the height of welfare reform, when low-income women were required to identify the fathers of their children in order to receive aid. We acknowledge the possibility that the identification of welfare-eligible children's biological fathers may have influenced parenting and partnering interaction between mothers and nonresidential fathers.

Ethnographic Methodology

Structured Discovery
The ethnography employed a method of structured discovery in which in-depth interviews and participant observation focused on specific topics but allowed flexibility to capture unexpected findings and relationships among topics (Burton, Skinner, and Matthews 2005; Winston et al. 1999). The interviews addressed child development, parenting, intimate relationships, health, experiences with TANF and other public assistance programs, education and work histories, family economics, support networks, family routines, and home and neighborhood environments. Ethnographers also accompanied mothers and their children to the welfare office, doctor, hospital, clinic, or workplace. Ethnographers met with each family once or twice each month for twelve to eighteen months, with follow-up interviews at six months and one year. Mothers were compensated with vouchers for each interview or visit. Pseudonyms are cited in this study.

Coding and Analyses

Multiple sources of data were used for our analysis of mothers' recruitment. Field ethnographers in each city wrote field notes, including transcribed interviews and observations from family interactions. Interview transcripts, field notes, and other documents were coded for entry into a qualitative data management (QDM) software application and summarized into a case profile for each family. The QDM program and case profiles enabled counts across the entire sample as well as detailed analysis of individual cases.

For this analysis, notes and profiles were reviewed for mothers' reports of efforts to involve men in children's lives. We identified these reports in general discussions of mothers' and children's interactions with men, as well as discussions of intimate relationships, social support, and kinwork. We enhanced data credibility and dependability (Lincoln and Guba 1985) through prolonged engagement in the field, repeat coding techniques, member checks with participants, and triangulation through multiple data sources and multiple methods of data collection.

Three waves of coding were conducted on complete sets of data for each family. First, field notes and family profiles were coded with common codes and sensitizing concepts. Next, coding patterns were examined within and across all families. We identified three contexts for kinscription in the initial years of relationships in these young families. First, single mothers look for examples of conventional fathers and partners, those men who fulfill women's beliefs about a normative "gold standard" of involved fathering. Second, mothers reconcile the overlap of maternal advocacy with the demands of intimate relationships with biological fathers and nonbiological partners. Third, mothers try to minimize risks to themselves and their children through subsequent monitoring of non-intimate father figures and legacies with paternal kin. In the final phase of selective coding, we identified kinscription as our core analytical category, with specific emphasis on how these three contexts shaped the processes of monitoring and recruitment (LaRossa 2005). We integrated patterns of variation in these processes across all 149 cases to develop theoretical insight into the broader process of kinscription of men in low-income families.

Findings

Complex Family Configurations and Needs

Mothers pursue support with nonresidential biological fathers, new partners in intimate relationships, male friends and family members in non-intimate relationships, and paternal kin, including paternal grandmothers. Across all

149 families, 299 men are identified as being involved with children (approximately two men in each family context). Two or more biological fathers are involved in about 40 percent of the families ($n = 61$). The majority of men that mothers identify in their families are biological fathers who live permanently outside of households (62 percent of all men, $n = 186$) or who move in and out of households frequently (14 percent, $n = 42$). Just under one-fifth of all involved men that mothers acknowledge (18 percent, $n = 53$) are their unmarried partners. By considering contributions of male friends and family members outside of intimate relationships (6 percent, $n = 18$), mothers locate additional supportive male figures for short-term and limited bridge care.

We noted three family needs that mothers hoped to address through recruitment of men to support the development of children: (1) material support, (2) trustworthy child care, and (3) emotional support and guidance. Material support, both financial and in-kind, is the most common goal for recruiting fathers (78 percent, $n = 116$). More than half of the mothers in the study (56 percent, $n = 83$) indicated that they look for trusted kin members to offer limited hours for child care. One-third of the mothers in this sample discussed the need for a father's emotional support as a co-parent and guidance as a role model for children (32 percent, $n = 47$). There were no significant differences by race/ethnicity for mothers' reports of family needs.

Given the complexity of family configurations and multiple family needs, we examined kinscription within three overlapping contexts: conventional father involvement, intimate partnering, and involvement of non-intimate men or family members. In the following sections, we explore each of these contexts, with an eye toward the dynamics of monitoring and recruitment processes for low-income mothers.

Search for Conventional Fathers and Partners

Low-income mothers aspire to conventional parenthood like other families in American society (Anderson 1990; Edin 2000). Given limited economic opportunities, however, some mothers find that parenthood not only precedes marriage but also occurs in the absence of a committed relationship altogether (Jarrett, Roy, and Burton 2002). In such a circumstance, mothers seek to recruit men who can fulfill some of the most basic expectations of fatherhood. However, after monitoring involvement over time, many mothers find that these men face multiple challenges as parents.

Legitimacy through "That Gold Standard"

Mothers refer to being brought up with traditional family values, with gendered divisions of work in their families. For example, Sonya, a twenty-four-year-old African American mother of three children living in Boston, was raised to aspire to "that gold standard, you know—that there should be a mother in the home, a father at work. She should cook, clean, and nurture the kids, while the man provided for his family and provided discipline." If fathers are recruited and maintain some level of involvement with their children, mothers believe that they could be "strong influences" who could emerge as role models for their children.

For poor mothers without partners, the mere presence of a father in the household conveys a strong sense of social legitimacy for themselves and their children. Yolanda, a forty-year-old mother in Chicago, tried repeatedly to involve Javier, the biological father of her infant son, through appeals to join her and become "a real family. . . . I want to have a normal family." Even after the father moved to New York, she intended to ask him to move back in with her and her son. She firmly believed that her son knew his estranged father by his smell, insisting "la sangre llama" (the blood calls) to children.

Mothers often refer to the standard of responsibility that biological fathers have to their children. They watch for men to consistently fulfill financial obligations to their children, which is one of the most common and important measures of "good fathering." Recruitment of responsible men is based in large part on what mothers perceive as evidence of men's abilities to act responsibly toward their children. Carla, a young Latina mother in Chicago with a four-year-old daughter and eighteen-month-old twin sons, was able to maintain a supportive relationship with her ex-husband. In addition to paying one hundred dollars in weekly child support, he remained integrally involved as a caregiver for his children. He stopped by at the family's apartment after work every day at four o'clock, ate dinner with the family frequently, and took his daughter to stay with him at his parents' house on weekends. Carla had emphasized that he needed to take care of the children "he had brought into this world."

Accountability for Involvement

Arrangements such as Carla's are typically short-lived. To be "responsible as a mother," women need to monitor men after recruitment and hold them accountable for their involvement with children. For example, it was commonly stated among mothers in the study that "[the biological father] has no right to see his children unless he's contributing." Since material support is the most urgent and common family need, it is also the breaking point for many young families. Samora, a Latina mother in San Antonio, regretted that she had to monitor the work activities of the biological father of her three-year-old son. She could not believe that "he's working [in a car lot] and he's six, seven months behind in payment. He doesn't act like a daddy." When recruitment of men grows volatile or too complicated, some mothers determine that their roles as coordinators are "too much hassle" for too little material support.

Beyond simple material support, paternal involvement requires a level of maturity and commitment from men. Gisella, a Puerto Rican mother in Chicago, held onto her high expectations and grew frustrated at the lack of responsibility of her baby's father. He moved back and forth to Puerto Rico repeatedly, without direction and with little ambition. Eventually, he served five months in jail, and he did not seem intent on maintaining his relationship with his infant daughter. Gisella adamantly refused to let him sign the birth certificate or to give the baby his last name, saying, "When he shows me that he can be a father, then he can sign."

Over the course of many months of monitoring, mothers realized that consistent contributions are a challenge for low-income men who do not have access to good jobs. Gold-standard expectations for conventional fatherhood can be set too high, and some mothers began to lower their expectations for men's involvement. Sabine, a twenty-three-year-old African American mother of two daughters, focused on the efforts rather than the contributions of the biological father. She described Earl as "a good man" when he took the girls shopping for clothes, shoes, and food, or when he "put money in a savings account for their future." Earl abused drugs on and off for seven years, but Sabine gave him credit for doing "the right thing" and giving what he could when he was "clean." Similarly, Juanita, a young mother of two preschoolers in San Antonio, settled for the efforts of her baby's father, despite his commitment to three other children. "Just as long as he sees his daughter," she said. "That's what's important. He's part of her life. I'd rather have him part of her life than giving me money and not coming around at all."

Cultural and Environmental Barriers to Fathering

A more extensive range of barriers to men's involvement reshaped mothers' monitoring efforts and constrained recruitment of potential fathers. Almost 20 percent of the families in the study report that at least one nonresidential father or intimate partner has been incarcerated. Despite their best efforts, most men cannot act responsibly—as conventional fathers—when they are in jail, in prison, or on work release. In addition, some mothers find that men are usually not committed to a single child but to multiple family members in multiple kin networks. Many men continue to live with their aging parents and are partially responsible for their parents' well-being. (In the study, this was especially common for older African American men, about 40 percent of whom lived with their own mothers or fathers.) This responsibility for well-being usually means caregiving (transportation to church or the store) rather than extensive financial support.

Mothers often feel that this commitment is wrongly placed when men have their own children. Moreover, mothers fear that support from successfully recruited fathers will grow tenuous if these men have children with a new partner. For example, one mother described her ex-partner as a "good father" who reliably contributed diapers, clothes, and other important resources, and who cared for his children nightly and during weekends. However, she was concerned that he would "wash his hands of us" and the demonstrations of support would end when his current partner gave birth.

Changes in family relationships because of immigration are perhaps the most complicated context for kinscription of fathers. The ambiguity of residency status, the search for jobs, and the return home to visit or care for family members across international borders leaves recruitment an unresolved question for many Mexican and Puerto Rican families. Even though Clarissa moved into an apartment in Boston with Alex, the biological father of their young son, she insisted, "He has done very little for us, but I let it continue because family is very important to me." For her, shifting cultural expectations for men's roles as partners and parents confuse what mothers accept as gold-standard conventions for recruitment of fathers: "Latino men learned American values when they [came to the States], so that [they believe], 'nobody can depend on me, what's mine is mine and what's yours is yours.' . . . U.S. culture makes men dismiss our traditional culture of supporting women. I don't want to *mantener* [support] a man. . . . If he leaves us, I will continue living."

After recruiting Alex to become an involved father, Clarissa began to understand competing pressures that could keep him from commitment to her son. Many Latina mothers believe that for men who have potential partners and children in two countries, "it is impossible to live in two different worlds." Alex, in fact, had an older son from a previous relationship, and he continued to send money to his sisters and to his son. A year later, he returned from a visit to Puerto Rico with his older son, who "had no one to care for him." Clarissa confronted him about the differences in how he treated his two sons, but he misinterpreted her comments, assuming that she did not want his older son to stay with them. Eventually, Alex returned to Puerto Rico with his older son, built a house, and cut off ties with Clarissa and their child.

For Clarissa, monitoring Alex's involvement as a parent was complicated by his movement back and forth between the cultural expectations and distinct job opportunities in these "two different worlds." Valerie, a young woman in Chicago, also worked hard to reconcile her relationship with the father of her child in distinct contexts. During the course of pregnancy and the birth of her daughter, she followed him twice—back and forth to Puerto Rico—as he sought employment. In Chicago, he did not live up to her and her mother's expectations of a good partner and father, yet in Puerto Rico, he fulfilled his own family's expectations as a breadwinner. Valerie was uncomfortable with the more traditional parenting roles in Puerto Rico, which placed the burden of daily care on her and freed her boyfriend from care work (particularly because his family was involved in watching his infant daughter). After months of "trying to do the right thing" by staying together, Valerie chose to return permanently to her own mother's house in Chicago.

The question of residential status for immigrant families further complicates the monitoring of men's involvement. In many families, fathers are not legal citizens and prefer to return to their home countries after work opportunities erode. After Alejandro, a young father in Boston, returned to Guatemala, his girlfriend, Luz, worked out a child-care arrangement with Alejandro's mother. When he returned to Boston, Luz took this as a sign of recommitment and broke up with a new boyfriend. However, in other families, a father's departure clearly means that future involvement is not an option. For example, the father of Marta's children became frustrated with trying to gain citizenship and decided to return to Mexico. After years of tracking his sporadic involvement, Marta realized that she could not wait for him to return. She filed for abandonment with legal aid in Chicago in order to qualify for any kind of public assistance for his children.

In sum, mothers try to recruit men based on gold-standard potential, but monitoring sporadic and constrained contributions leads them to more realistic assessments, often based on effort and not actual time with children or financial contributions. For most mothers, some involvement is better than none. They take advantage of what one mother described as "what was offered, when it was offered." Men who even try to achieve conventional success as fathers put their families a step closer to legitimacy. As one mother argued, "Any help is welcome, from any of these men. I need to bring them all along." In effect, many mothers feel that they have little choice but to recruit a complicated configuration of men, even if they acknowledge the inconsistent contributions that lead to ambiguity and conflict in their lives.

Implications for Intimate Relationships

If "bringing [men] along" as involved *parents* proves problematic, kinscription has even more complicated implications for men as potential intimate *partners*. As DiLeonardo (1987) suggests, the early stages of kinwork (in this case, monitoring and recruitment of fathers) unfold in fits and starts, competition and cooperation, guilt and gratification. Negotiation over men's involvement leaves open the question of how participation in children's lives leads—or does not lead—to intimacy, companionship, and long-term commitment. For some mothers, advocacy for children's well-being is infused with self-interest as the promise of a conventional father folds into the promise of a conventional partner.

In this section, we examine implications for relationships with biological fathers and intimate partners separately. Mothers' recruitment of partners is closely linked to subtly different forms of monitoring, often focused more on leveraging involvement with children as a prerequisite for intimacy.

Investments in and Settling for Biological Fathers

Mothers often noted the significant investment of work and emotion, often over many years, on the part of their children's biological fathers. Due to this "history," most mothers give priority to the recruitment of biological fathers who had fallen out of their children's lives. However, reinvolvement of biological fathers opens negotiation over intimate relations, and mothers struggle to redefine their relationships. Clarissa found that her relationship with Alex, her son's father, could not be defined with conventional descriptions of marital partner or co-parent:

> Marriage is what women dream about, society asks that of a woman, or the economic situation, or love, but more than anything, to get married by God's law is a serious compromise. But [Alex] is my *marido*—like a companion or a boyfriend. . . . In Latino countries, the man gets a house for the woman, but things are different here—a man moves into a woman's house. The relationship has changed now—it's like a schedule, I get up, clean, he goes to work, I cook, take care of Justin. . . . I'm trying to hold the relationship together for Justin. I'm not confident we'll remain together.

When mothers appeal to biological fathers for involvement with their children, as Clarissa did, their appeals could imply that intimate relationships are back on track. However, such implications are often unintended. Karen, a forty-five-year-old European American mother of two young children, relied solely on her own father for child care while she worked. Upon his death, she regrettably appealed to her ex-husband for help:

> I work at night, and I needed to find someone new. It's easier for him to move back in. I'm not entirely happy with the situation—it's more economical, more for the kids than for me. Our relationship has not really improved but Beth and Brian are happy to have him around. Unless he makes changes—stop drinking, his swearing, his work ethic—I don't actually see myself with him. But I don't have time to meet anyone new. I really just need his help. I'm tired of worrying about having enough money and resources for my kids. I tried living on my own, went on welfare for a few months, but I can't make ends meet. I went into credit debt and thought about filing bankruptcy. I just don't know how single mothers are supposed to work full-time and take care of children.

By stipulating that her children's father must "make changes," Karen indicates how mothers monitor men's lives and can negotiate conditions for their involvement. As a type of ultimatum, they can make their relationships contingent on men fulfilling expectations as good providers and caregivers. One mother in Chicago asked her baby's father to move in even after he cheated on her. But she insisted, "We're not really 'together' together. I told him, 'The only way you're going to stay here is if you pay all the bills, do everything.'" If mothers see that a man's potential for financial contribution has faded, they often end relationships. After her children's father lost his job at the tail end of four years of engagement, Katherine, a European American mother in Boston, ultimately decided not to marry him and ended the relationship.

Although these mothers describe clear-cut offers to "pay to stay" (Edin and Lein 1997), the daily process of monitoring men's involvement as partners is actually quite open-ended. Most mothers have few alternatives to their heavy investments with biological fathers, and they cannot readily anticipate the consequences of their appeal for paternal involvement. Rejection of biological fathers means letting go of the chance of legitimacy with fathers as well as the promise of marriage with a partner. Yesenia was a young Chicago mother with five children, and she secured a restraining order for eighteen months against the children's biological father after he served three months in jail for a domestic violence offense. However, she still needed someone to watch her children when she was at work during the day:

> I'm trying to give him a second chance. We've been doing well since he came back, we're much happier. He's promised not to drink. But that

makes his temper short, and I don't want him to lash out, so we don't talk very much. He's helping more around the house, doing things that needed to be done for some time now. I want this to work out, for the kids' sake. He's a great father and the kids love him. I don't mind him being back, and they really missed him.

Looking for "More" with Intimate Partners

Men who are not the biological fathers of children do not carry a history of disappointments. They represent the chance to start again with the potential for legitimacy. The standards for involvement are similar; as one mother said, "A relationship with me is not an option if [the guy] doesn't support my kids—they come first." However, mothers have to look elsewhere for solid examples of these men's efforts at parenting. For example, Valerie completed an Alcoholics Anonymous (AA) course after splitting up with the father of her sons. She began to develop a relationship with another AA member who lived in sober housing. "He's divorced, with two kids, a good job," she said. "And I like spending time with him—he's intelligent, he's a good conversationalist." Valerie could not see her partner's contributions, but she took his word that "he supports his children too, he hasn't run out on them. That's good for my kids. He's a good catch."

Material support from intimate partners can end reliance on inconsistent contributions or conflict with biological fathers. New partners give mothers renewed confidence as well as scarce resources needed to nurture children. Eva, a young Latina mother of three preschool-age children in San Antonio, left her abusive former partner, who threatened to pursue custody. Her new fiancé's consistent financial contributions and offers to help with child care allowed Eva to avoid contacting her former partner for financial support or child care.

Monitoring men's involvement, however, also leads some mothers to compare contributions between intimate partners and biological fathers. The result can be more critical assessments of relationships with intimate partners. Kate, a European American mother of a two-year-old son, began to receive formal child support and regular child care from the father of her child, and her live-in partner contributed little. She tolerated her partner's lack of commitment for a few months before ending their relationship "for not offering anything to me and my kids." Kim, an African American mother in Boston, reflected on the necessity of companionship. She did so in the context of limitations of both biological fathers and potential partners.

I'm lonely. . . . But I've learned that no man can destroy me. Men don't see my heart—they're just looking to take from me. With all my kids' fathers, what got me first was they'd give me money and take me out. But then that ended, and it was more as if they were another one of my children. I'm not having it, I can't grow with someone like that. It's not my responsibility to believe in my kids' fathers and make them constantly accountable to their children. Men can get away with it—they do me like that.

As Clarissa noted, some mothers are propelled by "society/economics/ love/God" to continue to seek men to support their children as well as themselves. The conflation of intimate relations and parenting often leads them to overlook risky behavior that could have been exposed by close monitoring. Kris, a mother of five children, reported that "when my kids needed a father figure, I tried to find one. . . . I tried to make sure that there is a man in my life that loved me and respected me and loved my kids." She was consumed with finding legitimacy and stability with a father and partner, and in turn entered into relationships with three men who abused her and her children. In retrospect, Kris blamed herself for bringing this damage into her family and for not insisting on her children's safety: "It was my fault maybe, and I'm sorry for ruining my kids' lives."

Reduction of Risks through Involvement of Father Figures

Father Figures as Alternatives
Negotiations to recruit biological fathers and intimate partners prove to be exhausting for mothers in low-income families, and these interactions often put women and children at risk of abuse or gaps in material or care-giving support. The recruitment of men in non-intimate relationships offers alternative choices. Although only 6 percent of all the men identified in the sample were non-intimate relations, they offered critical short-term and "bridge" care options for mothers. When mothers interact with men in online chat rooms and at work, parties, and neighborhood gathering places, they develop and assess friendships with potential role models for their children. Once involved, the loss of these father figures can be just as devastating as the loss of a child's biological father. Lucy, a pregnant Mexican American mother of four, lost her home and moved into a family shelter. At the shelter, a new friend, Sean, convinced her not to put her baby up for adoption, and three years later he had assumed the title of "father" to her daughter. He died unexpectedly, leaving Lucy without the person who she insisted was "the only constant in my life." Likewise, when she had few reliable men in her family life, Yesenia turned to an older grandfather figure for child care and occasional financial aid. This older man's poor health removed him from this

role, and she and her children felt his absence "like the loss of my father or uncle."

By maintaining a network of fathers and father figures, mothers secure a consistent web of support that will not put their children at risk for lack of resources. Emma, a fifty-year-old European American grandmother in Boston, agreed that "Daddy" was a complicated concept for Sunny, her four-year-old custodial granddaughter. Sunny did not live or interact regularly with her biological father or her mother's new boyfriend, but Sunny's uncle and her step-grandfather were both "Daddy" because they shared a household with her. At a picnic on Father's Day, Emma celebrated the efforts of fathers in the extended family, including these four men as well as seven other men with children (Emma's father-in-law, her husband's brother and his son, a son by her first husband, her brother, her nephew, and her next-door neighbor). Paternal involvement with Sunny was shared among a number of men, most of whom were non-kin father figures. Monitoring their involvement is by nature different than monitoring the involvement of biological fathers. Expectations for their involvement are limited and short-term based on who is there and which needs arise. For many mothers, even a network of untapped but potential father figures represents security and support. With a complex array of father figures, Emma flexibly tailored parenting needs to the demands of shifting residence, employment, and care arrangements.

In the aftermath of dissolved relationships with biological fathers and intimate partners, many mothers only trust men in their family. Some mothers and their male siblings set up reciprocal care arrangements. Crystal, a forty-five-year-old African American mother in Chicago, turned to her older sons to care for her younger children, whose biological fathers were incarcerated. In Boston, Jamilla, a young single African American mother, recruited her godfather to care for and play with her child. After a few months, her boyfriend and the child's biological father returned to the neighborhood, and her godfather's obligations faded out. Again, the commitments of father figures typically are limited in focus and short-term in duration. Relatedly, keeping tabs on these men takes less time and energy: men of the family are typically trusted and familiar figures who do not need to live up to unattainable standards for contribution.

Involvement and Legacies of Paternal Kin

After growing tired of biological fathers' low levels of involvement, some mothers opt to recruit paternal kin. Mothers make direct appeals for housing or financial assistance to paternal kin who feel obligated to children through biological ties. Some young mothers live with paternal grandparents in order to remain in school during the early years after giving birth. When biological fathers completely fall out of their children's lives, paternal kin often feel compelled to take up responsibility for care and support of their youngest family members. Mothers recruit and assess paternal grandmothers, usually without much initial monitoring, as participants in an "as-needed" optional day care network as well as purchasers of clothing and sole custodians of children during emergency situations. Mothers noted how men's brothers and sisters serve as confidantes on parenting, jobs, and money matters, and also how they serve as caregivers who can offer children weekend visits to households filled with cousins.

The act of establishing paternity often activates the involvement of paternal kin (Stack 1974), and mothers often work to secure a paternal family legacy and ongoing resources for their children. For example, Yolanda photocopied the DNA test results that confirmed Javier's biological ties to their son and mailed them to his mother and sisters in Mexico. She explained that "esto es por si todavía dudan" (this is in case they still doubt [who the father is]). Francesca, a twenty-two-year-old European American mother in Boston, maintained a strong relationship with the family of Roberto, her daughter's father. She kept in touch through regular phone calls to them in the Dominican Republic and eventually saved enough money so that she and her daughter could visit them. Francesca wanted her daughter to know her five-year-old half-brother and agreed to have him come visit her and her daughter for periods of time as he grew up.

The involvement of paternal kin does not reintroduce unwanted intimacies and is often more reliable, in part due to the commitment of the women in the family. However, kinscription of paternal kin can become problematic and even unproductive for some mothers. Some mothers in paternal kin networks grew critical when the kin care and contributions to children enabled biological fathers to be seen as "involved parents," when in fact they were not involved. Cassandra, a young European American mother in Chicago, was separated from the Puerto Rican father of her two children, and she minimized her former partner's contributions, saying, "He's a chicken daddy—his family watches my baby, and he gets the credit."

In the midst of kinscription of men as parents and partners and kinscription of alternative family figures, mothers are engaged constantly in a process of minimizing risks for their children. Lorena, a twenty-nine-year-old Puerto Rican mother of three, moved to Boston after a string of abusive relationships with the biological fathers of her children. She chose not to rely on her new partner for financial support, however, and found that friends and her children's paternal kin offered inconsistent support at best. After a few years, Lorena moved south to look for better jobs. In a new community, the exhausting and often risky process of monitoring, assessing, and recruiting fathers and father figures was no longer an option. Instead, Lorena relied solely on her own employment and personal resources for her children. For the 30 percent of the Three-City Study families who did not have nonresidential fathers or father figures, and who were therefore not involved in this analysis, mothers may have opted out of the involvement of fathers and father figures for similar reasons.

Conclusion

In this chapter we discussed paternal monitoring and recruitment as critical dimensions of mothers' kinscription efforts to involve nonresidential fathers in the lives of their children. Our goal in presenting this work is to conceptually extend current knowledge on women's labor in paternal involvement. In our sample we outlined a model of three related contexts for the kinscription of fathers by low-income single mothers. First, mothers seek legitimacy through recruitment and monitoring of men as conventional fathers and partners. For single mothers in nontraditional family structures, involved fathers offer a chance for social legitimacy. Second, mothers negotiate how kinscription reshapes potential intimate relationships. As single parents, negotiation of intimate relationships is particularly contested. As was the case for Yesenia, Karen, and Gisella in our analysis, mothers often struggle to understand how the search for ideal fathers is linked to the status of these men as partners. Some men cannot live up to conventional expectations as fathers and are risks as partners as well. Finally, mothers try to minimize risks to their children at every step of kinscription. If mothers are unable to secure conventional fathers or to find intimate partners who contribute to their families, they often turn to non-intimate friends and acquaintances, men in their own families, or paternal kin as options for involvement. In effect, kinscription of fathers is a way for single, economically disadvantaged women to be "good" mothers.

This model of kinscription contributes to new theory development about parenting and partnering. First, it offers insight into two linked contexts in low-income families. This study confirms that low-income mothers initially pursue recruitment of biological fathers, and they subsequently pursue recruitment of intimate partners, non-intimate father figures, and paternal kin members. Findings also suggest that mothers' power in families comes into play during the process of monitoring men's involvement. Often, studies of monitoring are unspecified as to the purpose or means of surveillance (Marx 2007). In low-income families, informal monitoring leads mothers to assess men's material contributions, commitment of time for care, and commitment to children and partners in often ambiguous relationship contexts. The goal of monitoring is clear: to protect children and to ensure positive involvement of men in families.

A sole focus on men's financial support in previous studies has resulted in limited understanding of mothers' strategies to enhance their children's well-being. In contrast to the rather clear-cut process of "pay to stay" (Edin and Lein 1997), we found that mothers are often unsure of the consequences of asking potential partners to contribute financially to their children or to care for their children. Moreover, it proves difficult to transform a relationship based on men's financial contributions into a parental commitment to emotional support, child care, or role modeling. Often, it is assumed that mothers are at fault when gaps emerge in caregiving practices for children (Garey 1999). Kinscription strategies aim to fill gaps in resources and care, and also to reallocate blame and ensure that a mother is not solely responsible for family well-being.

Kinscription also challenges us to reconsider the concept of maternal gatekeeping. Despite the frustration of not being able to count on men's support, women often do not "give up" on fathers and continue to encourage their efforts. Similar to studies of emotion work in father-child relationships (Seery and Crowley 2000), mothers praise the involvement of men and craft positive images for fathers. Their most basic efforts to solicit and cultivate father involvement indicate that they value inclusion, but also that they recognize the need to monitor men in order to both reassess and maintain their involvement over time. This chapter reflects recent literature on an expanded conception of women's efforts to both include and exclude men in care networks (Hansen 2005; Nelson 2006).

Second, low-income single mothers have to negotiate men's involvement, and these negotiations lead to complex family configurations. A structured discovery approach allowed us to consider a full range of relationships without making assumptions about who performed paternal roles. For example, kinscription is not confined to marital relationships; often, when mothers exclude nonresidential fathers from involvement, they monitor and recruit other men or paternal kin to support children's well-being. By identifying conditions in which biological fathers, intimate partners, male friends and family members, and paternal kin participate as kinworkers, this study extends theory development on men's fulfillment of normative roles (Townsend 2002) for a single biological child. It also supports the suggestions of Garey et al. (2002) to direct attention to patterns of interdependence within families in order to reconceptualize caregiving in contemporary families.

Monitoring and recruitment are shaped by life circumstances for low-income fathers as well. In particular, men's immigration patterns (Portes and Sensenbrenner 1993) force mothers to shift and supplement their strategies to secure material support across international borders and multiple family systems. Incarceration removes many potential fathers and father figures from children's lives (Arditti, Lambert-Shute, and Joest 2003; Nurse 2002). Paternal kin step up often during incarceration, as do other biological fathers for children within the same family. Men's job instability, physical abuse, and substance use increasingly lead mothers to assess how the risks might outstrip the benefits of often inconsistent paternal involvement (Sano 2004).

This model is attuned to specific historical and developmental contexts in the first stages of kinscription. These were not long-standing relationships between mothers and biological fathers, and these men and women were often unfamiliar with what would be demanded of them during the first few years of co-parenting with young children. These fragile relationships unfolded under new systems designed to monitor men's involvement under welfare reform in the late 1990s. Future analyses and other studies must detail the "next steps" of kinscription. By considering more than a year or two of data on family relationships, we can more systematically examine kinscription strategies, particularly how monitoring may change as mothers maintain, supplement, sanction, and dissolve men's involvement over time.

Findings may help to guide large-scale survey research on parenting in low-income families, suggesting a range of effective kinscription strategies that may result in paternal involvement and, ultimately, in promotion of child well-being. Moreover, these findings may offer ways to clearly conceptualize the separation of intimate relations from childbearing. They suggest the need for further exploration of how tensions emerge during negotiated connections of men as partners and co-parents in low-income families.

This study has important policy and program implications for unmarried mothers, nonresidential fathers, and economically disadvantaged children. Formal monitoring systems that lead to paternity establishment and child support may divert or even harm mothers' informal strategies to monitor and make recruiting decisions (Roy 1999). Less intrusive (and more forgiving) methods of marking fathers' involvement may encourage men to participate as active fathers. State and federal agencies attempt to secure finances through child-support regulations, but policies and programs aimed at poor, nonresidential fathers are usually punitive in nature and force mothers to identify fathers in order to qualify for welfare assistance (Edelman, Holzer, and Offner 2006). Consequently, children and their mothers see little money from child support, as poor fathers are unmotivated to divert scarce resources to reimburse state outlays of welfare benefits (Johnson, Levine, and Doolittle 1999). Recent tax initiatives in New York, in which nonresidential fathers can receive earned income tax credits for their children, may motivate some fathers to contribute financial support (Kaufman 2005). However, social policy has failed to offer job training and placement services by which recruited fathers can support mothers as well as children.

Although men's guidance, time, and attention may be vital for children's development, these contributions do not translate into dollars, and few programs since 1990 have recognized and encouraged alternatives to financial provision (e.g., in-kind contributions; Pirog-Good 1993). The study suggests that a sense of belonging through family and family-like relationships drives some aspects of mothers' recruitment of fathers. It also suggests that families expect different commitments from different men. Although nonbiological fathers may not compensate for financial support of biological fathers (McLanahan and Sandefur 1994), they may compensate for other aspects of paternal involvement, such as caregiving. We need to explore systematically the contexts in which compensation may occur—and how to promote such compensation to maximize resources and supports for children and their families.

Finally, care responsibilities, particularly in low-income and minority families, extend beyond the relationship of biological parents to obligate both maternal and paternal kin. Although current policy initiatives encourage paternal involvement and support through funding for marriage promotion among low-income couples, marriage focuses exclusively on partnering processes. Paternal involvement requires broader child-centered parenting processes embedded in extended kin systems. In many families, the interdependence of extended family members' kinwork can be at odds with welfare reform policy goals of locating biological fathers. Instead, social policies that work to stabilize and strengthen adults' lives through good jobs, child care, health care, and housing will be more effective in cultivating more parental figures to support children in low-income families.

Note

This study was conducted with support from the National Institute for Child Health and Human Development under Project No. 5 R03 HD 42074-2, and from the Purdue Research Foundation at Purdue University. We gratefully acknowledge the funders of the ethnographic component of Welfare, Children, and Families:

A Three-City Study, including the National Institute of Child Health and Human Development; the Assistant Secretary for Planning and Evaluation, U.S. Department of Health and Human Services; the Social Security Administration; the Henry J. Kaiser Family Foundation; the Robert Wood Johnson Foundation; the W. K. Kellogg Foundation; and the John D. and Catherine T. MacArthur Foundation. We extend special thanks to our 210-member ethnographic team, and particularly to the Penn State team, whose members provided the infrastructure, organization, and data management for the multisite ethnography. Most important, we thank the families who have graciously participated in the project and have given us access to their lives.

References

Allen, Sara, and Alan Hawkins. 1999. Maternal Gatekeeping: Mothers' Beliefs and Behaviors That Inhibit Greater Father Involvement in Family Work. *Journal of Marriage and Family* 61: 199–212.

Anderson, Elijah. 1990. *Streetwise: Race, Class, and Change in an Urban Community.* Chicago: University of Chicago Press.

Arditti, Joyce, Jennifer Lambert-Shute, and Karen Joest. 2003. Saturday Morning at the Jail: Implications of Incarceration for Families and Children. *Family Relations* 52: 195–204.

Burton, Linda M., Debra Skinner, and Stephen Matthews. 2005. Structuring Discovery: A Model and Method for Multi-site Team Ethnography. Workshop presented at the annual meeting of the American Sociological Association, August 13–16, Philadelphia.

Byng-Hall, John. 1985. The Family Script: A Useful Bridge between Theory and Practice. *Journal of Family Therapy* 7: 301–5.

Carlson, Marcia, Sara McLanahan, and Paula England. 2004. Union Formation in Fragile Families. *Demography* 41: 237–61.

Crosbie-Burnett, Margaret, and Edith A. Lewis. 1999. Use of African-American Family Structures and Functioning to Address the Challenges of European-American Postdivorce Families. In *American Families: A Multicultural Reader,* edited by Stephanie Coontz, 455–68. New York: Routledge.

DeLuccie, Mary. 1995. Mothers as Gatekeepers: A Model of Maternal Mediators of Father Involvement. *Journal of Genetic Psychology* 156: 115–31.

DiLeonardo, Michaela. 1987. The Female World of Cards and Holidays: Women, Families, and the Work of Kinship. *Signs: Journal of Women in Culture and Society* 12: 440–53.

Dominguez, Silvia, and Celeste Watkins. 2003. Creating Networks for Survival and Mobility: Social Capital among African-American and Latin-American Low-Income Mothers. *Social Problems* 50: 111–35.

Edelman, Peter, Harry Holzer, and Paul Offner. 2006. *Reconnecting Disadvantaged Young Men.* Washington, DC: Urban Institute Press.

Edin, Kathryn. 2000. What Do Low-Income Single Mothers Say about Marriage? *Social Problems* 47: 112–33.

Edin, Kathryn, and Maria Kefalas. 2005. *Promises I Can Keep: Why Poor Women Put Motherhood before Marriage*. Berkeley: University of California Press.

Edin, Kathryn, and Laura Lein. 1997. *Making Ends Meet: How Single Mothers Survive Welfare and Low-Wage Work*. New York: Russell Sage Foundation.

Fagan, Jay, and Marina Barnett. 2003. The Relationship between Maternal Gatekeeping, Paternal Competence, Mothers' Attitudes about the Father Role, and Father Involvement. *Journal of Family Issues* 24: 1020–43.

Garey, Anita Ilta. 1999. *Weaving Work and Motherhood*. Philadelphia: Temple University Press.

Garey, Anita Ilta, Karen V. Hansen, Rosanna Hertz, and Cameron Macdonald. 2002. Care and Kinship: An Introduction. *Journal of Family Issues* 23: 703–15.

Gibson, Christina, Kathryn Edin, and Sara McLanahan. 2005. High Hopes But Even Higher Expectations: The Retreat from Marriage among Low-Income Couples. *Journal of Marriage and Family* 67: 1301–12.

Hansen, Karen V. 2005. *Not-So-Nuclear Families: Class, Gender, and Networks of Care*. Piscataway, NJ: Rutgers University Press.

Jarrett, Robin, Kevin Roy, and Linda M. Burton. 2002. Fathers in the "Hood": Insights from Qualitative Research on Low-Income African-American Men. In *Handbook of Father Involvement: Multidisciplinary Perspectives*, edited by Catherine Tamis-LeMonda and Natasha Cabrera, 211–48. New York: Lawrence Erlbaum Associates.

Johnson, Earl, Ann Levine, and Fred Doolittle. 1999. *Fathers' Fair Share: Helping Poor Men Manage Child Support and Fatherhood*. New York: Russell Sage Foundation.

Kaufman, Leslie. 2005. Unmarried Fathers Gain Tax Incentive in Pataki Proposal. *New York Times*, January 17.

Kotchick, Beth, Shannon Dorsey, and Laurie Heller. 2005. Predictors of Parenting among African-American Single Mothers: Personal and Contextual Factors. *Journal of Marriage and Family* 67: 448–60.

LaRossa, Ralph. 2005. Grounded Theory Methods and Qualitative Family Research. *Journal of Marriage and Family* 67: 837–57.

Lincoln, Yvonna, and Egon Guba. 1985. *Naturalistic Inquiry*. Thousand Oaks, CA: Sage.

Marx, Gary T. 2007. Desperately Seeking Surveillance Studies: Players in Search of a Field. *Contemporary Sociology* 36: 125–30.

McLanahan, Sara, and Gary Sandefur. 1994. *Growing Up with a Single Parent: What Hurts, What Helps*. Cambridge, MA: Harvard University Press.

Mincy, Ronald, Irwin Garfinkel, and Lenna Nepomnyaschy. 2005. In-Hospital Paternity Establishment and Father Involvement in Fragile Families. *Journal of Marriage and Family* 67: 611–25.

Nelson, Margaret K. 2000. Single Mothers and Social Support: The Commitment to, and Retreat from, Reciprocity. *Qualitative Sociology* 23: 291–317.

———. 2005. *The Social Economy of Single Motherhood: Raising Children in Rural America*. New York: Routledge.

———. 2006. Single Mothers "Do" Family. *Journal of Marriage and Family* 68: 781–95.

Nurse, Anne. 2002. *Fatherhood Arrested: Parenting from within the Juvenile Justice System*. Nashville: Vanderbilt University Press.

Pirog-Good, Maureen. 1993. In-Kind Contributions as Child Support: The Teen Alternative Parenting Program. In *Young Unwed Fathers: Changing Roles and Emerging Policies*, edited by Robert Lerman and Theodora Ooms, 251–66. Philadelphia: Temple University Press.

Pleck, Joseph, and Brian Masciadrelli. 2004. Paternal Involvement in US Resident Fathers: Levels, Sources, and Consequences. In *The Role of Fathers in Child Development*, 4th ed., edited by Michael Lamb, 222–71. Hoboken, NJ: Wiley.

Portes, Alejandro, and Julia Sensenbrenner. 1993. Embeddedness and Immigration: Notes on the Social Determinants of Economic Action. *American Journal of Sociology* 98: 1320–50.

Roy, Kevin. 1999. Low-Income Fathers in an African-American Community and the Requirements of Welfare Reform. *Journal of Family Issues* 20: 432–57.

Roy, Kevin, and Linda M. Burton. 2007. Mothering through Recruitment: Kinscription of Non-residential Fathers and Father Figures in Low-Income Families. *Family Relations* 56: 24–39.

Roy, Kevin, Carolyn Tubbs, and Linda M. Burton. 2004. Don't Have No Time: Daily Rhythms and the Organization of Time for Low-income Families. *Family Relations* 53: 168–78.

Sano, Yoshi. 2004. The Unanticipated Consequences of Promoting Father Involvement: A Feminist Perspective. In *Sourcebook of Family Theory and Research*, edited by Vern Bengtson, Alan Acock, Katherine Allen, Peggye Dilworth Anderson, and David Klein, 355–56. Thousand Oaks, CA: Sage.

Seery, Brenda, and M. Sue Crowley. 2000. Women's Emotion Work in the Family: Relationship Management and the Process of Building Father-Child Relationships. *Journal of Family Issues* 21: 100–127.

Stack, Carol B. 1974. *All Our Kin: Strategies for Survival in a Black Community*. New York: Random House.

Stack, Carol B., and Linda M. Burton. 1993. Kinscripts. *Journal of Comparative Family Studies* 24: 157–70.

Strauss, Anselm, and Juliet Corbin. 1998. *Basics of Qualitative Research: Techniques and Procedures for Developing Grounded Theory*, 2nd ed. Thousand Oaks, CA: Sage.

Torpey, John. 2007. Through Thick and Thin: Surveillance after 9/11. *Contemporary Sociology* 36: 116–19.

Townsend, Nicholas. 2002. *The Package Deal: Marriage, Work and Fatherhood in Men's Lives*. Philadelphia: Temple University Press.

U.S. Department of Health and Human Services. 2002. Federal Register, vol. 67, no. 31, February 14, 6931–33.

Waller, Maureen, and Sara McLanahan. 2005. "His" and "Her" Marriage Expectations: Determinants and Consequences. *Journal of Marriage and Family* 67: 53–67.

Waller, Maureen, and Raymond Swisher. 2006. Fathers' Risk Factors in Fragile Families: Implications for "Healthy" Relationships and Father Involvement. *Social Problems* 53: 392–420.

Winston, Pamela, Ronald J. Angel, Linda M. Burton, P. Lindsay Chase-Lansdale, Andrew J. Cherlin, Robert A. Moffitt, and William J. Wilson. 1999. *Welfare, Children, and Families: Overview and Design.* Baltimore, MD: Johns Hopkins University.

Zuriek, Elia. 2007. Surveillance Studies: From Metaphors to Regulation to Subjectivity. *Contemporary Sociology* 36: 112–15.

Part IV

Monitoring inside the Family

Internal family monitoring occurs at all stages of life, and the essays in this section cover various stages of development from infancy and childhood through emerging adulthood. (Although the essays do not include discussions of adults monitoring other adults, it is interesting to note that some of the mechanisms used for infants and small children, such as baby monitors and electronic bracelets, are now used to monitor the elderly.) Two of the chapters explore new technological devices, such as baby monitors and cell phones; the other two chapters focus on more traditional monitoring approaches. Taken as a whole, this section demonstrates that parental monitoring does not depend on the new technology, but that the new technology might alter that practice.

Although the distinction between care and control may blur at any of the levels of monitoring discussed in this collection, the difficulty in distinguishing care from control is most evident in the monitoring that occurs inside the family. The chapters in this section explore the manner in which family relationships, gender, and sexuality are all shaped and reshaped by daily practices of monitoring and surveillance.

11

Watching Children

Describing the Use of Baby Monitors
on Epinions.com

Margaret K. Nelson

Contemporary popular culture is replete with descriptions of a new stance of anxiety that appears to prevail especially among middle-class parents who, it is said, worry all the time about both the safety and the development of their children and who, it is said, monitor them more closely than ever before. Parenting books (Anderegg 2003; Warner 2005), journalists (Marano 2004; Applebome 2006), and even academics (Stearns 2004; Hulbert 2003) comment and occasionally offer advice on this phenomenon that Katz (2001) calls "hyper-vigilance."[1]

Popular and ad hoc explanations for these specific new attitudes suggest a variety of immediate causes. Some argue that since 9/11, the world has become—or has appeared to be—a more dangerous place, and parents are "simply" responding to that new danger—or to that perception of danger (Starr 2003). Others point to the widely publicized stories of kidnapping, Internet pornography, and sexual predators (Anderegg 2003). Still others suggest that the downsizing of the 1980s combined with the shrinking of the middle class has led to heightened anxiety about children falling behind and dropping below the accomplishments (and income) of their parents (Middlebury College Public Affairs 2006). Finally, some note simply that as parents have fewer children, each one becomes ever more precious (Zelizer 1985; Beck 1992).[2]

Adapted from Margaret K. Nelson, "Watching Children: Describing the Use of Baby Monitors on Epinions.com" (© *Journal of Family Issues*, 2008), by permission of Sage Publications Ltd.

Theoretical accounts of the rise of a more generalized "anxiety" rest on the work of Giddens (1999) and Beck (1992) regarding the emergence of a "risk society." Giddens (1999, 3), for example, notes that although the world has not necessarily become more hazardous, the absence of tradition leads to a preoccupation "with the future (and also with safety)." When dangers are redefined as risks and thus "viewed as the product of human action and decision-making rather than of fate" (Lupton and Tulloch 2002, 318), individuals might hold themselves ever more responsible for ensuring both their own safety and that of their dependents.

A growing body of empirical work notes that as the dangers facing children are interpreted as risks to be managed, parents come to limit the mobility of their children, leading ultimately to a more circumscribed existence (Backett-Milburn and Hardin 2004; Valentine 1997a, 1997b; Valentine and McKendrick 1997). Much of this research considers the issues facing parents of children who might be old enough to have their own conceptions of danger and safety and thus notions about the degree of mobility appropriate for them. Less research concerns the attitudes among the parents of very young children for whom mobility is not yet an issue (Martens, Scott, and Uprichard 2006). This chapter takes a first step toward filling that gap by exploring how the parents of very young children discuss parental anxiety as they describe the purchase of products that they view as reducing the risks facing their children. More specifically, this chapter examines consumer reviews of baby monitors on Epinions.com and demonstrates that the reviews constitute a site of popular culture in which parental anxiety is treated as an everyday occurrence to be addressed through a particular practice of consumption.

The particular product under consideration, baby monitors, ties this chapter to a second set of concerns. Some commentators explicitly link issues of monitoring and surveillance to issues of "risk society" (Haggerty and Ericson 2006; Lyon 2001). Other commentators leave these links implicit, as, for example, when Staples (2000, 155) simply notes that the "imperative of more and more social control is . . . a function of fear." For the most part, however, the burgeoning literature on the "new surveillance" (Marx 2002)—which brings new populations and "not just the official 'deviant'" (Staples 2000, 6) under the "watchful gaze" of others—finds its theoretical roots in the work of Foucault (1977) rather than that of theorists concerned with risk such as Giddens or Beck. And the bulk of this literature concerns practices of surveillance and monitoring that operate in the public sphere (e.g., by the state and its agents, by business and corporations) rather than in the private, personal realm. Increasingly, however, scholars note that these practices have become part of our daily lives and occur within personal and social relations. To the extent that this expansion of "everyday surveillance" (Staples 2000, 3) disciplines "people into acting in ways that others have deemed to be lawful or have defined as appropriate or simply 'normal,'" some believe it threatens the very groundwork of our society: "Taken together, these 'small acts of cunning' constitute the building blocks of what I would argue is a rapidly emerging disciplinary society; a society increasingly lacking in personal privacy, individual trust, or viable public life that supports and maintains democratic values and practices" (Staples 2000, 153).

Other scholars note that surveillance does not just threaten, but that it also protects. Lyon (2001) writes, for example, that although new monitoring technologies obviously can be used in the interest of power, they can also be used in the interest of care: we engage in surveillance of those about whom we care in order to reduce the risks to which they are exposed. Hence "the same process . . . both enables *and* constrains, involves care *and* control" (3; emphasis added).

As noted in the introduction to this volume, little empirical work to date has addressed the private (family) surveillance that employs the new technologies. Thus questions remain about the balance between care and control that characterizes the use of these technologies; questions remain also about the effects these technologies of surveillance have on the individual employing them as well as on those toward whom they are directed. This chapter represents a modest first step in consideration of these issues as well. I explore how those who monitor their babies (in response to their anxieties about risks) describe their experience of that practice. More specifically, I ask how that practice is linked to a vision of a child as being at risk (and therefore in need of care) as well as how that practice is linked to a vision of a child as being out of control (and therefore in need of correction). Finally, I ask how parents experience the relationship with a child when that relationship is mediated by a new technology of monitoring.

I take the reviews on Epinions as public utterances that, in the process of commenting on a specific product (in this case the baby monitor), articulate specific attitudes toward appropriate activities for parents. As reviewers participate in the promotion of consumer goods, they also participate in the "selling" of anxiety and of attitudes toward the appropriateness of careful monitoring—or surveillance—of children.

In what follows, I first describe my method of content analysis and then turn to a discussion organized around three sets of findings that emerge from a consideration of parents' comments regarding baby monitor use. Finally, I consider how the introduction of a monitor into a parent's relationship with her or his child affects that parent's freedom and skill development. In the conclusion I link the discussion back to the broader issue of parental anxiety and the solution of close monitoring as practices in society today.

Methods

Data Collection

Baby monitors vary widely in type and form: some transmit sound alone, some transmit both sound and lights, and some transmit video pictures. Some monitors allow for two-way communication (like an intercom or walkie-talkie), and some systems detect movement (to ensure that a baby is still breathing). These various types are combined for the purpose of analyzing the reviews.

The data for this chapter were obtained by coding 102 product ratings for baby monitors on Epinions.com. I selected every fifth baby monitor review (out of 510 on the site as of October 2005) and studied both the information contained in the respondent profiles attached to those reviews and the reviews themselves.

Epinions.com and Its Reviewers

Posting on Epinions is relatively straightforward; although there are rules to follow about word count and writing standards, anyone can post a review, and anyone who lands on the site can read the opinions there. A visitor to the site can also find out something about at least some of those who write the reviews. Epinions, in fact, prides itself in transparency:

> Epinions goes to great lengths to highlight the people behind the reviews so that you know exactly whom to trust. In addition to user biography pages, review lists, and the ability to comment on reviews, Epinions has introduced "tickets" to flag users who have violated our User Agreement. This mechanism allows shoppers to discount certain members' advice accordingly, and to stop seeking advice from these members.

Although they are given the opportunity to describe themselves, most reviewers offer little personal information on the biography pages. They do, however, reveal additional information in their reviews. Drawing on this information, I found that 88 percent of reviewers are women, a fact that is not surprising since women do much of the consumption work attached to households in general, and especially the consumption work attached to babies and children (de Grazia and Furlough 1996). The median age of these women is twenty-nine, and the vast majority (98 percent) of these women are married. (Reviewers indicate neither race/ethnicity nor sexual orientation.) Sixty-two percent of the women have one child, and 64 percent of those are expecting another. The average number of children is 1.6, and the median number is one. The reviewers come from twenty states and Canada. In terms of regions of the country, the Midwest is especially under-represented (relative to its total population), while both the South and, less significantly, the Northeast are over-represented. Most (59 percent) of the women describe themselves as "stay-at-home mothers," or, as they put it, SAHMs. The vast majority (92 percent) have more than a high school education.[3] In short, this is not a group representative of the U.S. population of mothers, although it may well be representative of the population of mothers among whom the attitude of parental anxiety is most prominent.

Making Sense of the Comments

Like other forms of content analysis (Berg 1998), this method is "unobtrusive" and does not generate the data with which it is concerned. The scholar becomes "relevant" in the analysis through the selection of the methodology and the interpretation of the data, but not through the generation of the data per se. These are utterances whose motivation lies outside the research context. Of course, it is hard to know just what these utterances mean. The Epinions authors are active consumers who, in one sense, become promoters of—or detractors from—particular products. In this chapter, although I am attentive to the context in which comments are written, ultimately what matters are the opinions reviewers offer in their accounts of monitors, because this is what visitors to Epinions can know. Hence, I explore here the practices encouraged by the public *discussion* of the technology of baby monitors.

The Normative Status of Parental Anxiety

Although baby monitors appeared on the scene only relatively recently, reviewers do not appear to think that they need to account for why they want or need a baby monitor.[4] Rather, they dive right in with a discussion of the benefits—and drawbacks—of the particular monitor they are reviewing. For example, one respondent said, "[This monitor] was a mother's dream. This is the monitor I wanted. . . . I researched them, spent hours in the baby stores, etc. I registered for this monitor, and received it." A casual reader of these reviews would thus learn that monitors are expected equipment: the central question is not whether to buy one, but rather which one to buy.

Routine Anxiety

When reviewers indicate *why* they asked for a monitor as a gift or purchased one themselves and, more frequently, when they discuss how they use their monitors, they explain what it is they are anxious about. Most often, they cite concerns about whether the configuration of their home or their own habits will allow them to hear their baby cry. These explanations indicate that the reviewers are motivated above all by a desire to satisfy anxiety through care and attentiveness: "When I first found out I was pregnant, I of course went to register for all the 'neat' things at the baby store! A definite necessity was a baby monitor so I could know when I was being 'paged.'" "I received the [monitor] as a baby shower gift. Being the ever careful, new mom, I knew that I would need one." "A monitor was definitely a necessity for the night-time being that we would never be able to hear a baby cry from that far away." Some reviewers suggest that they did not initially view a monitor as a necessity, but over time came to feel the need to respond to their own anxieties about their infant's care. For some, this change occurred after having received a monitor ("little did I know the fears of a new parent"); for others it followed moving the child to a separate room ("Eventually I wanted to move her to the crib in her room. I found this to be a BIG STEP. I was nervous about not seeing and hearing her every move").[5] One parent said that she had chosen not to follow medical advice and allowed her new baby to sleep on his or her stomach; she said she then needed a monitor because she and her husband "were nervous wrecks because of the SIDS risk."[6]

Implicitly, and sometimes explicitly, reviewers thus indicate that only by being aware of the baby at all times—by hearing the baby and occasionally even also seeing it or having a sensor ready to tell you if it stops breathing—can they achieve anything approximating peace of mind. Without that awareness, the reviewers suggest they would have no way to alleviate their anxieties. As the reviewers write about the motivations underlying their use of the monitors, they normalize anxiety and suggest its (partial) resolution through heightened surveillance. Indeed, they identify anxiety as a part (and perhaps an essential part) of what it means to be a parent, especially the first time around, and they implicitly give *other* parents permission to experience the same anxiety and to respond similarly by keeping a close eye on the baby: "Being new parents, we are, of course, checking about every 30 seconds to make sure our baby is still breathing." Anxiety, then, is never interrogated; rather it is accepted as a routine part of the everyday condition of parenting.

Enhanced Anxiety

Interestingly, the parental anxiety the baby monitor is meant to relieve turns out to be broadened by the technological solution: once a monitor is in place or available, a variety of activities which might otherwise not have been occasions for attentiveness (or might have been occasions on which one chose explicitly not to be attentive) now become occasions on which one has to be—or at least must consider being—attentive. As one woman said, with a monitor "you don't have to worry about not being able to hear your baby when you are doing laundry or even taking a shower."

Moreover, as monitors become commonplace (and are assumed to be essential) in the homes of (at least some) parents of young children, "necessary" attentiveness reaches ever deeper. It is no longer sufficient to hear the baby; you now have to be able to hear every breath it takes and the slightest mewl or whimper: "I used the monitor because, even though I could probably hear him, I wanted the added security of hearing *exactly what was going on*" (emphasis in original). In writing about some monitors—namely, those that show pictures and those that send out an alarm if the baby stops breathing—reviewers suggest that hearing alone may be insufficient: an attentive parent observes a baby's every activity and ensures that it is alive. One woman revealed just how insidious the practice of relying on a sensor had become, and how monitoring had created the fear of *not* monitoring, when she debated whether or not to wake her baby who had chosen to nap in a playpen rather than in his crib.

In short, as the reviewers describe the virtues of their monitors, they make parental anxiety the expected state of parenthood. Ironically, the solution they put in place to alleviate that anxiety both extends and intensifies it. If the price of monitoring is the expansion of attentive care and the elimination of the option of *not* being attentive at certain times or to certain sounds, two questions arise. First, why do babies need to be monitored? And second, what effects does monitoring a baby have on a parent's development of her or his own role? I address each of these in turn below.

Monitored Babies

The answer to the first question demonstrates that baby monitoring, like other surveillance techniques, can encompass both care and control.

Babies in Need of Care

The perceived need for monitoring rests on an image of babies as being intensely vulnerable, at risk, and in need of parental intervention: they may stop breathing and a parent will not be aware, and they may need or want attention that is not forthcoming. I am not arguing that this is not the case—after all, babies do stop breathing, babies require solicitous care, and babies do want their parents near them when they wake from naps. But I do want to suggest that rather than viewing the baby as "essentially" okay, or more likely than not to be able to sustain its own life or even to entertain itself, the monitor discussions reenvision the baby so as to emphasize its fragility and neediness; they then suggest that the proper stance is heightened attention and the ready responsiveness of "intensive mothering" (Anderegg 2003; Hays 1996; Lareau 2003; Warner 2005): "Some people I know say since their house is so small, they don't need [a monitor]. My house isn't very big, but I know that in order for me to hear her, she has to scream, and it is not very good for babies to have to work up into a full scream in order to be tended to."

Babies in Need of Control and Adjustment

As I discuss further in the conclusion, this care is, in and of itself, a kind of discipline in the broader sense that the word implies of producing some behaviors even as others are restrained (Foucault 1977). Interestingly, babies also turn out to need "discipline" as the concept is used in everyday speech, to imply correction and change. Even babies, it seems, are capable of getting into trouble. One woman, referring to her infant still in a crib, wrote: "The [monitor] does what it ultimately intends to do, give you piece [sic] of mind that you can leave your baby alone for a little while and be able to hear her if she gets into mischief."

The notion of the potential for mischief becomes more pronounced as infants mature into toddlers, and even more so as they become school-age children. Baby monitors play a role here, too.[7] Some parents say that they rely on monitors to hear just what it is their youngsters are doing in the playroom, and they rely on intercom systems to get those children to change their behavior when they become too rambunctious: "This is also a great monitor to hide in the playroom. I can put the transmitter in the room and when I hear them getting too rowdy, I just push the button and tell them to simmer down. It's great because they think God told me they were acting up and I don't have to walk all the way upstairs!"

Of course, this control would not be necessary if infants and children

were perfect to begin with. But babies and children turn out to be very im-
perfect creatures. Not only do they cry, but they cry loudly; they also sleep
when parents want them to be awake, and they wake when parents want
them to sleep. Interestingly, reviewers suggest that the monitor put in place
to relieve the anxiety of having a highly vulnerable (and potentially mischievous) baby creates a new possibility: that of adjusting the baby to meet speci-
fications. That is, parents suggest that as a "by-product" of using a monitor,
they get technological control over an "unsatisfactory" baby. One woman
expressed delight about her newfound capacity to control input: "I love the
fact that if I want to I can switch to the 'on' position and hear every breath or
I can switch to 'voice activated' position and only hear [the baby's] cries or
talking."

Although the basic use of the monitor is to get *more* information than
would be possible if one relied on one's senses alone, monitors also provide
the option of getting *less* information and thus reducing the "annoyance" of
having a new baby in the home:

> Our baby is LOUD in his sleep. He snores, he grunts, he wiggles, he passes
> gas. On the regular setting it was too much for either my husband or my-
> self to get any sleep. Once we switched over to the voice-activated setting
> we were much happier. Now we hear him if he talks or needs us, but we
> are not kept up constantly by his flatulence.

> Say you're on the phone and baby is sleeping in the next room. You can
> turn the volume down . . . but you can still see if baby is crying because the
> light bars will go across the monitor. . . . It's a nice way to keep tabs on baby
> without listening to every single little sound coming from that room.

Sound reduction and light substitution turn out to be especially handy for an
anxious mother who has a cranky baby she does not want to hear or for an
attentive mother who has decided to let her baby cry and would rather not
live with those consequences:

> Our son was very colicky the first few months, and it was nice having the
> option of just watching him wake up or fall asleep rather than hearing
> him—a little break for Mommy's ears, but I'm still completely "tuned in" to
> the little guy.

> When the baby would cry and cry, and we would try to let her cry it out
> and put herself to sleep . . . [it] was easier if we didn't have to actually hear

her. So, we would turn the volume on the monitor all the way down, but we would still be able to see the lights. . . . The lights let us still be aware of the intensity of her crying, and also let us know when she had stopped, so we could sneak in and look at our sleeping angel and give ourselves a pad [*sic*] on the back.

Parents thus can decide just how much information they want. A parent with a monitor equipped with a sensor explained that there is a switch that allows an audible "tick" every time the baby moves or even breathes. Ultimately, she found that she did not want to live with a ticking baby: "I think I used the tick for about five minutes before it got too annoying and [I] shut it off." Another woman, however, "loved" her new toy and her capacity to be reassured by the "ticking sounds": "In fact, it is BECAUSE of the 'tics' that I am able to sleep so peacefully. Every time I wake up in the middle of the night, I just listen for the tics and then fall back asleep."

Although the adjustments actually involve tinkering with the monitor itself, parents sometimes write as if the monitor *is* the baby. Instead of saying that they have heard the baby cry, they comment that the monitor lights themselves tell them that something is amiss. Recall the woman quoted above who said that she enjoyed "having the option of just watching him wake up or fall asleep rather than hearing him" when what she was "watching" was not the baby at all but a row of lights on her monitor.

As the conflation between baby and monitor proceeds, the positive emotions associated with the baby become attached to the monitor: "I received [the monitor] and I fell in love . . . I am so very happy with this monitor." "I LOVE this monitor." "These little guys are in one word exceptional!" Negative emotions are conflated as well: one woman, with a note of deep sadness more appropriate to a failed adoption, wrote regretfully, "We wanted to love this monitor but it just broke our hearts." Another said, "Out of the 4 monitors we have owned I HATE this one the most." To be sure, some of the immoderate language is a product of the forum in which these comments are being produced. The Epinions writers are trying to convince others that they know what they are talking about; they are also trying to persuade others to share their feelings and to trust them as a source. Moreover, from reading reviews of other products on Epinions, it is clear that not only monitors are "loved" and "hated." Advertising teaches us to wax hyperbolic about products. Hence it might not be surprising that reviewers exaggerate the perfections—or failures—of the particular monitors they have purchased (Chen, Fay, and Wang 2003). But whether or not this language is driven by the medium itself, it reflects the transfer of affection from the baby to the technology associated with the baby, and it indicates a fetishistic attitude similar to that attached to other baby paraphernalia (as when parents bronze a child's first pair of shoes or save each tooth as it comes out). When parents anthropomorphize the monitors, they place themselves in the position (at least verbally) whereby they need merely to confront a machine rather than a live infant. Control thus becomes easier.

Monitoring Parents

As reviewers write about monitors in sharply evaluative language, they reveal that as new parents they both have a capacity to change *and* are resistant to change. Parents are willing—in fact, perhaps, eager—to become attentive in order to participate in what they believe is risk reduction. They are less willing, however, to give up their mobility or to adapt themselves (rather than adapt the baby) to achieve this attentiveness. The new technology of surveillance allows them to retain old behaviors; it might also have its own costs and teach parents some new skills.

Freedom's Pleasures, Freedom's Costs

Reviewers comment that they value monitors because they give the literal gifts of freedom of movement and of making noise while enabling them to achieve the peace of mind that results from remaining attentive to vulnerable babies. Reviewers commenting on the use of monitors write frequently about these freedoms, cherishing the fact that they can go outside to mow the lawn, vacuum, take a shower, relax with the sound of music turned up high, enjoy a movie with a partner, or even throw a noisy party. As one reviewer said in characteristically hyperbolic language, "For my family, [the monitor] is a miracle. The system gives us independence."

Of course, there is a literal price to be paid for these literal "freedoms." That price includes not only the cost of the monitor and the slight hassles associated with setting it up, but also a willingness to accept being tethered. (Indeed, so tethered are parents that they almost invariably conflate the machine with themselves and refer to the mobile component of the monitor as the "parent unit.") The newfound mobility has strings attached. Some reviewers, having had a taste of freedom, want still more: they want to go next door to talk with a neighbor, to wander into the basement of a large apartment building, or to have sufficient battery power to use the monitor while camping. The technological limits are not easily accepted.

The Status of Skill

In other ways as well, parents appear to expect the monitor to make necessary adaptations for them. Whereas "traditionally" new parents comment on how they learn to sleep less soundly than they did before, reviewers suggest that with baby monitors it might not be necessary to develop this skill. One woman, for example, noted that she relied on the monitor to do the listening for her: "I kept using that monitor though because I didn't want to risk using nothing and not hearing my son if he woke up in the night. I am a very hard sleeper, so that worried me." Another wrote, "My husband and I are both deep sleepers so a monitor is a must for us to be on the listen for our son at night."

But reliance on this technology is not "free," either. As parents learn to rely on the monitor they might need to develop a new set of skills, even though they are less explicit about these. In an interesting article, Sandelowski (2002) writes about how the new "virtual geography" of nursing has changed the tasks of the nurse, the skills they develop, and the medium through which they experience their patients:

> No longer simply encountering their patients directly as manifestly physical presences, they now increasingly encounter them indirectly as virtual presences on screen and over telephone lines. . . . In the burgeoning field of telephone nursing . . . nurses and patients rely on a "mono-sensory device" to communicate with each other. . . . Telephone nurses are compelled to "infer from reduced data" the conditions and intentions of their patients. (67)

Similarly, it could be argued that parenting with the assistance of a monitor involves experiencing one's child as a "virtual presence," receiving communication from a "mono-sensory device," and thus needing to make greater inferences from reduced data. And reviewers do suggest that in time they become adept at interpreting the row of flashing lights and distinguishing the intensity of a child's cry from the monitor static.

In addition, in cases where the monitor allows for two-way communication, another set of skills might be developed. As Sandelowski (2002) notes about nurses,

> Telephone-mediated encounters "vastly reduce the richness of the presence" of the nurse to patient, as each party is only partially present to each other as a voice and thus without the full range of "sensory presence" occurring in face-to-face encounters. . . . Moreover, as telephones "incline"

users towards interactions involving the communication of information, nurses must work around the telephone to convey the fullness of attentive care. (67)

In the same vein, when parents communicate to their children through the use of the intercom, they might need to invest their voices with the "fullness of attentive care" they might previously have conveyed through their presence or physical touch: "When he starts crying, he wants to hear my voice, [so] I will sing to him on the intercom and he will fall right back to sleep. Just knowing that I am right there with him." "I can be in another room and talk into the parent unit and my baby will hear me on the nursery unit. . . . Sometimes when she would wake up at night, as long as she could hear my voice, she would go right back to sleep."

In short, I am suggesting that reliance on a baby monitor may encourage the development of a somewhat different set of skills than would exist if parents relied on their senses alone. Instead of learning to sleep lightly, parents learn to listen for the squawk of a monitor; instead of directly observing their children, they learn to interpret their children's needs through the medium of the flashing lights; and instead of communicating comfort with their presence, they rely on oral communication.

Interestingly, the technology users also become adept at some unusual skills unrelated to care. Technology has traditionally been seen as highly gendered and as a male preserve (Fox Keller and Longino 1996). But women write these reviews and explore the technology associated with the monitors. While none of that technology seems overly complex, monitors do require multiple adjustments. Women as well as men seem eager and ready to develop ingenious tests for the equipment and to mold it to their purposes. (For example, one user described putting a stack of books on a sensing monitor to see if it could actually tell the difference between an inert weight and a live one.)

In addition, monitor users also gain new experiences of "voyeurism" and come to view stealth observation as both an appropriate and an enjoyable practice. For example, reviewers write about the enormous pleasure of listening to a baby who is putting herself to sleep without directly intruding on or disrupting that process, and about the delights of getting to know what their children are doing when the children believe themselves to be unobserved.

As the monitor mediates the relationship between the parent and the baby, and as the parents rely on the monitor to represent the baby in virtual space, perhaps it is not surprising that sometimes parents speak as if the monitor has become alive, and even as if it is an independent *substitute* caregiver. Monitors interact with cell phones ("The monitor has bonded with one of my . . . cordless phones that is plugged into the same outlet as the receiver"); monitor lights act autonomously ("There have been a few times when I thought the baby was sleeping too long only to look up and see the lights going nuts"); and monitors listen ("I have peace of mind knowing there's an ear, or *two* listening in on my son"). Indeed, the monitor even makes its own decisions:

> When the monitor is set to "voice activated," it eliminates this faint noise. It simply shuts the speaker off when there is no noise. However, as soon as [my daughter] makes the slightest peep, the speaker belts out with the peep. . . . If [my daughter] is starting to rouse, *the monitor will turn on at first but then assume that the consistent (minor) noise is background noise and filter it out.* As [my daughter] gets slightly louder and louder, *the speaker will continue to filter the noise out.* Finally, *the speaker will decide that [my] little [daughter] is indeed awake,* but by then, she's pretty hacked off and making quite a racket. :) (emphasis added)

As Epinions reviewers assess products, they proffer considerable information that allows a window into their preoccupations. They suggest that parental anxiety is normal and that vigilance is an appropriate response to that anxiety. Indeed, there appears to be very little resistance to this central notion. Only one reviewer among the over one hundred examined suggested that a monitor was unnecessary and that parents would do better to be somewhat *less* attentive:

> I registered and received the [monitor] for a shower gift when I was pregnant with my first child. I thought this would be something we couldn't do without but found out differently. . . . If your baby doesn't sleep very well, our pediatrician tells you to put the monitor away because you jump at every noise you hear or you get them up when perhaps they might comfort themselves back to sleep.

The almost uniform requirement of attentiveness rests on the notion that babies are simultaneously fragile (and thus in need of surveillant care) and capable of mischief (and thus in need of surveillant control). In addition, the reviewers suggest that babies are also adjustable and that those adjustments can protect parents from incurring some new obligations of parenting, even as they accept tethering in the name of freedom and acquire some new skills and some new pleasures.

Conclusion

The Epinions monitor reviewers are often self-conscious about their descriptions and their product ratings. They are also occasionally self-conscious about their parenting practices: a reviewer who said that she let her baby cry added, in parentheses, "I know some may not agree with my process of getting my little one to sleep, but please don't rate on that." However, reviewers are not particularly self-conscious about parental anxiety itself: they appear to view anxiety not as a problem that needs to be nipped in the bud, but rather as an acceptable (if intolerable) position that requires a technological fix. And they do not appear to have the same concerns as those who write about the spread of surveillance in our society and its problematic features. That is, parents using monitors do not worry about whether they are engaged in "meticulous rituals of power" (Staples 2000), in threats to autonomy or democracy, or even in invasions of privacy. This lack of self-consciousness suggests that parents believe they have both a "right" and a moral obligation to know what is going on with their own child. Indeed, as noted above, monitor users believe it is necessary to "hear every breath," and they experience the "voyeurism" associated with surveillance as an appropriate and enjoyable practice. However, we might ask some questions (and speculate about some issues) that monitoring the baby raises, even if parents themselves assert a kind of unself-conscious acceptance of anxiety and ease with this new technology purchased to alleviate it.

One question is whether parents fail to develop trust in their own observational skills so that they become dependent on technology to do the observing for them. That is, we might wonder whether postmodern parents are "underdeveloped" with respect to their own capacities for attentiveness (e.g., light sleep, keeping an "ear" out for noise). Although the answer might be "yes," and that answer might not be troublesome, concerns clearly arise at unforeseen moments when monitoring parents cannot rely on the technology (e.g., if the electricity fails or the monitor breaks). More significantly, the consequence of underdeveloped skills of attentiveness may be the inability to watch over children without a monitoring device and a failure to develop the confidence to do so.

This raises a second, related issue of whether parents who rely so extensively on monitoring come to distrust their children's capacities for *self*-monitoring (Salmon 1999). Recall that some parents use monitors to keep track of babies as they mature into toddlers and even older children. One parent asked—albeit jokingly—whether it would be possible to slip a monitor into her children's rooms when they became teenagers. To the extent that monitoring rests on a notion of children being simultaneously fragile and mischievous and relies on the capacity of monitors to observe and adjust, it might be that these parents will want to use other devices for similar purposes later on. These monitor users might be tempted by walkie-talkies for young children, cell phones for older children, global positioning systems in the cars of teenage drivers (LaGesse 2005), "smart cards" to tell them what their children have ordered for lunch in school (Yee 2005), and at-home drug testing (Moore and Haggerty, Chapter 3). And while some of these devices enable children to expand and negotiate their own range of movement (Fotel and Thomsen 2004), others invade personal space and bodily privacy (Lyon 2001; Staples 2000).

Third, we might ask whether children who are always monitored not only might be *perceived* as being less capable of monitoring themselves but actually might *become* less capable of doing so. Do "fragile" babies who are monitored get less exposure to practices that would make them less fragile? And does that fragility mean that parents must monitor ever more closely and assiduously? The lone resisting reviewer, for example, suggested that her pediatrician believed in the capacity of children to "comfort" themselves. The bulk of the reviewers, however, appear to believe that children want and need an immediate response to distress. Does the reliance on the technology encourage the "helicopter" mothers or "hovercraft" parents, who swoop down (by cell phone or in person) to help children solve their momentary crises and thereby create children who are unable to solve their crises themselves (Young 2002; Hofer et al., Chapter 14; ABC News 2005)? Are developmental tasks of increasing autonomy and self-reliance thus put at risk?

In short, we might ask whether monitoring becomes a vicious cycle, with more monitoring leading to ever more monitoring both because parents trust neither themselves nor their children and because more monitoring actually produces children who require this form of external control. If this is the case, we all stand in danger: when we assume the relevance of monitoring for all people, and when those who have been monitored cannot be trusted to act so as to merit the privilege of *self*-control, that privilege might be eroded for us all.

But I return from this apocalyptic vision to a more sober and modest conclusion, which rests on my findings rather than (mere) speculation. I found that Epinions constitutes an interesting site of popular culture which gives access to an understanding of how widespread and normal parental anxiety has become, that the solution of monitoring simultaneously rests on a view of children as vulnerable to danger and as being dangerous themselves, and that engagement in monitoring has the potential to transform parents even as it "protects" children.

Notes

The author thanks Yelizavetta Kofman for her help in coding and for her interest in the topic; the author thanks as well the anonymous reviewers for, and the editor of, the special issue of *Journal of Family Issues* in which this essay first appeared.

1. Newspaper columns on the topic engender a vociferous response. See, for example, the website Marano has entitled "A Nation of Wimps" (*www. nationofwimps.com*) and the many letters generated by Applebome's article in the *New York Times* ("Readers Respond" 2006).

2. Whatever the cause, commentators are ready to offer solutions. Some suggest that the problem of parental anxiety could be "solved" if there were more social responsibility for children (Warner 2005). For a more "academic" version of this argument, see Katz (2001) and Moore and Haggerty (2001). Those with a more conservative point of view suggest the solution might be found in having more mothers leave the workplace to watch children themselves and to practice "appropriate" family values ("Readers Respond" 2006).

3. There are other clues about the class location of the respondents. Many of the respondents said that they requested a specific monitor when they registered for gifts to be given at a shower or upon the birth of the baby, suggesting ease with that practice (and a community of friends who could afford to purchase gifts off a registry). Moreover, not only do these respondents have access to a computer and the Internet, both of which are tied to income (Newburger 2001), but over half (54 percent) of the twenty-two reviewers who mentioned that they had hobbies indicated that these included some form of computer technology or activity on the Internet (e.g., Yahoo! Groups or eBay). In addition, one-third of the women who listed hobbies specifically mentioned scrapbooking, a practice which prevails among individuals "who have a family-oriented culture, are economically upscale, are well educated, and have an extensive communications network with others involved with the hobby" (Fram 2005, 215).

4. The first reference I have been able to find to baby monitors occurred in July 1984 (Cable 1984).

5. By and large, monitors are used when babies sleep in a separate room from their parents. Of course, this practice is, in and of itself, a cultural phenomenon.

6. The reviewer here is referring to the recent public health campaign encouraging parents to place children on their backs to sleep in order to discourage Sudden Infant Death Syndrome (SIDS).

7.   Advertisements for other monitoring devices are even more explicit about the trouble children can get into if they are not closely watched. A wrist bracelet like those worn by people under house arrest keeps young children from wandering off in the mall; although some of the threat is identified as coming from the outside (predators), advertisements also suggest that the device will stop children from playing "hide and seek" without permission (*www.familyonboard.com/angelalert.html*, accessed December 2005). A global positioning device, SkyGuard, lets you know "*your kids are where they should be*, or avoiding areas where they shouldn't go" (emphasis in original). Devices to monitor and filter Internet use exist to keep children from predatory interactions in virtual space. However, the advertisement for the devices also suggests that boys "are aggressive downloaders" of pornography, music, and movies "invested with viruses, worms, and Trojan Horses," and that girls will use names in chat rooms which might inspire predators (*guardiansoftware.com*, accessed December 2006).

References

ABC News. 2005. Do "Helicopter Moms" Do More Harm Than Good? *ABC News Internet Ventures. abcnews.go.com/2020/print?id=1237868*.

Anderegg, David. 2003. *Worried All the Time: Rediscovering the Joy in Parenthood in an Age of Anxiety.* New York: Free Press.

Applebome, Peter. 2006. How We Took the Child out of Childhood. *New York Times*, January 8, New York/Region section.

Backett-Milburn, Kathryn, and Jeni Hardin. 2004. How Children and Their Families Construct and Negotiate Risk, Safety and Danger. *Childhood* 11 (4): 429–47.

Beck, Ulrich. 1992. *Risk Society: Towards a New Modernity.* London: Sage.

Berg, Bruce L. 1998. *Qualitative Research Methods for the Social Sciences*, 3rd ed. Boston: Allyn and Bacon.

Cable, J. C. 1984. Bringing Home Baby—and Monitor Too. *American Baby* 46: 18–21

Chen, Yubo, Scott Fay, and Qi Wang. 2003. Marketing Implications of Online Consumer Product Reviews. Working paper, Department of Marketing, University of Florida, Gainesville.

de Grazia, Victoria, and Ellen Furlough. 1996. *The Sex of Things: Gender and Consumption in Historical Perspective.* Berkeley: University of California Press.

Fotel, Trine, and Thyra Uth Thomsen. 2004. The Surveillance of Children's Mobility. *Surveillance and Society* 1 (4): 535–54.

Foucault, Michel. 1977. *Discipline and Punish: The Birth of the Prison*, trans. by Alan M. Sheridan. New York: Pantheon.

Fox Keller, Evelyn, and Helen E. Longino. 1996. *Feminism and Science.* New York: Oxford University Press.

Fram, Eugene H. 2005. The Booming Scrapbooking Market in the USA: Despite Phenomenal Growth, the Future's Unclear. *International Journal of Retail and Distribution Management* 33 (3): 215–25.

Giddens, Anthony. 1999. Risk and Responsibility. *Modern Law Review* 62 (1): 1–10.

Haggerty, Kevin D., and Richard V. Ericson. 2006. *The New Politics of Surveillance and Visibility.* Toronto: University of Toronto Press.

Hays, Sharon. 1996. *The Cultural Contradictions of Motherhood.* New Haven, CT: Yale University Press.

Hulbert, Ann. 2003. *Raising America: Experts, Parents, and a Century of Advice about Children.* New York: Knopf.

Katz, Cindi. 2001. The State Goes Home: Local Hyper-vigilance of Children and the Global Retreat from Social Reproduction. *Social Justice* 28 (3): 47–56.

LaGesse, David. 2005. My Car, the Informer. *U.S. News and World Report*, March 21.

Lareau, Annette. 2003. *Unequal Childhoods: Class, Race, and Family Life.* Berkeley: University of California Press.

Lupton, Deborah, and John Tulloch. 2002. "Risk Is Part of Your Life": Risk Epistemologies among a Group of Australians. *Sociology* 36 (2): 317–34.

Lyon, David. 2001. *Surveillance Society: Monitoring Everyday Life.* Philadelphia: Open University Press.

Marano, Hara Estroff. 2004. A Nation of Wimps. *Psychology Today* (November–December). *www.psychologytoday.com/articles/pto-20041112-000010.html.*

Marx, Gary T. 2002. What's New about the "New Surveillance"? Classifying for Change and Continuity. *Surveillance and Society* 1 (1): 9–29.

Martens, Lydia, Sue Scott, and Emma Uprichard. 2006. "Safety, Safety, Safety for Small Fry": Children and Safety in Commercial Communities of Parenthood. Statens institutt for forbruksforskning. *www.sifo.no/files/Lydia_Martens.pdf.*

Middlebury College Public Affairs. 2006. Do Cell Phones and Email Impede College Students' Transitions to Adulthood?, April 17. *www.middlebury.edu/about/ pubaff/news_releases/news_2006/news632808647373657799.htm* (accessed June 4, 2006; no longer available).

Newburger, Eric C. 2001. *Home Computers and Internet Use in the United States: August 2000.* Current Population Reports No. P23–207. Washington, DC: Department of Commerce, U.S. Census Bureau, September.

Readers Respond: Taking the Child Out of Childhood. 2006. *New York Times*, January 14, New York/Region section.

Salmon, Jacqueline L. 1999. Out of Trust, Some Parents Turn to Spying. *Washington Post*, February 28.

Sandelowski, Margarete. 2002. Visible Humans, Vanishing Bodies, and Virtual Nursing: Complications of Life, Presence, Place, and Identity. *Advances in Nursing Science* 24 (3): 58–70.

Staples, William G. 2000. *Everyday Surveillance: Vigilance and Visibility in Postmodern Life.* Lanham, MD: Rowman and Littlefield.

Starr, Alexandra. 2003. "Security Moms": An Edge for Bush? *Business Week* December 1: 60.

Stearns, Peter N. 2004. *Anxious Parents: A History of Modern Childrearing in America.* New York: New York University Press.

Warner, Judith. 2005. *Perfect Madness: Motherhood in the Age of Anxiety.* New York: Riverhead Books (Penguin).

Valentine, Gill. 1997a. "My Son's a Bit Dizzy," "My Wife's a Bit Soft": Gender, Children and Cultures of Parenting. *Gender, Place and Culture* 4 (1): 37–62.

————. 1997b. "Oh Yes I Can," "Oh No You Can't": Children and Parents' Understandings of Kids' Competence to Negotiate Public Space Safely. *Antipode* 29 (1): 65–89.

Valentine, Gill, and John McKendrick. 1997. Children's Outdoor Play: Exploring Parental Concerns about Children's Safety. *Geoforum* 28 (2): 219–35.

Yee, D. 2005. What Is Junior Eating at School? System Allows Parents to Monitor. *Associated Press*, May 29.

Young, John G. 2002. Parenting the Creatively Gifted. Adventures in Creativity Publications. *www.adventuresincreativity.net/1Parenting%20the%20 Creatively%20Gifted.htm.*

Zelizer, Viviana A. 1985. *Pricing the Priceless Child: The Changing Social Value of Children.* New York: Basic Books.

12

Policing Gender Boundaries

Parental Monitoring of Preschool Children's Gender Nonconformity

Emily W. Kane

In their review of the literature on parents, children, and gender, Coltrane and Adams (1997) conclude that parents "establish different learning environments for boys and girls and expect them to do different things" (245). Like other scholars offering broad overviews of the literature on gender and parenting (e.g., Maccoby 1998; McHale, Crouter, and Whiteman 2003), they reveal myriad ways in which parents gender their children, some of which are unconscious. In this chapter, I draw on data from qualitative interviews with parents of preschool-age children to explore how parents consciously monitor their children's gender performance and subsequently police gender boundaries by discouraging gender nonconformity. I argue that although many parents make efforts to stray from and thus expand traditional conceptions of gender, they do so within limits, balancing these efforts with conscious attention to producing socially acceptable gender performances, especially for their sons. This balancing act is evident among many parents I interviewed, regardless of their gender, race/ethnicity, social class, sexual orientation, and partnership status. But within that broader pattern of balancing, I also document notable variations. Heterosexual fathers play a particularly central role in monitoring their sons' masculinity and, in the process, reinforce their own as well. Their expressed motivations for that monitoring and boundary work often involve personal endorsement of traditionally de-

This chapter draws on material from a previously published article: Emily W. Kane, "'No Way My Boys Are Going to Be Like That!': Parents' Responses to Children's Gender Nonconformity," *Gender and Society* 20 (2006): 149–76.

fined masculinity. Heterosexual mothers and gay parents, by contrast, are more likely to report motivations for monitoring and boundary work that invoke fear of monitoring by others as they craft their sons' masculinity.

Parents and the Social Construction of Gender

Decades ago, literature on gender and parenting indicated that new parents may perceive male and female newborns differently, even when there are no actual differences in their appearance or behavior (Rubin, Provenzano, and Zella 1974). More recent literature documents a variety of practices, from first impressions on, through which parents construct and reproduce gender as a social category (e.g., Coltrane and Adams 1997; Maccoby 1998; McHale, Crouter, and Whiteman 2003). Some researchers highlight subgroups of parents who actively seek to disrupt traditional gendered expectations for their children (e.g., Risman and Myers 1997; Risman 1998; Stacey and Bibliarz 2001). But as a whole, the literature provides evidence of definite parental tendencies toward gendered treatment of children. For example, research indicates differential treatment of sons and daughters in terms of parental selection of toys and activities (Wood, Desmarais, and Gugula 2002; Beets et al. 2007); clothing (Cahill 1989); and decor for children's rooms (Pomerleau et al. 1990). Parents also treat sons and daughters differently in their degree of vocalization to young children (Clearfield and Nelson 2006); emphasis on emotions versus autonomy in telling family stories (Fiese and Skillman 2000; Reese, Haden, and Fivush 1996); styles of play (Lindsey and Mize 2002); and expectations for children's household chores (Raley and Bianchi 2006). Along with documenting gender-typing by parents, this literature highlights two additional patterns. First, fathers appear to engage in more differential treatment of sons and daughters and more enforcement of gender boundaries than do mothers; second, for both mothers and fathers, such boundary maintenance appears to be more evident in the treatment of sons than daughters (Antill 1987; Coltrane and Adams 1997; Maccoby 1998).

Quantitative research that relies on such methods as experiments, closed-ended surveys, and counting the frequency of various parental behaviors features prominently in the extensive literature on gender-typing by parents. This literature is valuable in establishing the role that parents play in gendering their children. However, it does less to explore the nuances of how parents make meaning around gender, to reveal what motivates parents as they participate in the social construction of their children's gender, and to illuminate how aware parents are of their role in these processes. Parents are clearly gendering their children, but what are the gendered outcomes they seek to construct, why do they seek to construct those outcomes, and how aware are they of that construction process? It is around questions like these that I orient my analysis of parental monitoring of young children's gender.

Doing Gender:
Accomplishment and Accountability

The interactionist approach to gender as accomplishment (e.g., West and Zimmerman 1987; Fenstermaker, West, and Zimmerman 1991; West and Fenstermaker 1993, 1995) provides a helpful framework for understanding what I heard about gender nonconformity in my interviews with parents of young children. This approach allows us to view parents not simply as agents of gender socialization but as actors involved in a more nuanced and complex process of accomplishing gender with and for their children. In some of the earlier work elaborating this "doing gender" approach, West and Zimmerman (1987, 128) assert that "gender is not a set of traits, nor a variable, nor a role, but the product of social doings of some sort." From this perspective, gender is a situated accomplishment constantly being produced and reproduced in interaction. As West and Fenstermaker (1993, 152) later note, "Conceiving of gender as an ongoing accomplishment, accountable to interaction, implies that we must locate its emergence in *social situations*, rather than within the individual or some ill-defined set of role expectations" (emphasis in original).

The notion of gender as accomplished is thus central to this theoretical approach, but equally central is the concept of accountability. Fenstermaker and West (2002, 212) note that accountability "leads people to manage conduct in anticipation of how others might describe it on a particular occasion," and Fenstermaker, West, and Zimmerman (1991, 294) also argue that such accountability, in relation to gendered expectations, is a key part of the process of doing gender: "Insofar as societal members know that their conduct is accountable, they will frame their actions in relation to how they might be construed by others in the context in which they occur. . . . An individual involved in virtually any course of action may be held accountable for her/his execution of that action as a woman or as a man."

Accountability, they argue, is relevant not only when people are doing gender in accordance with the expectations of others but also when they resist or stray from such expectations. This claim, present in West and Zimmerman's 1987 formulation, is one to which Fenstermaker and West (2002) return in defending the approach against criticism that it does not allow for resistance and social change. They argue that their focus on the *process* by which gender is accomplished places activity, agency, and the possibility of resistance in the foreground: "Within the dynamic nature of the accomplishment of categorical difference reside the seeds of inevitable change" (219). But the accomplishment of such change takes place within the context of, and is constrained by, accountability to gendered assessment.[1]

As the results presented here demonstrate, many parents feel accountable for enforcing gender boundaries, monitoring their children's gender performance in order to live up to their own personal expectations and to respond to the assessments (potential or real) of generalized and specific others. Such accountability and assessment are evident for both young sons and daughters, but are particularly frequent and particularly intense in the case of sons.

Interviewees, Interview Process, and Analysis

In my analysis, I draw on data from forty-two interviews with a diverse sample of parents, each of whom has at least one preschool-age child (between the ages of three and five years). Interviews focused on parents' perceptions of their children's gendered attributes and behaviors. I emphasize the preschool age range because this is the period when most children begin to develop a clear understanding of the gender expectations around them and to engage in more gender-typed patterns of behavior (Maccoby 1998). Interviews were conducted primarily in southern and central Maine (with a small number conducted elsewhere in New England) over a three-year period ending in the fall of 2002. I recruited participants through postings in local child-care centers, parents' resource organizations, community colleges, local businesses, and public housing projects. I also recruited participants through personal networks (although none of the participants were people I knew prior to the interviews).

The process of participation began with a brief written questionnaire, followed by a semistructured interview. I placed particular emphasis on a focal child between the ages of three and five, although I also asked questions about any other children with whom the respondent lived. My major focus in the interview questions was on the current activities, toys, clothes, behaviors, and gender awareness of the focal child, as well as the parents' perceptions of the origins of these outcomes and their feelings about their children's behaviors and characteristics in relation to gendered expectations. The interviews were taped and transcribed, and generally lasted from one to two hours. I conducted most interviews, although a research assistant conducted some as well. I paid participants a modest honorarium for their time and participation and ensured them complete confidentiality.

The forty-two interviewees include twenty-four mothers and eighteen fathers. Interviewees come from a diverse range of family types (single parent and two-parent families, with some of the latter being blended families); class locations (based on self-identification and ranging from low income to upper middle class); racial/ethnic groups (thirty-five white, four Asian American, and three African American interviewees); and sexual orientations (thirty-seven heterosexual and five gay parents). These parents' children include biological children, adopted children, stepchildren, and foster children. Interviewees' educational backgrounds range from having completed less than a high school education to holding a doctorate, with the average level of formal schooling falling between high school graduate and college graduate. Ages range from twenty-three to forty-nine years, with the average age at thirty-five. Interviewees have, on average, 2.5 children (with the mode being two), and the children on whom interviews focus include twenty-two sons and twenty daughters.

For the particular topic of this analysis, my interest is in whatever parents themselves perceive as gender nonconformity on the part of their child, whether actual or potential. Therefore, I began by identifying all text in the transcripts in which a parent comments on items, activities, attributes, or behaviors as more typical of a child of the other sex. Among such mentions, I focus on those for which the parent reports some response, whether positive or neutral (e.g., "I love it"; "it's fine with us"; "we just go ahead and let him do it"; "I try hard to encourage that") or negative (e.g., "I worry about . . ."; "it bothers me when . . ."; "I tell him he can't do that"; "we just say no"). Many of the interview questions specifically address whether the parents consider their child's toys, clothes, activities and attributes to be stereotypically gender-linked, but I do not identify particular activities or attributes as stereotypically male or female. Instead, I document what parents themselves view as atypical. Given my focus on accountability to others, I also code all mentions of monitoring a child's gender performance in response to others noting gender noncomformity, whether by specific others or as a more generalized sense of social expectations.

The analyses presented in this chapter focus on parental monitoring and policing of gendered boundaries. Thus, although I offer a brief overview of positive responses some parents have to behavior or interests they consider atypical, I focus on negative responses. Negative responses toward children's gender nonconformity vary by gender of child and gender of parent. But they do not vary consistently by parents' racial/ethnic background or class location.[2] Therefore, although I indicate the race, class, and sexual orientation of each parent quoted, I only discuss variations by gender and sexual orientation, and only when my analysis revealed such variations.

Positive Responses to Gender Nonconformity for Daughters and Sons

Mothers and fathers, across a variety of social locations, often celebrate what they perceive as gender nonconformity on the part of their young daughters. They report enjoying dressing their daughters in sports-themed clothing, as well as buying them toy cars, trucks, trains, and building toys. Some describe their efforts to encourage, and their pleased reactions to, what they consider traditionally male activities, like tee-ball, football, fishing, and learning to use tools. Several note that they make an effort to encourage their young daughters to aspire to traditionally male occupations and comment favorably on their daughters as "tomboyish," "rough and tumble," and "competitive athletically." Altogether, about two-thirds of parents of daughters offer at least one positive or neutral response to evidence of gender nonconformity in their children.

Parents also offer a substantial number of positive or neutral responses to gender nonconformity on the part of their young sons, again with about two-thirds of parents who have at least one son offering such a comment. A large number report allowing or even encouraging traditionally female toys like dolls, doll houses, kitchen centers, and tea sets. With respect to these toys, parental neutrality or positive responses often revolve around a desire to encourage nurturance, sensitivity, emotional openness, empathy, and nonviolence as attributes parents consider nontraditional but desirable for boys. Mothers and fathers express with similar frequency these kinds of efforts to accomplish gender differently for their sons, but fathers are less enthusiastic and more likely to include caveats, such as age limits (e.g., "it's OK, up to a certain age, I guess") or qualifiers (e.g., "maybe if there's nothing else to do").

Negative Responses: Monitoring and Enforcing Gender Boundaries for Daughters

A few parents offer negative responses that indicate a monitoring of their daughters' gender nonconformity and a policing of femininity, although these tend to be general and offered with little strong sense of concern. For example, an African American, low-income, heterosexual mother offers some positive responses to what she perceives as gender nonconformity on the part of her daughter, but also notes limits: "I wouldn't want her to be too boyish, because she's a girl." Much as parents of children who appear to be of a different race/ethnicity than themselves are sometimes accosted by strangers curious about the family relationships (see Jacobson, Chapter 4), so too are some parents questioned in public about the gender performance of their children:

> She had this outfit, I remember when she was about three months old, it was black leggings and a little black sweater. . . . I was holding her at a bakery, and someone said, "What a cute fellow!" And I said "Oh, it's a girl, but thank you." . . . And the person said "Well, why are you putting her in black? That's why the sexes are all mixed up today!" (White, upper-middle-class, heterosexual mother)

Another mother reports feeling accountable to others in relation to her daughter's gender performance and, as a result, monitoring and restricting that performance:

> I'm a lot less tolerant of noise and aggression, just because I know that especially out in public, like if we're in church, if it's a little boy grabbing things or making noise people kind of, well, they kind of smile, you know, they want them to quiet down but they kind of smile first. If it's a girl, they're more standoffish, I do notice that . . . and I want her to feel that what she's doing is right, for her not to feel like she's different. (White, working-class, heterosexual mother)

This mother specifically reports an attempt to enforce gender boundaries by doing gender conventionally with her daughter in response to her experience of how generalized others react to her child's public behavior. This sort of monitoring and adjustment in response to the expectations of others is also evident in parents' reports about clothing and other aspects of appearance:

> When she was a baby, there were a couple of times when we took her out, where even though she was wearing pink, you know, people were like, "Oh, you've got a cute little boy there." . . . So I think we made a conscious effort to dress her a certain way, so they knew she was a girl. (White, middle-class, heterosexual father)

Thus, parents of daughters describe some degree of parental monitoring and enforcement of gender boundaries. But even the handful of parents who offer such comments do so in combination with at least one positive response to something they characterize as gender atypical. It is possible that as girls reach adolescence, parents may be more concerned about perceived departures from traditional femininity. However, in my interviews with parents of much younger girls, that concern is uncommon.

Negative Responses: Monitoring and Enforcing Gender Boundaries for Sons

The situation regarding sons is quite different. Many parents of boys express at least some concern or discomfort regarding what they perceive as gender nonconformity, with the most common mentions involving items, activities, or attributes that could be considered icons of femininity or associated in some way with homosexuality. In addition, while variations by parents' gender and sexual orientation are not evident in responses to daughters, parental monitoring and accountability motivations do vary by both gender and sexual orientation in responses to sons. For some parents, these motivations are personal and involve monitoring how well a son lives up to the parent's own preference for normative masculinity; these motivations are most common among heterosexual fathers. For other parents, motivations involve concerns about accountability to gender assessment by peers, other adults, and society in general; these motivations are most common among heterosexual mothers and gay parents (whether mothers or fathers).

Monitoring Icons of Femininity: Pink, Ballet, and Barbies

Wearing pink or frilly clothing; wearing skirts, dresses, or tights; and playing dress up in any kind of feminine attire are among the activities that elicit expressions of concern among parents of sons. A number of parents note concern over nail polish, reporting discomfort about young sons wanting to have their fingernails or toenails painted. Dance, especially ballet, and Barbie dolls are also among the traditionally female activities some parents of sons note negatively. Looking across all thirty-one parents of sons (the twenty-two for whom the son is the focal child plus an additional nine for whom the focal child is a girl but who have a son as well), twenty-three mention negative reactions to at least one of these icons.

In relation to objects like clothing and toys, the following response is typical of the many concerns parents raise and the many indications of actions they take to monitor gender boundaries with and for their sons:

> If we go into a clothing store . . . I try to shy my son away from the Powerpuff Girls shirt or anything like that. . . . I would steer him away from a pink shirt as opposed to having him wear a blue shirt. (Asian American, middle-class, heterosexual father)

Barbie dolls are an especially interesting example. Although many parents regard baby dolls positively, viewing them as encouraging nurturance and helping to prepare sons for fatherhood, Barbie, an icon of femininity, strikes many parents of sons as problematic. Barbie is often mentioned when parents are asked whether their child has ever requested an item or activity more commonly associated with the other gender. Four parents—three mothers and one father—indicate that they had purchased a Barbie at their son's request. But more often parents of sons note that they would avoid letting their son have or play with Barbie dolls, echoing one white, low-income, heterosexual mother who notes that "there's not many toys I wouldn't get him, except Barbie."

Some parents report that they have attempted, or would attempt, to compromise in ways that strike me as designed to minimize Barbie's iconic status. These instances are particularly pointed examples of carefully crafted parental policing of gender boundaries: "I would ask him, 'What do you want for your birthday?' . . . and he always kept saying 'Barbie' . . . so we compromised, we got him a NASCAR Barbie" (white, middle-class, heterosexual mother). Another father reports that his five-year-old son likes to play Barbies with his four-year-old sister, and expresses relief that his son's interest is more in Ken than Barbie:

> He's not interested in Barbie, he's interested in Ken. . . . He plays with Ken and does boy things with him, he has always made clear that he likes Ken. . . . If he was always playing with dolls and stuff like this, then I would start to worry and try to do something to turn it around. But he plays with Ken and it doesn't go much further than that, so I'm fine. (White, upper-middle-class, heterosexual father)

These parents carefully monitor "how far" things go, balancing an openness to some crossing of gender boundaries (Thorne 1994) with careful limits, as the father in the previous quote indicates when he says that he would "do something to turn it around" if his son's interest were in Barbie rather than Ken.

Along with material markers of femininity, parents express concern about excessive emotionality and passivity in their sons. They also report actions they have taken to discourage frequent crying (like telling a son to "stop crying like a girl") and to encourage sons to fight for what they want. These various examples indicate the work many parents are doing to police and enforce gender boundaries for their sons, distancing those sons from any association with femininity.

Motivations for Monitoring Icons of Femininity

Some parents express negative feelings about a son's perceived gender non-conformity that are personal, invoking a sense of accountability not so much to other people as to their own moral or normative framework. Twice as many fathers refer to this kind of feeling as refer to accountability toward others. For example, one white, middle-class, heterosexual father refers to this general issue in two separate portions of the interview. These comments are in relation to his four-year-old son's interest in what the father considers "girly" toys:

> *Father:* I don't want him to be a little "quiffy" thing, you know . . . it's probably my own insecurities more than anything. I guess it won't ruin his life. . . . It's probably my own selfish feeling of, like, "No way, no way my kids, my boys, are going to be like that."
> *Interviewer:* Is it a reflection on you as a parent, do you think?
> *Father:* As a male parent, yeah, I honestly do.

This comment conveys the interviewee's belief that fathers are responsible for enforcing gender boundaries and crafting appropriately masculine sons. Sometimes this invocation of a father's own sense of normative gender for his son is offered more casually, as in the case of an Asian American, middle-class, heterosexual father, who says about his four-year-old son, "I wouldn't encourage him to take ballet or something like that, 'cause I guess in my own mind that's for a girl."

Some heterosexual fathers explicitly judge their success as fathers on the degree to which they are raising adequately masculine sons, suggesting that passing along that normative conception to their sons may be part of how they accomplish their own masculinity. Not only their sons' masculinity but also their own execution of fatherhood are at risk of gender assessment. The following interviewee raises this issue, with specific reference to being accountable to others for his performance as a father:

> There's this particular construction worker [when we were remodeling the kitchen], his name was Fred . . . he and I would sit down in the back and have a beer and talk about, you know, the day. And you'd see [my son] walk by, playing dress up in his sister's Cinderella outfit, and I'm thinking, "What must Fred be thinking of this?" . . . That's a stigma I have to live down, I suppose. (White, upper-middle-class, heterosexual father)

Here, the father is expressing concern not so much for how his son will be judged in the world but for how he (as the father) is being judged.

Heterosexual mothers and gay parents execute a similar process of monitoring and enforcing gender boundaries in relation to icons of femininity for their sons. But their expressed motivations more frequently invoke accountability to *others*, and specifically invoke fear for how their sons may be assessed by others if they do not approximate social ideals. That is, these parents more often focus on the child and the others to whom they assume their son's gender performance will be accountable, rather than on themselves. (Some heterosexual fathers also express concern about accountability to others, but, as noted previously, such concerns are outnumbered two-to-one by their references to their own normative framework.) Among both heterosexual and lesbian mothers, two-thirds express fear that their sons might be treated negatively by adults or peers if they do not avoid icons of femininity. One mother indicates that she would encourage her three-year-old son to wear styles and colors of clothing typically associated with boys, explaining her reasoning in terms of her fear for how her son would feel if others treated him negatively: "This stupid world cares about what we look like, unfortunately. . . . You know, it shouldn't, probably shouldn't matter. It's a piece of cloth, but that's the way the world is, and I wouldn't want him to feel out of place" (white, low-income, heterosexual mother).

About half of the mothers making such comments refer in this way to society in general, or to the adult world, while the other half refer to the child's peers. The following quote is typical of the various responses invoking the risk of gender assessment within a son's peer group: "I would worry if he had too many feminine characteristics, that would worry me. I just want him to be a boy and play with the boys, not to like girl things. If he did that, the boys would think he's weird, and then he'd be lonely" (African American, low-income, heterosexual mother).

Another mother offers a particularly dramatic example of her sense of accountability to others, in this case expressing concern for both her son and herself, by describing an incident that occurred about a year before the interview. Her son, two years old at the time, sustained an injury while playing dress up with his older sister. He was dressed in a pink princess costume, and once they arrived at the hospital the mother began to feel anxious about the monitoring power of the hospital staff:

> People can be so uptight about things, I was worried they were going to think I was some kind of nut, and next thing you know, send a social worker in. . . . You never know what people will think, and in a hospital, someone has the power to go make a phone call to a social worker or someone, someone who doesn't realize he's two years old and it doesn't matter. . . . It was totally obvious that it was a little boy dressing up in silly clothing but there are people out there who would think that's really wrong, and I was afraid. (White, upper-middle-class, heterosexual mother)

Also notable among the comments expressing accountability to others are reports by gay and lesbian parents who feel under particular scrutiny in relation to their sons' (but not their daughters') gender performance. Although my sample is diverse in terms of parents' sexual orientation, all five of the gay and lesbian parents interviewed are white and partnered, and they identify as middle- or upper-middle-class. In most ways, their responses to gender nonconformity parallel those of heterosexual parents. But there are two particular ways in which heterosexual parents differ from gay and lesbian parents. Only heterosexual parents raise fears or concerns about their sons' eventual sexual orientation (which I discuss below). In addition, four of the five gay and lesbian parents I interviewed have at least one son, and all four of those report feeling especially accountable for their sons' gender conformity. One white, upper-middle-class, lesbian mother of two sons notes that she feels "under more of a microscope," and that her sons "don't have as much fluidity" because she has "loaded the dice . . . in terms of prejudice they will face because of who their parents are." Another interviewee expresses similar sentiments:

> I feel held up to the world to make sure that his masculinity is in check or something. . . . It's a big rap against lesbian parents, how can you raise sons without a masculine role model in the house, and that's something I always feel up against. (White, upper-middle-class, lesbian mother)

A gay father of a three-year-old son invokes a similar concern:

> I mean, I think we have to be a little bit conscious of going too far, you know, as gay men the last thing we want to do is put him in anything that's remotely girly. (White, middle-class, gay father)

Some past research has emphasized the lack of any variation in gender-typing by parents' sexual orientation (Golombock and Tasker 1994; Gottman 1990; Patterson 1992). Among more recent research, Stacey and Bibliarz (2001) offer a compelling case that gay and lesbian parents tend to allow their children more freedom in terms of gendered expectations. But the parents I interviewed express a concern that indicates yet another social price they pay in a homophobic society, and it is one that arises about sons more than about daughters. Based on only four interviews, I cannot offer conclusive claims about how gay and lesbian parents feel about gender conformity. However, the fact that all of the gay and lesbian parents with sons spontaneously mention this sense of additional accountability regarding their sons' masculinity strongly suggests that gay and lesbian parents feel that they are under particular scrutiny.

Along with this sense of accountability to others, heterosexual mothers reveal another intriguing pattern, one that indicates the unique role that heterosexual fathers play in monitoring their sons' gender performance. I asked no specific questions about each interviewee's partner or ex-partner, but twelve of the fifteen heterosexual mothers of sons spontaneously mention either actual or potential negative reactions by their son's father to the boy's gender nonconformity. These mothers report negative responses similar to those previously described by heterosexual fathers themselves. For example, one white, low-income, heterosexual mother reported, "My son, when he gets upset, he will cry at any child, boy or girl, and my husband has made the comment about that being, you know, a girl thing, crying like a girl." In another example, a white, middle-class, heterosexual mother recounts defending her clothing purchases to her husband after a stranger assumed her then-infant son was a girl:

> I had a few people think the baby was a girl, which is kind of irritating, because I would think, "Oh my God, am I buying clothes that are too feminine looking?" The first time it happened I went right to [my husband] and said, "I bought this in the boys' department at Carter's, I'm telling you, I really did."

Another heterosexual mother, this one a white, working-class parent, reports not just defending her actions to her husband but making a purchase decision based on what her husband might think. When her five-year-old son asked for a Barbie suitcase at the store, she told him, "No, you can't have that; your father wouldn't like it." This mother may be steering her son in a direction that avoids the need for his father to become aware of, or react to, gender-atypical preferences in his son. I have noted the direct action many fathers take to monitor and enforce gender boundaries for their sons, but the accountability to fathers reported by some mothers indicates another, indirect path through which heterosexual men may further influence that boundary enforcement.

Monitoring Sexual Orientation: Searching for Signs?

Linked to these icons of feminine gender performance is another clear theme among some parents' negative responses to their sons' perceived gender nonconformity: fear that a son is gay (or will face the perception from others that he is). In their comments about daughters, parents do not spontaneously connect gender nonconformity and sexual orientation, nor do gay and lesbian parents make this connection for either sons or daughters. But seven of the twenty-seven heterosexual parents discussing sons do spontaneously connect gender noncomformity and sexual orientation. For example, an Asian American, middle-class, heterosexual father of two sons notes actions he takes, and that he assumes other fathers take, to discourage homosexuality. These actions involve encouraging gender conformity in sons: "Well, I hope he's heterosexual. So I guess maybe in the back of my mind, and I'm sure a lot of other guys' minds, that's why they'd push their children to the blue shirt over the pink shirt and things like that."

Another parent suggests parental responsibility to monitor and "correct" non-heterosexual tendencies in a son:

> *Mother:* If a boy really wants to dance, I would encourage that. I would
>   never discourage their dreams.
> *Interviewer:* So if your son wanted dance lessons you'd let him?
> *Mother:* Yeah. Yeah. If he was acting feminine I would ask and get
>   concerned on whether or not, you know, well, I would try to
>   get involved and make sure he's not gay. (White, low-income,
>   heterosexual mother)

Rather than implying that dancing might encourage her son to become gay, this interviewee implies that an interest in dance might indicate an underlying tendency toward homosexuality, one that she would then try to monitor by "get[ting] involved and mak[ing] sure he's not gay." She is the only mother interviewed who implies she might work to craft a heterosexual orientation for her son. But this implication is apparent in five responses from heterosexual fathers. As in the example above regarding pink versus blue shirts, these fathers suggest that relatively mundane cross-gender activities might increase the likelihood of homosexuality. For example, a white, middle-class, heterosexual father indicates that he discourages his son's occasional requests for toys or activities more commonly associated with girls because he fears "his sexual orientation may get screwed up." He goes on to note that it is "probably stupid" of him to worry that playing with girls' toys will make his son gay, but concludes, "Hey, I don't know, so why risk it?" As in the previous example, the implication is that sexual orientation will develop in part on the basis of childhood activity, and thus the activities that parents allow will shape their child's sexual orientation at least somewhat.

Parallel to the examples noted previously in which fathers report judging their own parenting on the basis of whether their sons avoid icons of femininity, a white, upper-middle-class, heterosexual father indicates that he would feel like "something of a failure as a dad" should his son be gay. Regarding his own role in shaping his child's sexual orientation, he notes that he would feel like a failure because "I am raising him to be a boy, a man," a response that implies that heterosexuality is one of the "products" crafted by successful fathering activity. Another father, this one also a white, upper-middle-class heterosexual, implies that it is his responsibility to monitor his sons' cross-gender interests after a certain age to minimize the risk of homosexuality:

> There's a certain age at which you have to remind them that there's a
> certain direction in which they're supposed to be going, and do what you
> can to steer them in that direction. . . . I don't think there's a need for any
> strict adherence to gender-related toys, but only up to a certain point, up
> to a certain age, you know, then [I'd start] worrying about my son being
> effeminate, or even more so, homosexual.

These reports of action taken to encourage heterosexuality are intriguing in at least two ways. First, they suggest that some parents, particularly heterosexual fathers, view heterosexuality as something they need to actively craft. Second, and related, many of these comments convey something akin to a search for signs, a monitoring for visible manifestations of some underlying tendency toward homosexuality or heterosexuality: "If he was acting feminine, I would ask and get concerned. . . . I would try to get involved and make sure he's not gay." Or, in the words of a father referring to how he would feel if his son were to ask for a pink shirt, "I'd have some reserve about that. . . . It'd put a spark in me." Another father, who mentions that once in a while he wonders whether his four-year-old son might turn out to be gay, refers to such signs when asked whether that concern is a strong one: "No, no, for him I, you know, I don't see him playing with dolls all the time. I mean he has Ken, but that's all. I don't see him playing with dolls, I don't see him being effeminate in his way of talking or acting or things like that. You know, he likes to be on his bike and he does boy things" (white, upper-middle-class heterosexual father).

Some parents express the view that sexual orientation is biological, but then continue on to report that they try to discourage homosexuality. A heterosexual parent may believe that sexual orientation is outside her or his control, but may nevertheless monitor outward gender performance as an indicator of a biologically determined, underlying sexual orientation. The focus on outward gender performance may then encourage such parents to begin policing the outward performance, "steering" (as one father put it) or "pushing" (in the words of another) their sons away from cross-gender interests in order to craft a heterosexual orientation.[3] Parents may thus negotiate the perceived links between gender nonconformity and sexual orientation in ways that reinforce both heteronormativity and homophobia in the process. These implications merit future inquiry.

It is only in relation to sons that parents raise the connection between gender performance and sexual orientation, and spontaneously mention the fear of homosexuality, whether in relation to gender performance or not. Theorists of hegemonic masculinity, most notably Connell (1987, 1995) and Kimmel (1994), argue that homophobia is at the heart of hegemonic constructions of masculinity in the contemporary West. Connell (1987) states this bluntly when he notes that "the most important feature of contemporary hegemonic masculinity is that it is heterosexual. . . . Contempt for homosexuality and homosexual men . . . is part of the ideological package of hegemonic masculinity" (186). My interviews document that for sons, even among those who are very young, heteronormativity appears to play a role in shaping parental responses to gender nonconformity, a connection that is also found in literature on older children and adults and is made more for males than females (Antill 1987; Hill 1999; Kite and Deaux 1987; Sandnabba and Ahlberg 1999). As McCreary (1994) argues based on experimental work on responses to older children and adults, "The asymmetry in people's responses to male and female gender role deviations is motivated, in part, by the implicit assumption that male transgressions are symptomatic of a homosexual orientation" (526). This implicit assumption appears to motivate at least some parental gender monitoring and performance management among heterosexual parents, especially fathers, even for children as young as preschool age.

Motivations for Monitoring Sexual Orientation

Just as in the case of icons of femininity, heterosexual parents express a sense of accountability regarding the reactions of others in relation to sexual orientation, and that expression varies by gender. When heterosexual mothers raise the issue, they are more likely to invoke fear regarding the reactions of others. In fact, all three mothers I coded as offering a negative response to the possibility of a son being gay or being perceived as gay include at least some reference to concern about the reactions their children might have to face from others. Typical of mothers' concerns is the following response, which refers to a son being perceived as gay if he does not conform to masculine expectations:

> If he's a nurse or something he must be gay, you know, [people] label you instantly that there must be something wrong with you if you're doing this because men should be, like, construction workers and women should be nurses, and things like that. Yeah, it's very difficult in society. . . . I don't want people to think something of me that I'm not. I don't want them to think that on my children either, I don't want my children to be hurt by that in the future, you know? (White, low-income, heterosexual mother)

This comment, and others like it, demonstrate that parents—especially mothers—feel accountable to others in fulfilling heteronormative expectations for their sons and expect that those others will link gender nonconformity and sexual orientation in their assessments.

By contrast, all four of the fathers I coded in this category include at least some reference to their own personal negative reactions. For example, the white, middle-class, heterosexual father who refers to his fear that his son's sexual orientation could get "screwed up" also states simply and unequivocally that his son could "turn out to be something I don't want." He focuses on his own desire, not on how his son might be treated by others, in explaining that fear.

Conclusion

The interviews I analyze here indicate that most parents in my study have no hesitation about labeling various activities, interests, and behaviors as gender typical or atypical, suggesting a strong acceptance of dichotomous views of gender. Although parents tend to celebrate "crossing" of gender boundaries by their young daughters, their dichotomous views are especially constraining in relation to sons. Most parents either endorse or feel accountable to definitions of masculinity that include limited emotionality and rejection of material markers of femininity, and most parents make efforts to monitor and shape their young sons' compliance with those definitions. Heterosexual fathers are especially likely to report *work* to accomplish this type of masculinity; heterosexual mothers and gay parents are especially likely to report *accountability* to approximate hegemonic masculinity. Some heterosexual parents also invoke sexual orientation as part of this conception of masculinity, commenting with concern on the possibility that their son might be gay or that others might perceive him as such.

Rather than assuming masculinity as biologically predetermined, or simply ignoring it while unconsciously shaping their sons' experiences in accordance with gendered expectations, many parents indicate that they take action to craft an appropriate gender performance for their preschool-age sons. The evidence I present here demonstrates that parents are often consciously aware of gender as something that they must monitor, shape, and enforce, at least for their sons. Parental openness to domestic skills, nurturance, and empathy as desirable qualities in their sons likely represents social change, and the kind of agency in the accomplishment of gender to which Fenstermaker and West (2002) refer. As Connell (1995) notes, hegemonic masculinity is historically variable in its specific content, and the evidence I present in this chapter suggests that some broadening of that content is occurring. But the clear limits evident within that broadening suggest the stability and power of hegemonic conceptions of masculinity. The monitoring and boundary maintenance work parents execute for sons represent crucial limits on boys' options and separate boys from girls. Through the specific content of that boundary maintenance, parents also devalue activities marked as feminine for both boys and girls, as evident in their encouragement of traditionally masculine activities for their daughters and discouragement of any traditionally feminine activities for their sons. In these various ways, the kind of parental monitoring and boundary work explored in this chapter bolsters gender inequality and heteronormativity.

The heterosexual world in general, and heterosexual fathers in particular, play a central role in this process. This is apparent in the direct endorsement of hegemonic masculinity many heterosexual fathers express, and in the accountability to others (presumably heterosexual others) many heterosexual mothers and gay parents express. Scholarly investigations of the routine production of gender in childhood, therefore, need to pay careful attention to the role of heterosexual fathers as enforcers of gender boundaries, and to the role of accountability in the process of accomplishing gender. At the same time, practical efforts to loosen gendered constraints on young children by expanding their parents' normative conceptions of gender need to be aimed at parents in general, but especially need to reach heterosexual fathers. The concern (and even fear) many parents, especially heterosexual mothers and gay parents, express about how their young sons might be treated if they fail to live up to hegemonic conceptions of masculinity represent a motivation for the traditional accomplishment of gender. But those reactions could also serve as a motivation to broaden normative conceptions of masculinity and challenge the devaluation of femininity, an effort that requires participation by heterosexual fathers for significant progress to be achieved.

Along with the role individual parents can play in questioning their own routine accomplishment of gender, it is crucial to keep in mind larger structural forces as well. West and Zimmerman (1987) highlight how interactional and institutional levels work together in the accomplishment of gender, and thus by extension reveal the accountability dilemma parents face if they attempt to do gender differently for their children:

> If we do gender appropriately, we simultaneously sustain, reproduce, and render legitimate institutional arrangements. . . . If we fail to do gender appropriately, we as individuals—not the institutional arrangements—may be called to account. . . . Social movements such as feminism can provide the ideology and impetus to question existing arrangements, and the social support for individuals to explore alternatives to them. Legislative changes . . . can also . . . afford the possibility of more widespread loosening of accountability. (146)

Childhoods less constrained by gender require change and critical reflection on the part of parents. But they also require organized efforts, at the level of social movements and legislative agendas, to loosen the rigid contours of hegemonic masculinity to which many parents feel accountable. As Connell's (1987, 1995) analysis documents, such loosening threatens the very structures of heterosexual male privilege, and the racial and class privilege from which they are inseparable. These are deeply entrenched structures. But many parents, especially heterosexual mothers and gay and lesbian parents, express fear and concern regarding the risks their young sons may face if they cross gender boundaries. Social movements and policy advocates can appeal to that concern in their efforts to chip away at these structures of privilege, offering institutional-level support to parents' interactional-level efforts to do gender differently not only for their daughters but, with greater difficulty, for their sons as well.

Notes

1. Fenstermaker and West (2002) have argued that accountability is "the most neglected aspect of our formulation. . . . Few of those who have used our approach have recognized the essential contribution that accountability makes to it" (212).
2. The size and geographic specificity of my sample are limited; therefore, this lack of variation among my interviewees does not necessarily indicate that no variation would be evident in a larger or more geographically diverse sample.
3. This brings to mind the process for which Max Weber argues in *The Protestant Ethic and the Spirit of Capitalism*. If salvation is considered divinely predestined, but earthly successes and qualities serve as outward signs of that predestination, people may work to control the outward signs of their destiny as if those signs are not indicators, but rather causes, of the final outcome.

References

Antill, John K. 1987. Parents' Beliefs and Values about Sex Roles, Sex Differences, and Sexuality. *Review of Personality and Social Psychology* 7: 294–328.

Beets, Michael W., Randy Vogel, Stanley Chapman, Kenneth H. Pitetti, and Bradley J. Cardinal. 2007. Parent's Social Support for Children's Outdoor Physical Activity: Do Weekdays and Weekends Matter? *Sex Roles* 56: 125–31.

Cahill, Spencer. 1989. Fashioning Males and Females. *Symbolic Interaction* 12: 281–98.

Clearfield, Melissa W., and Naree M. Nelson. 2006. Sex Differences in Mothers' Speech and Play Behavior with 6-, 9-, and 14-Month-Old Infants. *Sex Roles* 54: 127–37.

Coltrane, Scott, and Michele Adams. 1997. Children and Gender. In *Contemporary Parenting*, edited by Terry Arendell. Thousand Oaks, CA: Sage.

Connell, R. W. 1987. *Gender and Power: Society, the Person, and Sexual Politics*. Stanford, CA: Stanford University Press.

———. 1995. *Masculinities*. Berkeley: University of California Press.

Fenstermaker, Sarah, Candace West, and Don Zimmerman. 1991. Gender Inequality: New Conceptual Terrain. In *Gender, Family, and the Economy: The Triple Overlap*, edited by Rae Lesser Blumberg. Thousand Oaks, CA: Sage.

Fenstermaker, Sarah, and Candace West, editors. 2002. *Doing Gender, Doing Difference: Inequality, Power, and Institutional Change*. New York: Routledge.

Fiese, Barbara H., and Gemma Skillman. 2000. Gender Differences in Family Stories. *Sex Roles* 43: 267–83.

Golombok, Susan, and Fiona Tasker. 1994. Children in Lesbian and Gay Families: Theories and Evidence. *Annual Review of Sex Research* 5: 73–100.

Gottman, Julie Schwartz. 1990. Children of Gay and Lesbian Parents. *Marriage and Family Review* 14: 177–96.

Hill, Shirley A. 1999. *African American Children: Socialization and Development in Families*. Thousand Oaks, CA: Sage.

Kimmel, Michael S. 1994. Masculinity as Homophobia. In *Theorizing Masculinities*, edited by Harry Brod. Thousand Oaks, CA: Sage.

Kite, Mary E., and Kay Deaux. 1987. Gender Belief Systems: Homosexuality and the Implicit Inversion Theory. *Psychology of Women Quarterly* 11: 83–96.

Lindsey, Eric W., and Jacquelyn Mize. 2002. Contextual Differences in Parent-Child Play: Implications for Children's Gender Role Development. *Sex Roles* 44: 155–76.

Maccoby, Eleanor E. 1998. *The Two Sexes: Growing Up Apart, Coming Together*. Cambridge, MA: Harvard University Press.

McCreary, Donald R. 1994. The Male Role and Avoiding Femininity. *Sex Roles* 31: 517–31.

McHale, Susan, Ann Crouter, and Shawn Whiteman. 2003. The Family Contexts of Gender Development in Childhood and Adolescence. *Social Development* 12: 125–48.

Patterson, Charlotte J. 1992. Children of Lesbian and Gay Parents. *Child Development* 63: 1025–42.

Pomerleau, Andrée, Daniel Bolduc, Gérard Malcuit, and Louise Cossette. 1990. Pink or Blue: Environmental Gender Stereotypes in the First Two Years of Life. *Sex Roles* 22: 359–68.

Raley, Sara, and Suzanne Bianchi. 2006. Sons, Daughters, and Family Processes: Does Gender of Children Matter? *Annual Review of Sociology* 32: 401–21.

Reese, Elaine, Catherine Haden, and Robyn Fivush. 1996. Gender Differences in Autobiographical Reminiscing. *Research on Language and Social Interaction* 29: 27–56.

Risman, Barbara. 1998. *Gender Vertigo*. New Haven, CT: Yale University Press.

Risman, Barbara J., and Kristen Myers. 1997. As the Twig Is Bent: Children Reared in Feminist Households. *Qualitative Sociology* 20: 229–52.

Rubin, Jeffrey Z., Frank J. Provenzano, and Luria Zella. 1974. The Eye of the Beholder: Parents' Views on Sex of Newborns. *American Journal of Orthopsychiatry* 44: 512–19.

Sandnabba, N. Kenneth, and Christian Ahlberg. 1999. Parents' Attitudes and Expectations about Children's Cross-Gender Behavior. *Sex Roles* 40: 249–63.

Stacey, Judith, and Timothy J. Biblarz. 2001. (How) Does the Sexual Orientation of Parents Matter? *American Sociological Review* 66: 159–83.

Thorne, Barrie. 1994. *Gender Play*. New Brunswick, NJ: Rutgers University Press.

West, Candace, and Sarah Fenstermaker. 1993. Power, Inequality and the Accomplishment of Gender: An Ethnomethodological View. In *Theory on Gender/Feminism on Theory*, edited by Paula England. Hawthorne, NY: Aldine de Gruyter.

———. 1995. Doing Difference. *Gender and Society* 9: 8–37.

West, Candace, and Don H. Zimmerman. 1987. Doing Gender. *Gender and Society* 1: 125–51.

Wood, Eileen, Serge Desmarais, and Sara Gugula. 2002. The Impact of Parenting Experience on Gender Stereotyped Toy Play of Children. *Sex Roles* 47: 39–49.

13

"I Trust Them but I Don't Trust Them"

Issues and Dilemmas in Monitoring Teenagers

Demie Kurz

Mothers and fathers are anxious about monitoring their teens because of what they see as the dangers of adolescence. Parents of teens worry about keeping their children interested in school, about the unprecedented amount of information that comes streaming into their homes every day on the Internet, about drug and alcohol use, about eating disorders and sexually transmitted diseases, and about car accidents and encounters with the criminal justice system. Many of these worries transcend class, location, and race. Some, like concerns about the ramifications of racism or teen pregnancy, are more likely to be of concern to specific groups of parents, such as parents of children of color or parents of girls.

In recent years, as surveillance and monitoring have become topics of wide societal concern, surveillance of teenagers by schools and by the criminal justice system has also increased (Dillon 2003; Dohrn 2000; Lyon 2001; New York Civil Liberties Union 2007; Polakow 2000). Parents have been urged to increase their surveillance efforts as well. In the media, in public spaces, and on the Internet, public service messages constantly ask, "Do you know where your children are?" The assumption embedded in such messages is that "good parents" are paying attention to their children at all times and always know where they are. The implication is that those who fail to supervise and discipline their children on an ongoing basis are "bad parents" who are not supervising their children's whereabouts and are failing to discipline and control them.

Despite the concern over monitoring teens in contemporary U.S. society, policy makers and the general public have little understanding of the work involved in monitoring children. The assumptions are that monitoring is a top-down, straightforward task that parents either do or don't do, and that parents entirely control whether or not monitoring takes place. "Good parents" monitor their children well, while "bad parents" do not. Mothers, who are seen as having primary responsibility for the welfare of their children, are particularly held responsible for perceived failures to monitor their teens (Garey and Arendell 2001).

Researchers, particularly in the field of psychology, have also traditionally assumed a top-down model of monitoring. Recently, however, some researchers have concluded that the monitoring process is more complex and less straightforward than originally assumed. Most important, research has demonstrated that because teens play a key role in the monitoring process through their willingness to disclose or tell parents what they are doing, the process is not just top-down. Indeed, psychologists now argue that information about the activities and whereabouts of teens is essential to monitoring, and that teenagers can be the crucial source of this information (Fletcher, Steinberg, and Williams-Wheeler 2004; Kerr and Stattin 2000; Stattin and Kerr 2000). Some researchers also demonstrate that the tenor of relationships with parents is critical and that teens are most willing to offer information when they have a warm relationship with their parents (Crouter and Head 2002). As a result of new findings about monitoring, psychologists have argued for the need for more research on the monitoring process—on what parents actually do in their monitoring and on the conditions under which teenagers do and do not disclose information to parents.

In this chapter I contribute to this area of research by presenting data on the challenges parents face in monitoring their teenage children. I interviewed parents about how they and their teens negotiate issues of monitoring. I also interviewed a smaller number of teens about their perspectives on their relationships with parents. These interview data provide the opportunity for a different kind of information than is found in existing research on teens and monitoring, which focuses on establishing statistical relationships between indicators of parent-child relationship quality, measures of parental monitoring and knowledge, and outcomes for teens (Crouter and Head 2002).

Although parents monitor teens in many areas, including educational choices and school work, physical and emotional health, and moral development, I concentrate my analysis on how parents monitor their teens' social lives. More specifically, I describe the monitoring of teenagers in the thirteen-to-sixteen-year-old age range, before teens gain greater independence through obtaining drivers licenses and holding part-time jobs.

The parents in my sample describe two major challenges in monitoring their teenage children. The first is how to monitor teens when they are away from parental or other adult supervision; the second is how to get accurate information about teen activities. In examining how parents, particularly mothers, confront these challenges, I focus on a set of shared concerns confronting all mothers and fathers. There are, of course, many variations in the experiences of parents. Although space does not permit an in-depth consideration of these differences, it is important to stress that class and racial/ethnic issues structure and shape the options available for managing environments. Low-income and minority mothers face special disadvantages. Unlike professional and middle-class parents, for example, many working-class mothers have to deal with unsafe neighborhoods. In addition, social class location can affect the time available for mothers to monitor their children. For example, some more-privileged mothers can afford to make major changes in their work schedules to monitor teens, such as cutting back on the time they spend at work. Alternatively, these mothers can continue to work long hours and hire substitute caregivers to ensure that their children are adequately supervised. Some of the middle-class mothers in my sample were also able to gain some flexibility in their positions as nurses and school teachers, professions that many women choose at least in part because they allow more scheduling flexibility than nine-to-five jobs. The lower a woman's income, however, the less likely she is to be able to work less and take a reduction in income or to convince employers to give her a more flexible schedule. Further, mothers raising children by themselves may need to work long hours to make ends meet. This leaves them less time for monitoring. These issues of different environments and different resources have largely been neglected in the study of parental monitoring.

Methods

My analysis of parental monitoring is based on interviews with eighty-eight mothers and fifteen fathers of adolescent children. I chose to interview primarily mothers because they are more involved with their children's daily activities than are fathers (Bumpass, Crouter, and McHale 2001; Crouter and Head 2002). The sample is diverse, including parents who are urban and suburban, black and white, and at a range of income levels. Thirty percent of the parents in the sample are single mothers. I have grouped the parents into three social classes: professional, middle class, and working class, based on education, occupation, and place of residence. In the interviews, I asked mothers and fathers open-ended questions about the tasks and challenges of parenting their teenage children, including how they monitor their teens.

To gain some idea of teenage perspectives, I also interviewed twenty high school students and twenty college students ages eighteen to twenty-one, and I held four focus groups with high school students. In the interviews and focus groups, I asked teenage and college-age young women and men to discuss their relationships with parents and other family members.[1]

Monitoring Teens in Their Environments

Controlling Environments

Parents worry a great deal about their adolescent children, particularly when they are away from adult supervision for long periods of time. Specific concerns vary with the neighborhoods in which families live and the resources of those neighborhoods. In the suburbs, parents are anxious about teenagers going to empty houses and drinking or using drugs. In the city, particularly in poorer neighborhoods, parents worry about unsafe neighborhoods and how teens could be victimized by gangs or violence. These concerns also vary by race/ethnicity. Minority parents have particular fears that their teenage boys could be unfairly treated by the police. African American parents worry especially about their sons. As one mother indicated, these worries cover a range of issues: "I worry about school, them finishing school, and that they're okay. And with a black male in this society . . . they want to prove themselves. They want to be a man. I'm constantly telling my son, 'You are your own person. You don't have to prove yourself. You don't have to do what the group wants. Walk away.' "

Parents' concerns also vary by the gender of their children. Parents have particular concerns that their daughters are vulnerable to sexual assault. For example, one Hispanic mother is particularly concerned about her fifteen-year-old daughter. Although she is also anxious about her seventeen-year-old son's safety, she sees her daughter as more vulnerable:

Respondent: I protect her [my daughter] more.
Interviewer: Why is that?
Respondent: She's more vulnerable, more could happen to her. And she has to consider her reputation.
Interviewer: You worry about her more than your son?
Respondent: Yes, although I worry about him too. He's six foot four, though.
Interviewer: So you don't have to worry as much about him?

Respondent: Well, sometimes I worry about what would happen to
him if somebody did attack him. They would have to do a lot to
him. [*groaning*] But women really have to put up their guard more.
They have more restrictions. They have their reputation.

Although parents find it especially difficult to monitor children who are away from home, parents also find monitoring their children to be difficult even when children are at home. Teens spend a lot more time alone in their bedrooms than do younger children; they also invite friends over and "hang out" in basement family rooms or bedrooms, where they are mostly unobserved even when their parents are home. Some parental concerns, such as those about watching too much television, drinking alcohol, using drugs, or having sex, may have changed little in recent years. Because both parents are now often in the workforce, however, many teens are home alone or with siblings after school for longer periods of time than they were in the past. The explosion of electronic media also presents some distinctly new challenges for monitoring teenagers both inside and outside the home. The Internet allows teens to "visit" more places; communication technology allows a greater range of interactions. Many of these activities are acceptable to parents, who see real benefits to them. For example, if their teen is shy or has unusual interests, parents might view electronic communication as a helpful way for a child to connect with others. However, parents also find it difficult to assess whether teens are seeing things on the Internet that may be harmful, or whether teens are meeting strangers online who might prey on youth.

Finally, parents worry about the influence of their children's peer groups. To be sure, parents know and accept that their teenage children want to spend a lot of time with their peers; they also worry if their teens do not have friends. At the same time, they have many concerns about peer pressure, which lead them to want more information about their teens' friends. However, mothers and fathers find that it can be difficult to learn about and monitor their teens' friendships. One respondent, a white, working-class mother with a fourteen-year-old daughter, distrusts one of her daughter's friends. Even though she doesn't have much evidence against her daughter's friend, the mother believes that this friend has done risky things and that her own daughter could be drawn into similar activities:

Interviewer: Have you ever disliked any of your daughter's friends?
Respondent: Yes, and I did tell her about it. I shouldn't say that I dislike
the kid. I like her, but I don't trust her. And I feel that she has a lot
of influence on [my daughter]. Like anytime [my daughter] asks

me to do anything with [the friend], like babysit or something, I tell her no, because I'm afraid this kid could be, well, I don't know her that well. She just comes on real strong. She seems to me like she's tried everything. Like sex, drugs. She may not have done none of this. I don't know. But it just scares me because she does a lot and this girl does have a lot of influence on [my daughter]. My daughter listens to this girl a lot. And it scares me.

As this example suggests, teens may or may not share their parents' concerns. Indeed, adolescence is a time when children begin to question their parents' view of what is safe and appropriate; adolescence is also a time when children develop their own views rather than seeing their parents as the sole authority on certain moral and social issues (Collins and Steinberg 2006). One white female, now a college student, explained how, as a younger teen, she had discounted parental advice and engaged in behavior she now considers to have been risky: "When you get all those lectures about how dangerous things are, you don't listen. You see that they are not dangerous. You see honor students smoking pot, and it's no big deal. It's not at all like what the adults are saying. You do some stupid things, yes, I see that now, maybe even some dangerous things I see now. But I never felt that way then."

Research also shows that, starting in adolescence, teens come to believe that they have the right to make more decisions about their lives than when they were younger (Smetana 1995). They may still grant their parents authority over some things, but they believe that in matters that affect them personally—their clothing and hairstyles, who their friends are, and where they can go—they should be able to make their own decisions about what to do. For parents, knowing that teens don't necessarily share their views of risk and danger increases their anxiety.

Strategies in Less Controlled Environments

Parents use a variety of strategies to observe and monitor their teenage children outside the home. Some try to put themselves in the physical presence of their children. For example, parents may volunteer to chaperone a dance to better monitor their children and their children's friends' activities. Similarly, they may volunteer to drive a group of teenagers places so they can observe what goes on. A white, professional mother with a nineteen-year-old daughter tells a story of accompanying her daughter to a social event when she was fifteen, although her daughter didn't want her to come and accused her mother of not trusting her:

> [Teenage children] are always a little ahead of us and they make us come
> along. My daughter would sometimes tell me I was inappropriate. But I
> had to know about things. Like my daughter was involved in theatre in
> high school. She started going to cast parties. She was fifteen years old. I
> realized there was beer at these parties, and older people, in their twenties.
> I said to her, "This isn't right." She said, "Yes it is, you don't understand;
> yes it is, it's fine." Finally I said, "I'm coming to one of these parties." My
> daughter said, "You can't do that. You're intruding on me. These are my
> friends. I can't have my mother coming to the party. You don't trust me." I
> said, "Well, I'm coming." So, I first went to the play, and then I went to the
> cast party. Well, it was a great group. I could see that the younger people
> and the older people had a lot in common. They really shared this interest
> in the theatre. And there was no question that the younger people would
> not drink the beer at all. So I said to my daughter, "This is great." Then she
> said, "Why didn't you trust me?" I said "Look, I had to know myself."

This mother achieved her goal of keeping an eye on her daughter's activities,
although it is not possible to tell from her story what the impact was on her
relationship with her daughter.

If mothers can't accompany teenage children to events, they may try
to inspect them when they come home, as does one working-class, African
American mother: "I sit up at night until they come home. I want them to
know that Mom is going to be there waiting. And we don't have an answering machine or a cell phone. I want to know who their friends are. I want
to know who's planning what." Alternatively, some families create space so
that home will be a desirable destination for their teens and their friends.
For instance, families might designate a room where teenage children have
priority use of a space, such as a "rec room" in the basement. One white,
middle-class mother with teenagers in junior high and high school states
that the inconvenience of making such adjustments is outweighed by the
benefits of knowing about her children's activities and friends: "Most of the
time kids are at our house. I let all his friends come over. I mean, my house is
always full of kids. I'd rather have all the neighborhood children in my house
and make a mess—I don't care, I'll clean it up, but I know where my kids are.
And I know they're not being bad. It doesn't bother me."

In addition to—or perhaps as a substitute for—the direct monitoring
of activities at home and elsewhere, some mothers try to get teens involved
in what they view as constructive activities after school and on weekends.
These activities include sports, church functions, and neighborhood groups.
One middle-class, African American mother is able to control many aspects
of her children's lives—such as television, movies, and friends—because the

teenagers' social activities all take place with church friends. As this mother said, "I just get them all into church activities. Fortunately, they like them." However, teens may not always want to engage in the activities their parents choose for them. One white, working-class mother explained that her fifteen-year-old daughter resisted her efforts to guide her choice of extracurricular activities: "I wanted her to join the softball team. She said no. I wanted her to join basketball at school. She said no. I wanted her to join those things because I think it's good that they get involved where their time's tied up. With their involvement, they can't get in trouble that way. [*laughing*] But she tried out for cheerleading, and then she didn't make it. Now she said she's supposed to try out for it next year again. So we'll see."

Another working-class, African American mother whose son just turned seventeen reports that her teenager wanted to stop going to a religious program. She found a similar program and, without her son's knowledge, is trying to finagle a way for her son to meet with the director in hopes that her son will want to join the program: "There's a guy who works with the [Teen Program] who knows Javon, but you know, Javon hasn't seen him since last year, but my sister Sandy was trying to find a way how they can have a meeting—like, not let Javon know that we set it up."

As another strategy, some parents send their children away to boarding school or to live with relatives in environments where they think their children will be better monitored. A few African American mothers mentioned trying to send their teenage children to relatives in the South, a practice found in some African American communities, to get them out of what they view as dangerous neighborhoods (Stack and Burton 1993).

Finally, parents find that cell phones can be extremely helpful in monitoring their teenage children. In recent years, cell phone use has grown rapidly among all segments of the population, including parents and teenagers (Hofer et al., Chapter 14; Holson 2008; Turkle 2007). One middle-class, African American mother explained that she had strict rules about answering calls: "My big rule is that you have to check in with me. I'm a worrywart. I can always get in touch with them. I could call my sixteen-year-old right now on her cell phone, and she would call me back right away. I don't want to call home on the land line and have no one be here. I have to know where you are. I have to know where everyone is." Other mothers said that they set rules for their teens to check in at specified times, and that if their children didn't call, they would do the calling.

In general, parents speak of cell phones giving them a great deal of relief in terms of monitoring and knowing that they can always connect with their teenager. This monitoring is not always restrictive, however. Parents also said that using a cell phone enabled them to give their teens more freedom than might otherwise have been the case. One white mother gave an example: "My son ended up at a party where there were not going to be adults. We found out this was going to happen ahead of time, but we thought the kids were responsible so we let him go. We gave him the cell phone and told him to call us if anything at all happened, anything, and we would come and get him." Similarly, another mother explained that the cell phone could enhance her child's freedom because it could be used as a safety device in difficult situations. She told about a friend of hers who has a "special code" she uses with her son. If he is at a party and wants to leave because there is drinking or other behavior with which he is uncomfortable, he calls his parents and says, "I forgot to tell you that Aunt Mary called." In this way he is spared any embarrassment that could occur if his friends found out he wanted to leave.

Cooperation and Resistance

Parents feel most secure when they can directly monitor their teens; get them into safe, supervised environments; or be in touch with them by cell phone. However, there are limits to these strategies. In the case of cell phones, for example, some mothers acknowledged the possibility for duplicity on the part of their teens. Because cell phones are not connected to a particular location, teens can say they are in one place when they are actually elsewhere. A middle-class, African American mother of a fourteen-year-old boy worries that her son might not be truthful in reporting his activities, even if he is reliable about calling her: "I worry. You never know when you're going to get a phone call. Especially with my son. He could get in trouble about a lot of things. I mean, that's my worldview; I see all these people getting into trouble. So I tell him, look, this is just the way I am, this is who I am. And how I deal with it is that he has the cell phone. And he has to call me every two hours. And if I'm not home, he has to leave messages. And I listen to the messages. Of course, he could be lying. . . . But I can't follow him everywhere."

Other mothers noted a different set of drawbacks. While cell phones make communication with teens easier, parents are less able to monitor telephone usage because the calls go directly to the teen rather than through a house phone. One woman said that she knew her older children's friends better because they used to call the house on the land line, which meant she could talk to them. Parents also worry when teens fail to answer their cell phone. One mother groaned and said that when her sixteen-year-old son "looks at the phone and sees it's me, he doesn't answer." Finally, some mothers wrestle with when to call their child's cell phone when their teen is with friends because they want to respect their teen's right to socialize without interruption by a parent.

The rhythm of teen life itself also creates obstacles to effective monitoring. When teens make last-minute decisions (a pattern abetted by cell phones), parents may not be able to do the necessary groundwork to assess the situation at hand. A white, middle-class mother described a situation in which her thirteen-year-old daughter got a call about an informal gathering among her friends to take place a few hours later, what the mother called a "spontaneous party." The daughter insisted that the gathering, which would take place at the home of one of her friends, would be attended by both female and male friends. The mother reported,

> So I called his mother, and she said she would be there. My daughter really wanted to go. She said kids were going there. So I drove her over and there were four boys there, no girls. And there was no mother! The parents are divorced. I guess she was there, and then she went out or something. Anyway, I immediately made a decision that I would let my daughter stay for an hour. I said, I'm going nearby to [a bookstore], and I'll come up and pick you up in an hour. Of course I was in a state the whole time. I felt like, what kind of bad parent am I, leaving my daughter with four boys? And I didn't know the boys. I got back the closest to when it wouldn't look like it was too early. Of course they hadn't raped her. Everything looked fine, they were hanging out, watching a movie. So then I took my daughter home. . . . I decided next time she gets invited to something, that before she says yes and before she hangs up the phone, I'm going to get on the phone with the parent—before she says yes.

In short, parents find that some strategies for directly monitoring their teenage children are reliable and give them confidence that they know what their teens are doing. These strategies have limits, however, and are neither foolproof nor available equally to all parents. Moreover, as recent research has begun to demonstrate (Fletcher, Steinberg, and Williams-Wheeler 2004; Stattin and Kerr 2000), monitoring does not begin and end with parental actions, but also depends on the cooperation of teens.

Getting Information from Teenagers

Getting information from teens can become more difficult in adolescence, a stage of life when teens begin to form their own identities (Collins and Steinberg 2006; Grotevant 1998; Lerner and Galambos 1998). Some parents and teens can come to a mutual understanding of guidelines and rules for what new things teens can and cannot do. However, many parents and teenagers experience difficult times in their relationships.

Trust is a key issue for parents in how well things go between themselves and their teenage children. Parents who trust their children to give them accurate information about where they are or what they are doing may feel less need to constantly monitor them. As one white, middle-class mother says, "I don't need to control them, because I trust them." Another white, middle-class mother says, "We have a lot of trust. I don't know what we would do if we lost that trust with any of the kids. If we found them smoking marijuana in their room or something."

Another white, middle-class mother of a fifteen-year-old daughter and thirteen-year-old son talks about how she can no longer assume she knows what her teenage children are doing, in part because she remembers that she herself didn't tell her parents certain things: "I have a few conflicts with my daughter. She occasionally is late for her curfews. I always worry, 'Where are they?' Like, she was at the sleepover last night. But I had a little thought: 'Is that really where she is?' I thought of calling up the girl's house, making up some stupid question, but I didn't. We don't have any real problems. I know her friends, I know their mothers. We compare notes. . . . I trust them, but, ah, I don't trust them. I think of myself and what I did. I'm sure they are doing things I don't know about: drinking, and not drugs, I hope." This mother expresses the difficulty shared by other parents when she says, "I trust them, but I don't trust them." Underlying her dilemma is the general challenge of how to monitor teenage children while also granting them some autonomy and a certain degree of privacy. Like many mothers, she feels caught between wanting to know things about her teenager and not wanting to be disrespectful or intrusive.

A working-class, African American mother explains that her children, ages fifteen and twenty, don't tell her much, and that she has to create opportunities for communication: "They don't really share with me what's going on too much in their life, the intimate details of their life. But I just, I try to leave the door open if, you know, they wanna talk." Many mothers describe times at the dinner table when they can't get their children to say much of anything. They tell stories about how their children respond to everything they ask with the answer "fine." Some mothers find that talking becomes a particular issue with their sons. One white middle-class mother talked sadly about how her thirteen-year-old son had just gone on a camping trip with friends. In the past, after returning from such trips, he always shared with her what he had done. This time he came home, picked up the telephone, and related the details of this camping trip to a friend. This mother very much missed hearing about her son's trip. She says, "He talks on the phone with girls a lot now—not girlfriends. Supposedly it's about schoolwork. His voice changed. And he just doesn't tell me things. He used to tell me all kinds of things. So I told his sister, 'When you come home from college, you need to know that your brother has become a teenager.' I just thought she should know."

Parents may have good reason to worry about the lack of communication. In my interviews with teens, some stated that although they tell their parents, particularly their mothers, about most of what they do, there are certain things they do not share with their parents. One nineteen-year-old college student from a white, middle-class family described a time when she was sixteen and lied to her parents: "That time I lied. But that kind of backfired. Like, I had this group of friends a couple of towns away. My parents didn't like them and didn't want me being with them. But I had a friend who lived near where these friends lived. So I told my parents I was going to her house. But then we would just walk to these guys' houses."

A fourteen-year-old black male from a working-class background flatly asserted that teens go ahead and do what they want to do, whether their parents approve or not: "Boys will be boys anyway. They gonna sneak and do what they gonna do. So it don't really matter. Girls will be girls too. Girls gonna sneak and do what they wanna do, too, behind their parents' back. Or if they got a boyfriend they want to be with their boyfriend. They gonna go with their boyfriend." A white teenage girl being interviewed in her home started to whisper when she talked about drinking alcohol: "My mom doesn't know; we're just experimenting, though. And I wouldn't tell my relatives because it would just get back to my Mom." Another teen, a sixteen-year-old Latina girl, one of the few who reported that she told her parents everything she did, acknowledged that she doesn't tell her parents everything her *friends* do:

> *Respondent:* I tell my mother everything. . . . Well, that's everything I
>   do. But I don't tell her some of what my friends do.
> *Interviewer:* Why not?
> *Respondent:* Because they would start worrying about me.

Because teens don't always tell their parents what they are doing or give them full information on a particular topic, parents experiment with different strategies for getting information. One set of strategies includes various mechanisms for changing the way they talk. For example, a parent might try to choose the right topic, something attempted by this white middle-class mother of a thirteen-year-old and a sixteen-year-old: "I found that if they don't want to talk and you want to find out what they are doing, you don't ask, 'How's school?' You ask something more specific, like, 'Did so-and-so get their braces off?' You use any kind of talk. You can always find something. It's good to have talk for its own sake. You can pick up a lot of things. Are they 'down'? 'OK'?" Another mother said, "I have to wait until the right moment to discuss things with him. You have to seize the moment when you can get your point in."

Some parents think ahead and choose locations to talk. As one middle-class African American mother said, "I'll tell you the perfect time to get my kids especially is in the car. I say, "We're going to have a talk. They are like, 'Oh!' I turn the radio off, and they be in the back seat, and they can't get away. Yes, it is the perfect time to say whatever you want to them." And some parents decide that one of them, rather than the other, might be more able to approach a child. One working-class African American mother thought that her husband could talk more easily with their teenage son: "If I see a situation coming, I tell my husband, 'Honey, when you get a chance could you talk to him about such-and-such a thing?' He can engage our son in a conversation."

Communication strategies can also involve *not* communicating fully and withholding judgment. Parents sometimes "bite their tongue" to get information. As one white middle-class mother said, "I try to keep my mouth shut and not try and say too much. Or else he might react to what I'm saying." A white professional who is the mother of sixteen-year-old twin girls similarly spoke about restraint and careful phrasing: "You really have to restrain yourself and resist saying things. You really have to bite your tongue. But you have to say things in a certain way, or they won't tell you things." Another white middle-class mother of a thirteen-year-old son and a nineteen-year-old daughter said that she, too, shapes her responses carefully and tries to avoid casual judgments: "When my kids have hung out with kids I didn't like, I talked to them and told them why I thought there was something problematic. I was trying to make that group seem less attractive. You can't prevent your child from seeing them, of course. I try not to be judgmental, but to talk about my fears."

Besides talk, parents develop certain unobtrusive strategies to monitor their teenage children so as to maintain at least the appearance of trust. One strategy they use is to keep track of what their teens have been doing by talking to other mothers and exchanging information with them about their teens' activities. One white, middle-class mother of a fourteen-year-old girl said that she calls the parents of her daughter's friends to check up: "This party she is going to tonight is a big deal. It's her first party. I made calls to different mothers of her friends, the ones I know, and I called the mother [hosting the party]. I made sure there weren't going to be any alcohol or drugs. The mom said, 'No, just a party in the backyard; we're going to have lights and things.'"

Another unobtrusive strategy is to watch children carefully for signs of alcohol and drug use. A white, working-class mother of three children ages seventeen, fifteen, and thirteen laughed as she talked about how, after her teenage children return home from social events with friends, she manages to smell for alcohol on their breath without their knowing:

> *Respondent:* I don't think they're doing anything. But how do you really know? And we all know what we did when we were young. Of course, I'm like a sergeant. When they come back, I look in their eyes and I see if I smell anything.
> *Interviewer:* Do they know you're doing that?
> *Respondent:* Well, sometimes I tease them and I say, "Oh, you've been hitting the bottle," or something like that, and they say, "Oh no, Mom." But I'm not sure they know I check up on them.

Some mothers say they are even more devious and that they eavesdrop or listen in on their teenage children as they talk on the phone or visit with friends at home. Eavesdropping leads some to wrestle with issues of privacy. A white, middle-class mother of three children ages nineteen, fifteen, and twelve says it is important to give children some privacy, and she says she will not read their diaries. She will, however, listen in on a conversation: "And you have to give them privacy. Including privacy they can have with their friends. It's better they be with their friends at home than at the mall. But then they get their space in the family room or out at the pool. Of course, I can hear a lot of what they are saying through the kitchen window. But if I go in their room to bring laundry or something and I see an open diary on their bed, I won't read it. I wouldn't open their drawers or their school bags either. That's private."

While this mother was firm about the fact that she will not read or look through her children's materials, not all parents have the same attitudes toward privacy issues. Some parents explain that they believe mothers and fathers have a right to information about their teens, and that reading a teenager's diary is acceptable. But most parents apply a more situational ethic, as did one white middle-class mother who said that she would read a diary or even look at her daughter's e-mail if she thought her daughter was starting to do something "serious," like use drugs.

Conclusion

Researchers have argued that we need more data on how parents monitor teens and on the monitoring process, in particular how parents obtain the information they need to monitor their children. The data presented in this chapter address these questions. For my analysis, I have focused on two challenges of monitoring. The first is how to monitor teens when they are out on their own, away from adult supervision. The second is how parents obtain information from their teenage children. The data presented about how parents cope with these challenges suggest that parents develop inventive ways—some direct, some indirect and unobtrusive—of monitoring. Researchers should continue to explore the possibilities and limitations of new technologies and the other types of monitoring that parents adopt, including changing the way they talk to their teenage children and managing the environments where teens spend their time.

The understanding that in all likelihood class and race/ethnicity affect the capacity of parents not only to ensure safe environments for their children but also to participate in ongoing monitoring has implications for public policy. Both the public and private sectors could acknowledge the challenges parents face as they seek to care for and monitor their children; the public and private sectors could also provide more social supports for parental efforts. For example, better after-school programs could allow monitoring of teens during after-school hours, a period when many go home to empty houses. Better coordination between family life and work life would also help the problem of unsupervised after-school hours. Public agencies and nonprofit organizations could also provide information sessions for parents. Some mothers in my interviews expressed an interest in workshops on how to communicate better with their teens: when to listen, when to monitor, and when to intervene. Such assistance to individual parents could supplement social policies that promote more structural changes in support of families.

Rather than deem mothers deficient if they are unable to control or ensure safety for their children, social policies could provide safer environments for teenagers who spend long periods of time away from adult supervision. Unfortunately, the monitoring issues that arise as a result of difficult social conditions are often viewed as private problems to be solved by the individual family. There is little government support for assisting parents or for creating safe conditions that would make monitoring easier, and parents are left on their own to figure out individualized solutions for monitoring their teens. Our society should take more collective responsibility for families, and the government should develop policies that create safer environments for teens.

Notes

The author would like to acknowledge the support of the Philadelphia Education Longitudinal Study and the MacArthur Family Study, Department of Sociology, University of Pennsylvania, in carrying out the research on which this chapter is based, and to thank the editors of this volume for their helpful comments.

1. For the purposes of this study, I chose samples from the city of Philadelphia and surrounding suburbs that would yield a diversity of parents to interview, based on class and race. I chose middle-class and working-class respondents from the following four samples: (1) The suburban sample was drawn randomly from the high school roster of a predominantly white, suburban community. The community was solidly middle class. (2) A first sample from the city was drawn randomly from citywide school records and included a few professional and middle-class mothers but was primarily composed of working-class mothers. (3) A second sample from the city was drawn randomly from census tracts that were chosen to represent primarily working-class households but also some lower middle-class households and some poor ones. There was an oversampling of African Americans. (4) The fourth sample was a snowball sample, a nonprobability sample in which the researcher asks the initial study subjects to refer or provide names of other potential subjects for inclusion in the sample. For this snowball sample I sought out professional mothers and fathers who did not know each other. I then asked each of them for several names of people whom they thought I could interview. These people agreed. From the four samples, I designated three different social-class groups based on education and occupation. Professional and higher-income women had post-college education and a professional occupation. Middle-class women had a bachelor's or associate's degree and an occupation requiring a college degree, or held a semi-professional position, including school teacher or nurse. Working-class women had a high school diploma, two years or less of post-high-school education or training, and an occupation not requiring a college degree, such as secretary or administrative assistant, sales clerk, security guard, day care worker, medical technician, or home health aide.

References

Bumpass, Matthew F., Ann C. Crouter, and Susan M. McHale. 2001. Parental Autonomy-Granting in Adolescence: Exploring Gender Differences in Context. *Developmental Psychology* 37: 163–73.

Collins, W. Andrew, and Laurence Steinberg. 2006. Adolescent Development in Interpersonal Context. In *Handbook of Child Psychology*, vol. 3, edited by William Damon and Richard M. Lerner, 1003–67. New York: Wiley.

Crouter, Ann C., and Melissa R. Head. 2002. Parental Monitoring and Knowledge of Children. In *Handbook of Parenting*, edited by Marc H. Bornstein, 461–83. Mahwah, NJ: Lawrence Erlbaum Associates.

Dillon, Sam. 2003. Cameras Watching Students, Especially in Biloxi. *New York Times*, September 24, Education section.

Dohrn, Bernadine. 2000. "Look Out, Kid, It's Something You Did": The Criminalization of Children. In *The Public Assault on America's Children: Poverty, Violence, and Juvenile Injustice*, edited by Valerie Polakow, 157–87. New York: Teachers College Press.

Fletcher, Anne C., Laurence Steinberg, and Meeshay Williams-Wheeler. 2004. Parental Influences on Adolescent Problem Behavior: Revisiting Stattin and Kerr. *Child Development* 75: 781–96.

Garey, Anita Ilta, and Terry Arendell. 2001. Children, Work, and Family: Some Thoughts on "Mother-Blame." In *Working Families: The Transformation of the American Home*, edited by Rosanna Hertz and Nancy L. Marshall, 293–303. Berkeley: University of California Press.

Grotevant, Harold D. 1998. Adolescent Development in Family Contexts. In *Handbook of Child Psychology*, vol. 3, edited by Nancy Eisenberg, 1097–149. New York: Wiley.

Holson, Laura. 2008. Text Generation Gap: U R 2 Old (JK). *New York Times*, March 9, Business section.

Kerr, Margaret, and Håkan Stattin. 2000. What Parents Know, How They Know It, and Several Forms of Adolescent Adjustment: Further Support for a Reinterpretation of Monitoring. *Developmental Psychology* 36: 366–80.

Lerner, Richard M., and Nancy L. Galambos. 1998. Adolescent Development: Challenges and Opportunities for Research, Programs, and Policies. *Annual Review of Psychology* 49: 413–46.

Lyon, David. 2001. *Surveillance Society: Monitoring Everyday Life*. Buckingham, UK: Open University Press.

New York Civil Liberties Union. 2007. *Criminalizing the Classroom: The Over-Policing of New York City Public Schools*. New York: NYCLU.

Polakow, Valerie. 2000. *The Public Assault on America's Children: Poverty, Violence, and Juvenile Injustice*. New York: Teachers College Press.

Smetana, Judith. 1995. Parenting Styles and Conceptions of Parental Authority during Adolescence. *Child Development* 66: 299–316.

Stack, Carol B., and Linda M. Burton. 1993. Kinscripts. *Journal of Comparative Family Studies* 24: 157–70.

Stattin, Håkan, and Margaret Kerr. 2000. Parental Monitoring: A Reinterpretation. *Child Development* 71: 1072–85.

Turkle, Sherry. 2007. Can You Hear Me Now? *Forbes*, May 7.

14

The Electronic Tether

Communication and Parental Monitoring during the College Years

Barbara K. Hofer, Constance Souder,
Elena K. Kennedy, Nancy Fullman, and Kathryn Hurd

Phoning was expensive and not private [when I was in college]. Writing letters was the way to communicate private thoughts, but it was more sharing than asking for advice. I made decisions with very little input from my parents.

My parents and I talked once a week by phone and a letter once a month. My daughter and I talk several times a day.

—Responses from parent surveys

In previous decades the movement away from home to attend college generally involved diminished contact between students and their parents. This has changed substantially in recent years, as the comments above from parents attest. Technological developments such as e-mail, cell phones, instant messaging, and text messaging make it possible for college students and their parents to communicate frequently, and this frequent contact may provide the means for parental monitoring to extend well into a period of emerging adulthood.

In this chapter we explore this "electronic tether" and its influence on psychosocial development based on a series of studies we conducted with college students and their parents. We examine the frequency and initiation of contact and how this communication is related to a number of constructs, such as autonomy development, self-regulation, self-governance, the nature of parent-student relationships, and satisfaction with various aspects of the college experience. We explore parental attitudes toward the tether, as well as how students have responded to the level of contact with parents made possible by new technologies. Finally, we consider what strategies students have developed for containing communication.

Theoretical Background: Framing Our Research Agenda

Among the central tasks in psychological development during adolescence and "emerging adulthood" (ages 18–25) (Arnett 2000) is the movement toward autonomy, self-governance, and self-regulation (Hofer, Yu, and Pintrich 1998). During this phase of life individuals generally become more differentiated from their parents, more independent in their decision making, more capable of mature judgment without parental intervention, and more competent at regulating both their behavior and their learning. In the United States, many individuals leave home during this period in order to attend college, and parental engagement is usually diminished, fostering a further progression toward autonomy. This movement toward autonomy does not mean that these relationships are severed, of course, as healthy psychological functioning involves both growing independence and sustained connection with parents (Steinberg 2001). Navigating that balance is a psychosocial challenge influenced by a multiplicity of forces.

Emerging Adulthood as a Distinct Phase of Life

The period of life that has been the focus of our studies is "emerging adulthood," a recent conceptualization of a developmental phase that links adolescence and adulthood. Psychologists have typically partitioned life into periods that are each marked by distinctive cognitive, biological, and social changes for the individual, and these periods are sociologically and historically situated. The idea of adolescence as a discrete stage between childhood and adulthood, for example, is little more than a hundred years old (Hall 1904). This period of life was conceptualized at a time when an increasing number of individuals were able to continue schooling and delay entering the workforce; these individuals appeared to no longer be children but were not yet assuming adult responsibilities. Over the past century the boundaries of this period have been fluid (particularly given the drop in the age of menarche), and today psychologists often consider adolescence to be the second decade of life, although there is variation in what constitutes an appropriate endpoint. The markers of adulthood are highly diffuse in the United States (e.g., individuals may vote or serve in combat at age eighteen but are legally prohibited from alcohol consumption until age twenty-one), further complicating the delineation between adolescence and adulthood.

Recently, developmental psychologists have begun to consider the transitional period between adolescence and adulthood as warranting its own nomenclature, and the term "emerging adulthood" has been used to describe the period from age eighteen to twenty-five (Arnett 2000). Observed primarily in industrial societies, this stage of life is characterized as a time when individuals are relatively transient; involved in an ongoing exploration of identity, values, and occupations; and often not yet fully responsible for themselves or for others. Increased schooling, delayed marriage (the average age for entering one's first marriage has risen to over twenty-five for women and over twenty-seven for men; Johnson and Dye 2005), and other demographic shifts have led to a lengthening transition between what has been more clearly marked as adolescence and what society views as adulthood. Acknowledging this time as a separate developmental period also facilitates the articulation of the psychosocial tasks that may be transitional hallmarks of the passage between adolescence and adulthood.

Developmental Tasks of Emerging Adulthood

Although autonomy has been perceived by psychologists as one of the psychosocial tasks of adolescence, particular aspects of the process continue well into emerging adulthood. Autonomy has multiple components, and in our studies we have addressed issues of emotional and behavioral autonomy (Steinberg and Silverberg 1986). One of the early manifestations of emotional autonomy is the acknowledgment that parents are no longer perceived as perfect; this process of "de-idealization" (Chen and Dornbusch 1998) begins early in adolescence. One of the final indicators is when individuals can see their parents as people with lives apart from parenting, a step that takes place much later, often during the late teens and early twenties (Beyers et al. 2005). Emotional autonomy includes two other factors beyond de-idealization and seeing one's parents as people: individuation and nondependence (Steinberg and Silverberg 1986). We have included these constructs in our research, while acknowledging that this definition of autonomy is both contested (Ryan and Lynch 1989) and culturally constructed, and therefore perhaps less likely to be as applicable in families with more collectivist and less individualistic cultural orientations. We have also employed other definitions and measures of autonomy, including those from motivational theorists who focus more on the support for autonomy that is provided by teachers and parents (Ryan and Deci 2000), as well as more recent conceptualizations by European psychologists (Beyers et al. 2005).

Autonomy is also an issue in the behavioral realm, and our research has examined the degree to which parents are involved in monitoring the behavior of children no longer living at home. Do parents remind their college age children to eat well, get enough sleep, clean their rooms, or limit their drinking, for example? How often does this occur? Many parents are accustomed to such roles when children are at home, but these roles were presumably less easy to sustain during the college years prior to the availability of inexpensive technological forms of communication.

In terms of academic behaviors, successful students are those who are self-regulating: they learn to take responsibility for their own studying, become strategic and metacognitive about learning, and develop habits that guide their academic engagement with little external intervention (Hofer, Yu, and Pintrich 1998; Winne and Perry 2000). We have been curious about whether frequent contact with parents impedes this growing sense of responsibility, particularly in families where students were highly regulated by parents during high school. Although there is considerable research on self-regulation (Boekarts, Pintrich, and Zeidner 2000), we found no research on the process by which individuals move from being other-regulated to self-regulated (Hofer, Kennedy, and Hurd 2006), and this set of studies was designed in part to address that gap.

Parent-Child Relationships during Emerging Adulthood

Although this research was motivated by concern that frequent contact might impede autonomy development, undergraduate members of the research team and other college students with whom we discussed our ongoing work often noted that there might be a positive side to their regular conversations with parents: improvement in the quality of relationship. In focus groups we often heard the term "best friend" in regard to parents (particularly, although not exclusively, by female students in reference to their mothers). This might have been considered pathological in previous generations, but the term is frequently used with confidence and pride by current college students. Accordingly, we decided to assess student-parent relationships. Existing research, however, focuses on relationships between parents and children of precollege age who are still residing at home (Aquilino 1999; Furman and Buhrmester 1985; Mayseless, Wiseman, and Hai 1998); thus we found it important to advance this research into the developmental period of emerging adulthood.

Overview of Methods

We have conducted an extensive set of studies on the phenomenon of the electronic tether, including research on the transition to college (Hofer, Kennedy, and Hurd 2006; Kennedy and Hofer 2007), studies of senior and sophomore year, longitudinal studies of students during the first year of college, and cross-sectional research across the college years (Fullman 2007). We have included both students and parents. Our research has primarily been conducted through web-based surveys, with scaled measures as well as open-ended questions. We also have utilized focus groups extensively at the initiation of each phase of research, providing us with the opportunity to listen to the phenomenological perspectives of students before shaping our surveys.

Participants

The participants in our first set of studies were first-year students at a small liberal arts college ($n = 158$) and their parents ($n = 39$). In our most recent research, we expanded our participants to include students across all four years at both a small liberal arts college ($n = 598$) and a large research university ($n = 320$). We then surveyed parents of student participants from the liberal arts college ($n = 163$). Although our initial study began with a link to the survey on the college's orientation website, we subsequently sent e-mail invitations to students containing the link and offering them the opportunity to participate in a raffle as compensation. In some cases we were granted permission to use the mailing list of the entire group of interest (e.g., seniors or the entire student body), and in others we used stratified random sampling techniques (with the large research university); we also used psychology subject pools to supplement samples during particular phases of the research. Parent participation was recruited through multiple means: flyers at first-year orientation, our transition-to-college study, and e-mails forwarded by students in our most recent study (with both students and parents entered into raffles).

For the most part, we conducted the surveys at the end of the term, seeking retrospective data. Because we were concerned about the accuracy of such reporting, during our first study we included a subset of students ($n = 50$) who responded weekly. Their data regarding communication did not differ significantly from those who responded only at the end of the term; thus we continued to employ end-of-term assessments only.

Focus Groups

We conducted focus groups of eight to ten students each, selected for a common stage in their college careers. For example, we had groups composed of first-year students, students interviewed in the summer between high school and college, sophomores, and students between junior and senior year. Within these groups we sought gender and ethnic diversity. We used a semi-structured set of questions that guided the conversation, but we also provided opportunities for further development of topics, and focus group leaders were trained to encourage openness and a range of opinions. These sessions were taped and transcribed, and lasted about an hour, which was generally when it appeared that no additional information was likely to be forthcoming.

Surveys

Our instruments have included a broad set of questions about the frequency, content, format, and initiation of student-parent communication. Another set of measures is psychological in nature, mostly employing Likert-type scales with instruments related to emotional autonomy (sample item: "Even when my parents and I disagree, my parents are always right"; Steinberg and Silverberg 1986; Beyers et al. 2005); parental academic regulation and self-regulation (sample items: "I manage my time well," "My parents edit the papers I write"; adapted from Hofer, Yu, and Pintrich 1998; Winne and Perry 2000); behavioral regulation (sample item: "Parents suggested that you limited your drinking"; adapted from Steinberg 1987); and satisfaction with various aspects of the college experience (e.g., academic performance, enthusiasm for learning, and social life). In addition, our research team designed a "Relationship with Parents Questionnaire" based on items from multiple instruments (Aquilino 1999; Furman and Buhrmester 1985; Mayseless, Wiseman, and Hai 1998), adapting items for this age group. This includes five scales, each with high internal consistency (α = .70 to .91): Companionship, Mutuality, Comfort and Understanding, Control, and Conflict. We have explored the role of various demographic variables in explicating the relations among these other variables and have included such measures as parental education and income, gender, ethnicity, and form of secondary schooling in all our studies.

Summary of Key Findings

One goal of this project was to collect descriptive data on a phenomenon that has been reported anecdotally in the popular press: the frequency of student-parent communication during college. A second goal was to understand the relation between the frequency of communication and a number of important developmental constructs, as described above. Although the detailed findings may be accessed elsewhere (Hofer, Kennedy, and Fullman, in preparation), results can be broadly described in four main areas: frequency of communication, parental perceptions of change, communication and psychosocial development, and resistance and negotiation.

Frequency and Initiation of Communication

We began our studies, as noted above, with focus groups of students at the end of their first year of college. To our surprise at that time, many students spoke of daily conversations with their parents. They were seemingly less concerned about this than we might have expected, conveying a sense that it was normative in this population. We were curious to know whether students expect this level of contact and involvement while attending college; therefore, our second set of focus groups was conducted during the summer with recent high school graduates who were preparing to leave for college.

Although the first-year college students in the initial focus group appeared to accept frequent communication with parents, the recent high school graduates who had not yet left for college had contradictory expectations. With considerable positive affect, they described their anticipation of less parental monitoring and involvement in day-to-day activities than they had experienced during high school. As one student said, "If you're always underneath your parents, you don't have the opportunity to screw up or do well." Some spoke specifically of a drive toward autonomy; for example, "I'm trying to have a realization with my parents that they're not always going to be the support system, the control system. I'm trying to create my own support systems." This contrast between the two groups led us to design our first study so that data collection would begin before students left home and conclude at the end of the first term, so that we might contrast expectations of parental communication with actual behavior during the first semester.

The primary findings of this transition-to-college study (Kennedy and Hofer 2007) were that the majority of students, queried a month prior to arrival at college, expected to communicate with their parents an average of once per week, but in actuality students and their parents conversed an average of 10.4 times per week (a sum of all forms of communication, such as cell phones, e-mail, and letters). Students reported that the contact was more often initiated by parents than by themselves, although only slightly more so. Parents reported that initiation of contact was roughly equal. Moreover, the vast majority of students expressed satisfaction with the frequency of communication, and 29 percent of those surveyed would have preferred *more* communication with their fathers. None of the parents surveyed wanted less communication than they had, and 13 percent would have preferred more. Just over one-third of the students had had a conversation with their parents prior to leaving home about how often they would communicate while at college.

Our most comprehensive research to date has been a cross-sectional study of students across all four years of college at two different institutions, a small liberal arts college in New England and a large research university in the Midwest. We designed this study in order to sample a more demographically diverse population and to increase the generalizability of our findings. We were concerned that the phenomenon of frequent contact that we had documented at a small liberal arts college might be either isolated or heightened in degree of intensity, perhaps characteristic of a particular income bracket or representative of students and families who choose small colleges. We were interested in the reported frequency of communication, as well as whether this differed by key demographic variables.

Our data show that these college students and their parents communicated almost twice a day, or an average of 13.4 times per week (all forms of communication combined). We found no meaningful difference between institutions (students communicated an average of 13.5 times per week at the liberal arts college and 13.2 times at the research university) or among years in college; indeed, the frequency of communication in this study, regardless of institution, varies little between the first semester of college and senior year. Thus what we had initially identified as an aspect of current behavior during the first semester of college appears to be far more ubiquitous.

We learned that communication takes place across a variety of modes, including cell phone, e-mail, instant messages, text messages, and Skype, with cell phone and e-mail being the most frequently used modes, averaging five times per week each. Student respondents at both institutions reported that parents are slightly more likely than students to initiate communication, with seven of the thirteen weekly contacts perceived as initiated by parents. But this is a small difference, and students are still doing their fair share of contacting their parents. As one student wrote, "I actually feel like I contact my parents too much, not the other way around." Almost three-quarters of participants reported that they are satisfied with the amount of communication they have with their parents. Students were more satisfied with the amount of communication with their mothers than with their fathers, results that were consistent with the first study.

We found no differences in frequency of communication by parental income, distance from college, ethnic and racial background, or type of secondary school attended. We did, however, identify some gender differences. Females communicated with parents slightly more often than did males, and female students were more likely than males to be the initiators of communication with parents.

Frequent Communication and Psychosocial Development

In the initial study of the college transition (Kennedy and Hofer 2007), students responded to a survey before leaving home and again at the end of the first term on measures of academic self-regulation and parental involvement, as well as frequency of communication. We found that frequent communication during the first semester of college was related to more regular advice seeking and receiving from parents, and to increased parental regulation of academics and behavior. For males in particular, frequency of communication was related to lower scores of independence from parents, a measure of emotional autonomy. Overall, students' scores on the subscales of "seeing parents as people" and "nondependence" were significantly higher at the end of the first semester than they were at the beginning, and students supported this change with comments such as, "They are less involved in my life . . . now that I am self-dependent. But if need be, I can always turn to my parents."

As predicted, student self-regulation had a significant positive correlation with satisfaction with the college experience; parental regulation did not. Moreover, parental regulation of students in high school, as reported by students, was strongly correlated with parental regulation during the first year of college. Continued frequent contact appears to facilitate a pattern that might once have been altered in leaving home but which now can be readily sustained with the technological tools available.

We continued this research with surveys of these same students at the end of their first year of college, a study of students who arrived mid-year rather than in September, and a study of college seniors, all at the same institution. These studies supported the prevalence of the patterns of the initial research and led us to design a more comprehensive study. In this study we refined measures of several of the psychological constructs and included the measure of student-parent relationships appropriate to this period of life.

This latter issue became increasingly salient as students continued to report their own impressions that frequent communication might actually be beneficial in the strengthening of relationships with their parents.

The primary psychological findings in this later study were consistent with our earlier research. A high frequency of communication was related to parental regulation of academics and behaviors, as well as to increased parental dependency (Fullman 2007). Similar to the earlier study (Kennedy and Hofer 2007), results of analyses using a three-way split in communication frequency (low, medium, high) indicated that students who report high contact with their parents relative to their peers may be less emotionally autonomous.

We found in focus groups that students spoke of parental monitoring of academics and behaviors with nonchalance, and we pursued further questioning about these issues in our surveys. One student in the focus groups, for example, mentioned that his mother had collected his course syllabi and called regularly to remind him of upcoming papers or to ensure that he was studying for an impending exam. Others mentioned sending drafts of their papers by e-mail for parental editing. Various comments of this sort led us to design measures for our survey that would capture the frequency of such behavior.

The results of our survey indicate that such academic regulation by parents is not uncommon. Parents proofing papers and editing papers were reported by 19 percent and 14 percent of students, respectively, and 8 percent of the students responded that "my parent contacts my professors or deans when I have a problem," although they do so infrequently. Some parents check to see whether the students are keeping up with homework (32 percent) and check to make sure that students have written papers that are due (14 percent). Parental regulation of academics was negatively correlated with autonomy development on three of the four scales: nondependence, individuation, and separation.

Overall, students reported a fairly positive evaluation of their relationships with their parents. In addition to assessing components of the relationship, we included a global measure, a rating of the relationship on a 1 to 10 scale. Across the more than 900 students surveyed, the average rating provided was a 7.8, with only 8 percent of those who responded rating their relationship on the bottom half of the scale.

In terms of factors that compose the relationship, we found that frequency of communication was positively related to companionship, mutuality, and comfort and understanding, particularly when the contact was more student-initiated than parent-initiated. High parent-initiated contact, however, was positively correlated with control and conflict. The issue of who controls the frequency of communication appears important for understanding the nature of these relationships in emerging adulthood.

Parents' Perspectives

Our most recent research involved surveying the parents of current college students. We were interested in parents' impressions of the frequency of communication as well as their perceptions of how communication has changed since they left home a generation ago. Accordingly, we asked student participants at the liberal arts college to forward the survey's link to their parents. Preliminary results of this study provide a dramatic contrast in communication patterns between the generations. Parents spoke of the independence college had provided them, the difficulty and expensive nature of phoning home from the single pay phone in the dormitory hall, and how regular letters had been the primary source of communication: "My mother wrote me a long letter every week ('Today I cooked butter beans for supper') even though we were just one hundred miles apart. That was the only way we communicated." Parents acknowledged that the lack of immediacy made it easy to be independent in decision making, a contrast to what some experience with their own children: "My daughter talks to me daily and tells me about her daily activities. She also asks my opinion on everything." A few parents noted that the expectation of immediacy that cell phones convey was problematic. One father noted, "I welcome any and all communication with my children and never feel that it has been too often. However, I do feel that the advent of the cell phone has raised expectations that contact is always instantaneous. Many times I am in meetings and can't answer the phone, and my children call back several times to try to reach me in a span of minutes."

Although some parents spoke of the dependency that frequent contact has created, when asked about how the topics of conversations and the relationships had changed since their child arrived at college, a good number of parents spoke of the growing progression toward independence. A mother of a senior commented succinctly, "We have moved from counsel and advice to check-ins and reports." Some also spoke of making attempts to foster autonomy and a more adult relationship: "We moved consciously from parent-child to stewardship (on my part) and now are moving more toward a friendship. As long as he is financially dependent it will never be an 'equal' relationship, but we have clearly restricted our financial help. . . . This achieved greater independence and forced a faster maturity and guaranteed better decisions on his part than anything else we could have done. . . . I love seeing the wind under his wings." Others commented similarly of learning to refrain from offering advice and instead practicing the active listening they would do with friends. They also spoke of growing mutuality, of the pleasure of learning to develop a relationship with an individual on the cusp of adulthood, and of the wide range of substantive topics that were now a part of conversation.

Many parents described their college-age students as "becoming more like friends," yet they also noted the differences. As one mother commented: "As close as we are, I am aware that she's my daughter and not a contemporary of mine. While I may talk to her about the topics listed, I don't go into the same depth for all of them. For example, I'd be more likely to say 'things are tight right now' when talking about finances rather than say 'we just lost a bundle on the stock market and our house is in danger.'"

Overall, parents remarked they are more involved in their children's lives at this age than their parents were when they were at a similar developmental period. Parents cited a number of factors for this change, particularly noting the decrease in number of children per family during these decades. The dramatic rise in college tuition (which perhaps leads some parents to see this as an investment that needs protection), the college admissions frenzy, and the self-perceived youthfulness of many current parents may also contribute to these changes, but these are areas that need further investigation.

Students' Resistance Strategies and Negotiations

Although the vast majority of students in all our studies generally reported being satisfied with the amount of communication with their parents, some are not. And even those who are content reported that they have techniques for evading unwanted communication and described boundaries around certain topics of communication. Perhaps the employment of these techniques helps mediate student satisfaction, a hypothesis we want to test in future work.

Focus group conversations had cued us to the fact that some students were active in the process of protecting their privacy; for example, one student remarked, "What don't I talk to my parents about? Thursday night through Sunday morning!" Some were strategic in limiting the amount of time allotted to conversations with parents, and we heard many comments similar to this one: "I only call on the way to the gym. That way I can say, 'Gotta go now—I'm here!'" Such comments led us to investigate where students draw lines around protected areas of their lives, how they restrict the amount of conversation, and whether they direct these processes overtly or through more subtle means. We asked focus group participants what they do if they think their parents are contacting them too much, and students quickly listed strategies: lie, whisper and pretend to be in the library, say another call is coming in, claim to be busy, don't answer the phone, or, with e-mail, wait a few days before responding. One primary motive seems to be to decrease the appearance of access and availability that the current technology promotes.

Although our survey results suggest that such strategies are prevalent, just under half of all respondents in the cross-sectional study report they have experienced too much contact from their parents. Of those who had, the most common strategy, utilized by 39 percent of students, was to tell parents they are "really busy." This is not to suggest that students are always misrepresenting the truth with such a response; a number of students added comments that they actually are too busy to talk at various times in the term and do not use that as an excuse. Not answering the phone (19 percent) or resorting to e-mail rather than the cell phone (14 percent) are more common than confronting the issue directly, with only 11 percent reporting that they have told their parents they are calling too often. And some students have simply moderated their own behavior. One issue that arose in several comments is a resistance toward the recent media presentation of college students as highly controlled by parents. As one parent noted: "I've been a little surprised that my daughter hasn't been in more contact with us this first year at college. But I've gotten the impression that she has tried very hard not to be one of the students who can't make a decision without calling mommy and daddy. (In fact, she has said as much.) So much has been written about helicopter parents and their children that I think my daughter's attitude is part of a backlash against kids in her generation who don't seem to be able to grow up and the parents who won't let them."

The content of student-parent conversations has also been an area of investigation, and students were asked how conversations have changed since coming to college. A common sentiment expressed by students is that the topics are more open and personal, rather than just daily reporting: "My family has become much more open in terms of 'adult' subjects (i.e., sex, drugs, political situations, my boyfriend). . . . I feel like I am more friends with my parents than they are an authority figure." Students also reported that the conversations are more reciprocal and more future-oriented. One participant summed up the change: "I have become more open to talking about my life with my parents, and enjoy talking to them about political/world topics more than I did before. Also, I am more comfortable talking to them as adults and about their lives than before. I think the relationship is more reciprocal now that I am older." Another wrote, "My parents treat me more like an adult now. I can have in-depth conversations with my mom but

I also feel comfortable telling her that I am busy and will have to talk to her later. She is also more willing to talk about her own life with me."

Boundaries do exist, of course. Students were asked how much they share with their parents about life at college, ranked on a scale from 1 ("nothing") to 5 ("everything"). The most common answer regarding communication with fathers was a 3 ("half") and for mothers a rating of 4 ("more than half, but not everything"). Responses were quite similar when asked how much they thought each parent shared with them, with the perception that mothers share more about their lives than do fathers. Students are equally likely to talk to their mother and father about topics such as academic plans, career plans, current coursework, and significant successes. More intimate topics, however, such as serious relationships, sex life, significant failures, lonely times, and problems with friends are much more commonly discussed with mothers than fathers. Although relationships do seem to be more open, students are clearly drawing boundaries at more personal topics and are drawing different boundaries for each parent.

Sometimes, however, parents try to cross these boundaries. Students report that they have multiple strategies for addressing this. Participants were asked what they do when their parents bring up topics they don't want to talk about. (Only 26 percent of respondents said they have not experienced this.) Some students reported that they will just talk about it anyway (24 percent), while others try to avoid the topic (31 percent) or simply tell their parents they don't want to talk about it (34 percent). Others reported that they resort to telling their parents what they want to hear, even if it's not the truth (13 percent). A common strategy to avoid an extensive conversation about the topic was expressed as follows: "[I] tell them enough to make them happy, but not more than I want to talk about, or more than I think they should know."

Many students chose to provide additional tactics in response to an open-ended question that solicited any additional responses or elaboration. Most of these involved changing the subject quickly; engaging minimally; being curt or evasive; truncating the conversation, sometimes under false pretenses ("pretend there is a someone on call waiting and never call him back"); as well as expressing irritation and annoyance. One student noted his method of perceived acquiescence: "I play the nodding game, although you can't exactly see a nod over the telephone. I just play along without displaying my side but also not lying and not standing up for myself." Another commented, "It varies on subject matter. I might act like something is not as meaningful to me as it is if I really don't want them to dissuade me about my plans." Finally, one student said: "My parents don't bring up topics that I'm uncomfortable with. I bring up topics that they are uncomfortable with."

Another aspect of communication where students often draw boundaries is in the area of advice. Students were asked to indicate how often they asked for advice on eight different topics (academic, social or interpersonal, career, lifestyle or health, religious, athletic, financial, and personal), as well as how much influence their parents' advice had on their decisions. Nearly half of the students surveyed reported that parents' advice had between a 25 and 50 percent influence on every topic except religious, athletic, and financial. For religious and athletic, the majority of students said their parents' advice has no influence on their decisions, but nearly half of the respondents indicated a 50 to 75 percent range of influence on financial topics. Frequency of communication plays a role in this process: those who communicated only a few times per week were more likely to report less parental influence on their social or interpersonal decisions than those who communicated multiple times.

Conclusion

Our research indicates that frequent contact between college students and their parents may be a pervasive phenomenon in this era, abetted by current forms of technology. Unlimited calling plans and the ease and availability of both e-mail and cell phones make it possible for parents and students to communicate inexpensively and frequently. Students in our studies report that they are communicating with their parents, on average, at a rate of nearly twice daily. For the most part, students and parents report satisfaction with this level of contact, and many students would actually like more contact with their fathers; mothers appear to be doing more of the work of maintaining communication during these years. The vast majority of students as well as parents seem satisfied with the type of relationship that is evolving during emerging adulthood.

Yet the frequency of communication has its costs in some cases. Parents who use their ongoing contact to continue intrusive monitoring may be hindering their children's movement toward autonomy, and students who call home too frequently may be over-relying on parents rather than learning to seek assistance elsewhere. Parents who were highly involved in regulating their children's behavior and academic work in high school appear likely to be continuing these practices, abetted by technology. Well-educated parents also may be using technology in ways that perpetuate a class divide in education, providing unauthorized and unacknowledged academic assistance, for example, by editing and proofing student work that can easily be sent back and forth by e-mail. This is an issue that needs further discussion among college officials, particularly in regard to what constitutes unauthorized aid on academic work.

Our findings suggest the importance of parents and prospective college students discussing the proposed frequency of contact before students leave home, as a basis for a continued discussion of how much is enough. What remains surprising is how little families seem to overtly discuss these issues. Both generations are learning to navigate this relatively new situation that technology has offered and are finding ways to mitigate the burden it might sometimes represent, but more dialogue is needed about what is desirable and how mutual goals can be negotiated. Parents might consider how to promote appropriate help seeking and problem solving rather than offering to intervene or leaping to provide solutions themselves. This period of emerging adulthood is critical in shaping the type of adult an individual becomes, and those from families who take the long view are likely to benefit.

Humans sometimes respond to technological change reflexively, without consideration of the potential for conscious choice. E-mail can disrupt productivity, for example, when the arrival of each new message is heralded with a beep, but remarkably few people mute the sound or constrain checking e-mail to limited time periods. Similarly, the relatively recent situation of carrying a phone on one's person does not necessarily demand that individuals always respond, or that they use the phone to make contact in moments of boredom. (As one student reported, "You can call your parents walking to the gym or class. Talking to them is like filler.") We do not yet know the cost of such actions, or the degree to which the potential for reflection, privacy, and contemplation may have been diminished, particularly in the lives of the current generation of college students. It is not uncommon to walk across a college campus today and see students leaving classes and immediately flipping cell phones open—arranging to meet friends at lunch, calling home to complain about an exam grade, or simply not wanting to be alone, or perhaps to not *appear* alone. The costs and consequences of these actions need further study, not only in relation to family dynamics, but also more broadly.

Future research might also focus on the development of autonomy among those individuals who leave home not for college but for a job, as well as among college students who continue to live at home. In addition, continued work is needed on the full developmental continuum of early adulthood and the role of the electronic tether after college. We need a more complete developmental model of parental engagement and monitoring; both are viewed as beneficial during earlier years, and yet we know too little about how parents can help their college-age students effectively make the transition toward emotional and behavioral autonomy while remaining supported and connected. This need is particularly acute now that technology makes it possible to extend a level of involvement that our research shows to be detrimental in some cases. In spite of the potential for continued monitoring, however, students in our study indicate that they are finding the means to resist more intrusion than they wish. Furthermore, both parents and their college-age students are forging positive adult relationships that appear changed in nature from the previous generation. It is our hope that our research can be of use to families who are navigating this new path toward emerging adulthood.

Note

The authors deeply appreciate the additional contributions of other members of the research team: Lacee Patterson, Glenn Bickley, John LoPresto, Christine Barratt, and Chak Fu Lam.

References

Aquilino, William S. 1999. Two Views of One Relationship: Comparing Parents' and Young Adult Children's Reports of the Quality of Intergenerational Relations. *Journal of Marriage and Family* 61 (4): 858–70.

Arnett, Jeffrey J. 2000. Emerging Adulthood: A Theory of Development from the Late Teens through the Twenties. *American Psychologist* 55 (5): 469–80.

Beyers, W., L. Goossens, B. Van Calster, and B. Duriez. 2005. An Alternative Substantive Factor Structure of the Emotional Autonomy Scale. *European Journal of Psychological Assessment* 21 (3): 147–55.

Boekarts, Monique, Paul R. Pintrich, and Moshe Zeidner, eds. 2000. *Handbook of Self-Regulation*. San Diego, CA: Academic Press.

Chen, Zeng-Yin, and Sanford M. Dornbusch. 1998. Relating Aspects of Adolescent Emotional Autonomy to Academic Achievement and Deviant Behavior. *Journal of Adolescent Research* 13 (3): 293–319.

Fullman, Nancy. 2007. Parents on Speed Dial: The Psychological Implications of Frequent Student-Parent Communication in Emerging Adulthood. Unpublished honors thesis, Middlebury College.

Furman, W., and D. Buhrmester. 1985. Children's Perceptions of the Personal Relationships in Their Social Networks. *Developmental Psychology* 21 (6): 1016–24.

Hall, G. Stanley. 1904. *Adolescence: Its Psychology and Its Relation to Physiology, Anthropology, Sociology, Sex, Crime, Religion and Education*. New York: Appleton.

Hofer, Barbara K., Elena K. Kennedy, and Nancy Fullman. In preparation. The Electronic Tether: Frequent Parental Contact and the Development of Autonomy and Self-Regulation in Emerging Adulthood.

Hofer, Barbara K., Elena K. Kennedy, and Kathryn Hurd. 2006. From "Other-

Regulation" to Self-Regulation: Parental Contact and Influence during the Transition to College. Paper presented to the American Psychological Association, New Orleans.

Hofer, Barbara K., Shirley Yu, and Paul Pintrich. 1998. Teaching College Students to be Self-Regulated Learners. In *Self-Regulated Learning: From Teaching to Self-Reflective Practice*, edited by Dale H. Schunk and Barry J. Zimmerman, 57–83. New York: Guilford.

Johnson, Tallese, and Jane Dye. 2005. Indicators of Marriage and Fertility in the United States from the American Community Survey: 2000 to 2003. Washington, DC: Population Division, U.S. Bureau of the Census, May. *www.census.gov/population/www/socdemo/fertility/mar-fert-slides.html*.

Kennedy, Elena K., and Barbara K. Hofer. 2007. The Electronic Tether: The Influence of Frequent Parental Contact on the Development of Autonomy and Self-Regulation in Emerging Adulthood. Poster presented to the Society for Research on Child Development, Boston.

Mayseless, Ofra, Hadas Wiseman, and Ilan Hai. 1998. Adolescents' Relationships with Father, Mother, and Same-Gender Friend. *Journal of Adolescent Research* 13 (1): 101–23.

Ryan, Richard M., and Edward L. Deci. 2000. Self-Determination Theory and the Facilitation of Intrinsic Motivation, Social Development, and Well-Being. *American Psychologist* 55 (1): 68–78.

Ryan, Richard M., and John H. Lynch. 1989. Emotional Autonomy versus Detachment: Revisiting the Vicissitudes of Adolescence and Young Adulthood. *Child Development* 60 (2): 340–56.

Steinberg, Laurence. 1987. Single Parents, Stepparents, and the Susceptibility of Adolescents to Antisocial Peer Pressure. *Child Development* 58 (1): 269–75.

———. 2001. We Know Some Things: Parent-Adolescent Relationships in Retrospect and Prospect. *Journal of Research on Adolescence* 11 (1): 1–19.

Steinberg, Laurence, and Susan B. Silverberg. 1986. The Vicissitudes of Autonomy in Early Adolescence. *Child Development* 57 (4): 841–51.

Winne, Philip H., and Nancy E. Perry. 2000. Measuring Self-Regulated Learning. In *The Handbook of Self-Regulation*, edited by Monique Boekaerts, Paul R. Pintrich, and Moshe Zeidner, 531–66. New York: Academic Press.

Contributors

Holly Blackford is Associate Professor of English at Rutgers University–Camden. She teaches and publishes literary criticism on American, children's, and adolescent literature. She is the author of *Out of This World: Why Literature Matters to Girls* (Teachers College Press, 2004).

Linda M. Burton is James B. Duke Professor of Sociology at Duke University. She directed the ethnographic component of Welfare, Children, and Families: A Three-City Study and is currently principal investigator of a multisite team ethnographic study (Family Life Project) of poverty, family processes, and child development in six rural communities. She is a recipient of the Family Research Consortium IV Legacy Award and the American Family Therapy Academy Award for Innovative Contributions to Family Research. Her research integrates ethnographic and demographic approaches and examines the roles that poverty and intergenerational family dynamics play in accelerating the life course transitions of children and adults.

Nancy Fullman graduated in 2007 from Middlebury College, where she investigated the psychological implications of frequent student-parent communication across the college years. Nancy has worked as a research assistant at the National Institutes of Health and at the O'Neill Institute for National and Global Health Law at Georgetown University. She now lives in Seattle, conducting global health research and working on her master's degree in public health at the University of Washington. Nancy has no partner, no children, and no pet, but she does aspire to save the world some day.

Anita Ilta Garey is Associate Professor of Human Development and Family Studies and Sociology at the University of Connecticut. She is the author of *Weaving Work and Motherhood* (Temple University Press, 1999) and co-editor (with Karen V. Hansen) of *Families in the U.S.: Kinship and Domestic Politics* (Temple University Press, 1998). Her current project is a coedited volume (with Karen V. Hansen) of essays organized around the concepts of

Arlie Hochschild (Rutgers University Press, forthcoming). She lives in Rhode Island with her partner, her granddaughter TyAnn, and their two cats.

Kevin D. Haggerty is editor of the *Canadian Journal of Sociology* and book review editor of *Surveillance and Society*. He is Associate Professor of Sociology and Criminology at the University of Alberta and a member of the executive team for the New Transparency Major Collaborative Research Initiative. He is the coauthor of *Policing the Risk Society* (Oxford University Press, 1997), author of *Making Crime Count* (University of Toronto Press, 2001), and coeditor of *The New Politics of Surveillance and Visibility* (University of Toronto Press, 2006).

Karen V. Hansen is Professor of Sociology and Women's and Gender Studies at Brandeis University. She is the author of *Not-So-Nuclear Families: Class, Gender, and Networks of Care* (Rutgers University Press, 2005), and she is editing a collection with Anita Ilta Garey (Rutgers University Press, forthcoming). She is also currently working on a historical study of community, kinship, and land taking, *Reservation Sagas: Scandinavian Settlers and Dakota Indians at Spirit Lake, 1900–1930.*

Rosanna Hertz is Luella LaMer Professor of Sociology and Women's Studies at Wellesley College. She is the 2010 President of the Eastern Sociological Society. Her recent books are *Single by Chance, Mothers by Choice: How Women Are Choosing Parenthood without Marriage and Creating the New American Family* (Oxford University Press, 2006) and *Working Families: The Transformation of the American Home* (edited with Nancy L. Marshall; University of California Press, 2001). She enjoys browsing mom websites and family blogs.

Barbara K. Hofer is Associate Professor of Psychology at Middlebury College, where she teaches and conducts research in the areas of developmental, educational, and cultural psychology. She is the author of several dozen articles and book chapters and the editor (with Paul Pintrich) of *Personal Epistemology: The Psychology of Beliefs about Knowledge and Knowing* (Lawrence Erlbaum Associates, 2003). She is currently working on a book on student-parent communication during the period of emerging adulthood.

Kathryn Hurd graduated in 2006 from Middlebury College, where she examined how frequent communication with parents during college was related to the quality of the parent-child relationship during this period of life. Currently she works as an assistant teacher in a Connecticut middle school.

Heather Jacobson is Assistant Professor of Sociology at the University of Texas at Arlington. She is the author of *Culture Keeping: White Mothers, International Adoption, and the Negotiation of Family Difference* (Vanderbilt University Press, 2008).

Emily W. Kane is Whitehouse Professor of Sociology, and a member of the Program in Women and Gender Studies, at Bates College. Her research focuses on beliefs about gender inequality, including quantitative analysis of such beliefs in the United States and cross-nationally, and on gender and parenting. She is currently working on a book based on the qualitative interview data included in her contribution to this collection.

Elena K. Kennedy graduated in 2006 from Middlebury College and is currently pursuing a master's degree in education from Lesley University. As a student at Middlebury, she conducted research regarding communication between parents and emerging adults during the transition to college, and she has presented her work at the Society for Research on Child Development and the Council for Undergraduate Research. She is currently working as a teaching fellow with a nonprofit educational organization, Citizen Schools, in Houston, Texas.

Demie Kurz is Co-director of Women's Studies at the University of Pennsylvania, with an appointment in the Sociology Department. She is the author of *For Richer, For Poorer: Mothers Confront Divorce* (Routledge, 1995) and a coeditor of *Child Care and Inequality: Re-thinking Carework for Children and Youth* (Routledge, 2002), as well as the author of articles on divorce, domestic violence, and parenting. She is currently writing a book on the work mothers do and the challenges they face as they manage their teenage children's passage through adolescence.

Dawn Moore is Assistant Professor in the Department of Law, Carleton University. She works in the areas of governance, moral regulation, drug regulation, identity, punishment, sexuality, and state mandated psychological interventions. She is the author of *Criminal Artefacts: Governing Drugs and Users* (University of British Columbia Press, 2008). Moore is currently working on a three-year study concerning gender in Drug Treatment Courts. She is also (with Aaron Doyle) working on an edited collection about the future of criminology.

Margaret K. Nelson is Hepburn Professor of Sociology at Middlebury College. Her recent books include *Working Hard and Making Do: Surviving in*

Small Town America (with Joan Smith; University of California Press, 1999) and *The Social Economy of Single Motherhood: Raising Children in Rural America* (Routledge Press, 2005). She is currently completing a book that is tentatively titled *Parenting out of Control: The Roots and Dynamics of Child Rearing among the Professional Middle Class* (New York University Press, forthcoming).

Rayna Rapp is Professor of Anthropology at New York University. She is the editor or coeditor of *Toward an Anthropology of Women* (Monthly Review Press, 1975), *Promissory Notes* (Monthly Review Press, 1989), *Conceiving the New World Order* (University of California Press, 1995), and *Articulating Hidden Histories* (University of California Press, 1995). The author of more than seventy articles focusing on the intersections of gender, reproduction, disability, and medicine, she is currently working with Faye Ginsburg on a fieldwork-based project on cultural innovation in special education.

Kevin Roy is Associate Professor in the Department of Family Science, School of Public Health, at the University of Maryland–College Park. His primary research focus is the life course of men on the margins of families and the workforce. Through a mix of participant observation and life history interviews, he explores the intersection of policy systems, such as welfare reform and incarceration, with parents' caregiving and providing roles. He has published in *Social Problems*, *American Journal of Community Psychology*, *Journal of Family Issues*, and *Family Relations*, and is coediter of *Situated Fathering: A Focus on Physical and Social Spaces* (with William Marsiglio and Greer Litton Fox; Rowman and Littlefield, 2005).

Constance Souder graduated in 2007 from Middlebury College, where she conducted research on student-parent communication. She currently teaches elementary school in Washington, DC, and is working on her master's degree in teaching at American University.

William G. Staples is Professor and Chair of Sociology at the University of Kansas, the oldest sociology program in the United States. His most recent books include *Everyday Surveillance: Vigilance and Visibility in Postmodern Life* (Rowman and Littlefield, 2000) and the *Encyclopedia of Privacy* (Greenwood Press, 2006). He currently serves as coeditor of the *Sociological Quarterly*.